# DEJA REVIEW™

## Obstetrics & Gynecology

## NOTICE

# DEJA REVIEW™

## Obstetrics & Gynecology

**Catherine J. Lee, MD**

New York University School of Medicine
New York, New York

**Emily S. Miller, MD**

New York University School of Medicine
New York, New York

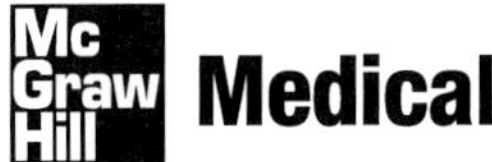


New York Chicago San Francisco Lisbon London Madrid Mexico City
Milan New Delhi San Juan Seoul Singapore Sydney Toronto

The McGraw·Hill Companies

**Deja Review™: Obstetrics & Gynecology**



1 2 3 4 5 6 7 8 9 0 DOC/DOC 0 9 8

ISBN 978-0-07-148122-9
MHID 0-07-148122-2

This book was set in Palatino by International Typesetting and Composition.

The editor was Catherine A. Johnson.

The production supervisor was Catherine H. Saggese.

Project management was provided by Vastavikta Sharma, International Typesetting and Composition.

The text was designed by Marsha Cohen/Parallelogram.

RR Donnelley was printer and binder.

This book is printed on acid-free paper.

**Library of Congress Cataloging-in-Publication Data**

Lee, Catherine J.
Deja review : obstetrics and gynecology / Catherine J. Lee, Emily S. Miller.
p. ; cm.—(Deja review)
Includes index.
ISBN-13: 978-0-07-148122-9 (pbk. : alk. paper)
ISBN-10: 0-07-148122-2 (pbk. : alk. paper)
1. Gynecology—Examinations, questions, etc. 2. Obstetrics—Examinations, questions, etc. I. Miller, Emily S. II. Title. III. Title: Obstetrics and gynecology IV. Series.
[DNLM: 1. Obstetrics—Examination Questions. 2. Female Urogenital Diseases—Examination Questions. 3. Gynecology—Examination Questions. 4. Pregnancy Complications—Examination Questions. WQ 18.2 L477d 2008]
RG111.L44 2008
618.1—dc22

2007033874

*To my family, friends, and teachers—thank you for being a constant source of light in my journey to becoming an excellent physician.*

*Catherine J. Lee*

*To all those who have taught me the art of medicine, inspired me to make change, and supported me throughout the process of becoming a physician.*

*Emily S. Miller*

# Contents

# Contributing Authors

**Jessica Maria Atrio, MD**
Department of Obstetrics and Gynecology
New York University School of Medicine
New York, New York
*General Obstetrics*

**Ricky Darnell Grisson II, MBA, MD**
Harvard Medical School
Boston, Massachusetts
*Women's Health*

# Illustrators

**Alex M. Kotylar**
New York University
College of Arts and Sciences
New York, New York

**Pavel Kotylar**
Touro College
Brooklyn, New York

# Faculty Reviewers

**Kristin L. Atkins, MD**
Assistant Professor
Division of Maternal Fetal Medicine
Department of Obstetrics and Gynecology
New York University School of Medicine
New York, New York
*Adolescent Development, Maternal-Fetal Physiology, Prenatal Care*

**Yoni Barnhard, MD, FACOG, MFM**
Vice Chairman
Department of Obstetrics and Gynecology
Lenox Hill Hospital
New York, New York
*Medical Conditions of Pregnancy*

**Jonathan S. Berek, MD**
Professor and Chair
Department of Obstetrics and Gynecology
Stanford University School of Medicine
Division of Gynecologic Oncology
Stanford Cancer Center
Stanford, California
*Ovarian Cancer*

**Stephanie V. Blank, MD**
Assistant Professor
Division of Gynecologic Oncology
Department of Obstetrics and Gynecology
New York University School of Medicine
New York, New York
*Cervical Cancer, Vulvar and Vaginal Cancer, Uterine Cancer, Fallopian Tube Cancer*

**Asaf Ferber, MD**
General Obstetrician-Gynecologist
Department of Obstetrics and Gynecology
Lenox Hill Hospital
New York, New York
*Benign Conditions of the Vulva and Vagina*

**Debbra A. Keegan, MD**
Associate Physician
IVF Florida Reproductive Associates
Margate, Florida
*Disorders of the Menstrual Cycle, Uterus, and Endometrium; Infertility; Osteoporosis; Perimenopause and Menopause; Hirsuitism, Viralization and PCOS*

**Chad Klauser, MD**
Assistant Professor
Division of Maternal-Fetal Medicine
Department of Obstetrics and Gynecology
New York University School of Medicine
New York, New York
*STDs and Pelvic Infections, Postpartum Care, Multifetal Gestation, Teratogens*

**Christina Kwon, MD**
Assistant Professor
Division of Urogynecology
Department of Obstetrics and Gynecology
New York University School of Medicine
New York, New York
*Urinary Infections, Pelvic Organ Prolapse, Urinary Incontinence*

**Ruth Lahti, MD**
Assistant Professor
Reproductive Endocrinology and Infertility Program
Department of Obstetrics and Gynecology
Stanford University School of Medicine
Stanford, California
*Endometriosis*

**Rachel Masch, MD**
Assistant Professor
Department of Obstetrics and Gynecology
New York University School of Medicine
New York, New York
*Menstrual Cycle, Family Planning*

**Victoria Ort, PhD**
Assistant Professor
Department of Cell Biology
New York University School of Medicine
New York, New York
*Female Anatomy*

**John C. Petrozza, MD**
Chief, Reproductive Medicine & IVF
Obstetrics and Gynecology Service
Massachusetts General Hospital
Harvard Medical School
Boston, Massachusetts
*Pelvic Pain*

**Michael Plakogiannis, MD**
Faculty Staff
Department of Obstetrics and Gynecology
Lenox Hill Hospital
New York, New York
*Late Complications, Postpartum Complications*

**Florencia Greer Polite, MD**
Assistant Professor
Department of Obstetrics and Gynecology
New York University School of Medicine
New York, New York
*Benign Masses*

**Ashley S. Roman, MD, MPH**
Assistant Professor
Division of Maternal-Fetal Medicine
Department of Obstetrics and Gynecology
New York University School of Medicine
New York, New York
*Labor and Delivery, Early Complications, Obstetric Infections, Abnormal Labor and Delivery*

**David Seubert, MD**
Associate Professor of Obstetrics and Gynecology
Director, Division of Maternal-Fetal Medicine and Medical Student Clerkship in Obstetrics and Gynecology
Department of Obstetrics and Gynecology
New York University School of Medicine
New York, New York
*Isoimmunization, Fetal Growth Abnormalities*

**Tomer Singer, MD**
Resident Physican
Department of Obstetrics and Gynecology
Lenox Hill Hospital
New York, New York
*Common Procedures, Medical Conditions of Pregnancy*

**Erin E. Tracy, MD, MPH**
Assistant Professor
Obstetrics, Gynecology, and Reproductive Biology
Harvard Medical School
Massachusetts General Hospital
Boston, Massachusetts
*Domestic Violence*

**Ming C. Tsai, MD**
Assistant Professor
Department of Obstetrics and Gynecology
New York University School of Medicine
New York, New York
*Sexual Dysfunction*

# Acknowledgments

The authors would like to thank all the contributors, artists, and faculty reviewers for their invaluable time and effort in contributing to this book and making it a useful resource for all medical students.

The authors would like to recognize all the faculty and staff at New York University School of Medicine, Harvard Medical School, Stanford University School of Medicine, and Lenox Hill Hospital for their endless commitment and dedication to educating medical students. We would also like to thank the students who used this text in preparation for the boards and provided essential feedback necessary to write an improved high-yield, comprehensive book. Finally, a special thanks to the editors and publishers at McGraw-Hill for their extraordinary patience and guidance at each step of the process to see this project through.

# Introduction

Thank you for using *Deja Review: Obstetrics & Gynecology* to assist you in your preparation for the core clerkship in Obstetrics and Gynecology, the in-service exam, and for the Ob and Gyn-related questions in Step 2 CK of the United States Medical Licensing Exam (USMLE). We have worked diligently to bring you a concise and rigorous review of obstetrics and gynecology. This book is a compilation of essential facts, organized into an easy-to-read question and answer format, with difficult concepts illustrated by figures and mnemonics. Furthermore, this review book encourages step-by-step logical problem-solving skills, necessary for good performance on the boards and success on the wards, by combining clinical scenarios with fundamental principles of these topics. Considering the huge volume of information that you must synthesize in order to perform successfully as a clinician, we recommend the use of all the books in the Deja Review series to help you form that required foundation.

## Organization

Section I includes Chapters 1–3, "Useful Facts for the Wards." These chapters include common laboratory values and essential knowledge of female anatomy and commonly performed procedures in obstetrics and gynecology.

Sections II and III are divided into several chapters that contain thorough and high-yield material on obstetrics and gynecology. It has been our goal to fulfill the third-year learning objectives recommended by the American Professors of Gynecology and Obstetrics (APGO) and the American College of Obstetrics and Gynecology (ACOG).

Section IV is dedicated to Women's Health Issues, which contains information on domestic violence, sexual assault, and ethics and law.

Section V of this book provides the reader with many clinical vignettes that students may face on the USMLE Step 2 CK and on the wards. This section encourages students to apply their knowledge of obstetrics and gynecology to relevant clinical scenarios.

Topics are covered in a question and answer format with buzz words highlighted in bold for each response. This format is designed for rapid review during the clerkship and before exams. Furthermore, we have included questions that require students to think about a problem in a logical and clinically appropriate manner.

It is our hope that this book will supplement topics learned in the clinical setting and will facilitate success on the clerkship shelf exam and the USMLE Step 2 CK. We also hope to stimulate interest in the fascinating fields of obstetrics and gynecology through exposure to some of the exciting clinical cases that are typical of this field.

## How to use this book

We recommend the use of this book alongside a standard textbook to test your comprehension of the material and to assist in the organization of these pertinent medical facts into a cohesive whole. When preparing for exams, this book can be used as a quick, last-minute review of high-yield facts. Please remember that while this book will be very useful for the USMLE Step 2 CK and for reviewing the fundamentals of medical science, this review book should neither replace standard medical texts or lecture notes, nor substitute for sound clinical judgment. Rather, it is intended to clarify difficult concepts, review high-yield topics, and to provide you with a small portable book that is easy to use to quiz yourself and classmates on these concepts.

We hope you will find this review book helpful during your preparations for the USMLE Step 2 CK and throughout your medical education. Thank you for letting us help with your medical education!

SECTION I

# Useful Facts for the Wards

CHAPTER 1

# Lab Values

## Common Lab Values in the Nonpregnant Woman and Their Change During Pregnancy

| Chemistries | Nonpregnant | Compared to Nonpregnant Woman |
|---|---|---|
| Sodium | 135–145 mEq/L | Decreased |
| Potassium | 3.5–5.1 mEq/L | Decreased |
| Chloride | 98–106 mEq/L | Decreased |
| Bicarbonate | 22–29 mEq/L | Decreased |
| Blood urea nitrogen (BUN) | 7–18 mg/dL | Decreased |
| Creatinine | 0.6–1.2 mg/dL | Decreased |
| Glucose | 70–115 mg/dL | Decreased |
| Calcium | 8.4–10.2 mg/dL | Decreased (due to decrease in albumin) |
| Phosphate | 2.7–4.5 mg/dL | Unchanged |
| Magnesium | 1.3–2.1 mg/dL | Decreased |
| Anion gap | 7–16 mEq/L | |
| Osmolality | 275–295 mOsm/kg | Decreased |
| Lipase | 10–140 U/dL | |
| Amylase | 25–125 U/dL | Unchanged |
| SGOT/AST | 7–40 U/L | Unchanged |
| SGPT/ALT | 7–40 U/L | Unchanged |
| GGT | 9–50 U/L | Unchanged |
| Alkaline phosphate | 38–126 U/L | Increased |
| LDH | 120–240 U/L | Unchanged |
| Uric acid | 2.0–6.9 mg/dL | |
| Free $T_4$ | 0.71–1.85 ng/dL | Unchanged |
| TSH | 0.32–5.00 mIU/mL | Unchanged |
| Free $T_3$ | | Unchanged |
| Total thyroxine, $T_4$ | | Increased |
| Free $T_4$ | | Increased |

*(Continued)*

## Common Lab Values in the Nonpregnant Woman and Their Change During Pregnancy (*Continued*)

| Chemistries | Nonpregnant | Compared to Nonpregnant Woman |
|---|---|---|
| | **Urinalysis** | |
| Color | Yellow | |
| Turbidity | Clear | |
| Specific gravity | 1.003–1.035 | |
| pH | 4.5–8.0 | |
| Ketones | Negative | Unchanged |
| Protein | Negative | Minimal increase |
| Blood | Negative | Unchanged |
| Glucose | Negative | Minimal increase |
| Nitrite | Negative | Unchanged |
| Leukocyte esterase | Negative | Unchanged |
| Osmolality | 50–1400 mOsm/kg | |
| Sodium | 40–220 mEq/day | |
| Potassium | 25–125 mEq/day | |
| | **Hematology** | |
| WBC | 4,700–11,000/$mm^3$ | Increased |
| RBC | 3.8–5.7 × 106/mL | Increased |
| Hemoglobin | 13.5–17.0 g/dL | Decreased |
| Hematocrit | 39–50% | Decreased |
| Mean corpuscular volume (MCV) | 80–96 fL | Increased |
| Mean corpuscular hemoglobin (MCH) | 27–33 pg/cell | |
| Mean corpuscular hemoglobin concentration (MCHC) | 32–36% hgb/cell | |
| Platelets | 150–400 × 103/mL | Decreased due to dilution increases |
| Erythrocyte sedimentation rate (ESR) | | |
| Red blood cell distribution width (RDW) | 11.0–16.0% | |
| Segs (neuts) | 35–73% | |
| Lymphocytes | 15–52% | |
| Monocytes | 4–13% | |
| Eosinophils | 1–3% | |
| Basophils | 0–1% | |

## Common Lab Values in the Nonpregnant Woman and Their Change During Pregnancy (*Continued*)

| Chemistries | Nonpregnant | Compared to Nonpregnant Woman |
|---|---|---|
| | **Coagulation** | |
| PT | 12.3–14.2 seconds | Reduced |
| PTT | 25–34 seconds | Reduced |
| Fibrinogen | 200–400 mg/dL | Increased |
| D-dimer | | Increased |
| Bleeding time | 2–7 minutes | |
| Thrombin time | 6.3–11.1 seconds | |
| | **Arterial Blood Gas** | |
| pH | | |
| 7.35–7.45 | | Increased (chronic, corrected respiratory alkalosis) |
| $Paco_2$ | 35–45 mm Hg | Decreased |
| $Pao_2$ | 80–100 mm Hg | Increased |
| $HCO_3^-$ | 21–27 mEq/L | Decreased |
| $O_2$ saturation | 95–98% | Unchanged |

CHAPTER 2

# Common Procedures

These tables list several of the most common procedures performed in obstetrics and gynecology. Procedures not listed here are reviewed in topic-specific chapters.

## Common Obstetric Procedures

| Procedure | Description | Indications/Contraindications | Benefits/Risks | Comments |
|---|---|---|---|---|
| Amniocentesis | Withdrawal of fluid from the amniotic sac to obtain fluid and cells for a variety of tests | Determine the presence of genetic diseases (e.g., Down syndrome, Tay-Sachs), fetal structural abnormalities (neural tube defects), fetal lung maturity, or intrauterine infection (i.e., chorioamnionitis) | 0.5% risk of fetal loss because of bleeding, infection, preterm labor, or fetal injury | Usually performed using ultrasono-graphic guidance to reduce the risk of fetal loss |
| Cerclage | It is the placement of a suture into and around the cervix to hold it closed | Used to prevent cervical opening in an incompetent cervix and prevent preterm delivery or miscarriage | It is controversial whether a cerclage reduces the likelihood of a preterm delivery | It is usually performed between 12 and 14 weeks and removed before labor begins |
| Cesarean delivery | It is the delivery of the fetus by making an incision through the abdomen and uterus | It is used when a vaginal delivery would be harmful to the mother or fetus or it can be requested by the patient (elective) | The mortality rate is less than vaginal delivery; however, complications include postoperative adhesion, infection, and problems with the next birth (i.e., placenta previa, uterine rupture) | The incision can be made in two ways: (1) Classical-midline longitudinal incision (2) Lower uterine segment section—transverse cut above the bladder; more commonly used and less bleeding |

| | | | | |
|---|---|---|---|---|
| Chorionic villus sampling (CVS) | A small cannula is passed through the cervix or transabdominally, and villus cells are aspirated for genetic analysis | Cells are taken for genetic studies | 0.5% risk of fetal loss. Usually reserved for patients with a greater than 0.5% chance of having an abnormality in the fetus | CVS is usually performed in early pregnancy to allow earlier decision making regarding possible pregnancy termination |
| Circumcision | It is the removal of the foreskin from the penis of a newborn male | It has been performed as part of religious and social customs, and health reasons | The same as for any surgical operation (bleeding, infection, surgical damage) | There is controversy over the health value of the procedure |
| Episiotomy | It is a surgical incision made through the perineum to widen the vagina and facilitate delivery | Used when there are signs of fetal distress while in the vaginal canal, when the baby's head or shoulders are too large to pass, to lessen perineal trauma and reduce postpartum pelvic floor dysfunction | It is controversial whether episiotomy may cause more morbidity (postpartum pain, trouble defecating, dyspareunia) | Perineal massage with oils beginning around the 34th week may help relax the perineum and avoid an episiotomy |
| External cephalic version | It is the application of constant gentle pressure (between 36 and 39 weeks) to the abdomen of the mother with a breech fetus to place it in cephalic presentation | To position a breech fetus into cephalic presentation | | Success rates are from 50–75%. Fetal monitoring is advised after the procedure as well as administration of Rh-immune globulin to Rh-negative women |

(*Continued*)

Common Obstetric Procedures (*Continued*)

| Procedure | Description | Indications/Contraindications | Benefits/Risks | Comments |
|---|---|---|---|---|
| Fern test (amniotic fluid crystallization test) | Vaginal secretion from the posterior vaginal pool is collected with a sterile swab and placed on a clean slide to dry | It detects ruptured membranes or the leakage of amniotic fluid from the membranes surrounding the fetus during pregnancy. It is helpful to diagnose premature rupture of membranes. If positive, the amniotic fluid will form a fernlike pattern of crystallization | | To be used in conjunction with the Nitrazine test (pH test to determine presence of amniotic fluid. pH paper will turn blue, demonstrating an alkaline pH) |
| Forceps delivery | It is an instrument applied to the fetal head used for assistance in vaginal delivery | Used to provide traction to augment and/or direct the expulsive forces during the second stage of labor (i.e., prolonged second stage of labor) | Maternal complications: lacerations of the cervix and birth canal, blood loss, and hematomas. Fetal complications: bruising, cephalohematomas, facial and head lacerations | Four types of forceps are classified as outlet, low, mid, and high depending on the station of the fetal head. High forceps is not recommended by American College of Obstetricians and Gynecologists (ACOG) |
| Pelvimetry | It is the assessment of the size of the female pelvis in relation to the space needed for the birth of a baby | It has been used to determine whether a natural or vaginal delivery is possible, or whether a caesarean delivery is indicated | | Can be performed by physical exam, radiography, or MRI |

| | | | | |
|---|---|---|---|---|
| Percutaneous umbilical blood sampling (PUBS) | A needle is placed transabdominally and fetal blood is obtained from the umbilical cord under real-time ultrasonographic guidance | Fetal blood gas and metabolic status, fetal hemogram, fetal blood chemistries, and fetal genetic studies can be performed | The risk is similar to that of an amniocentesis (0.5%). There may also be bleeding at the umbilical puncture site | Also referred to as *cordocentesis* |
| Tubal ligation | It is a permanent form of female sterilization where the fallopian tubes are severed, sealed, or "pinched shut" to prevent fertiliztion | It is used when fertility is no longer desired | No major complications | Tubal reversal is possible.<br>Tubal ligation does not affect hormone production, libido, or menstrual cycle |
| Ultrasound imaging | Specific parts of the body are exposed to low-energy sound waves which produce images reflective of the structure and movement of the body's internal organs | Establish the presence of a living embryo/fetus, estimate the age of the pregnancy, diagnose congenital abnormalities, evaluate the position of the baby, evaluate the position of the placenta, determine if there are multiple pregnancies, determine the amount of amniotic fluid around the baby, check for opening or shortening of the cervix or mouth of the womb | It is a painless procedure and does not involve any ionizing radiation | Doppler ultrasound can be used in conjunction to evaluate blood flow through a blood vessel |
| Vacuum extraction | It is a suction cup device that is applied to the fetal head to help in delivery | Indications are similar to that of forceps delivery | Less complications as compared to forceps delivery, but hematomas and abrasions to the fetal scalp can occur | |

## Common Gynecologic Procedures

| Procedure | Description | Indications/Contraindications | Benefits/Risks | Comments |
|---|---|---|---|---|
| Angiography | It is a medical imaging technique in which a radiographic contrast medium is injected into the blood vessel and an x-ray picture is taken to visualize the blood vascular system | It can be used to locate the source of continued bleeding from postoperative procedures, visualize bleeding from sites infiltrated by cancers, help assist in the embolization of the uterine arteries in hematomas, and to reduce the size of uterine myomas | | |
| Bimanual pelvic examination | Two fingers are placed in the vagina and the flat of the opposite hand is placed on the lower abdominal wall. Gentle palpation and manipulation should delineate the position, shape, mobility, tenderness, and size of the uterus and adnexal structures. See Figure 2-1, page 22 | Part of routine pelvic exam and part of investigation for gynecologic pathology. Tenderness may be elicited on direct palpation or on movement/ stretching of pelvic structures (i.e. acute salpingitis or pelvic inflammatory disease [PID]) | Difficult to elicit any information on obese patients or uncooperative patients | |
| Cervical conization | It is a surgical procedure that involves excising a cone-shaped sample of tissue that includes the entire cervical | It is used for either diagnostic or therapeutic reasons. The test is done when results of a cervical biopsy indicate precancerous cells in the area or cervical | An early complication is excessive bleeding. Infrequent complications include cervical stenosis or incompetence | Conization can be performed using a knife (cold knife cone), laser excision, and |

| | | | | |
|---|---|---|---|---|
| | transformation zone and a portion of the endocervical canal. The sample is then examined for any signs of malignancy | cancer. It may also be done if the cervical biopsy has not revealed the cause of an abnormal Pap smear | | electrocautery (large loop excision of the transformation loop electrosurgical excision procedure [LEEP]) |
| Colposcopy | It is the direct magnified inspection of the surface of the cervix, vagina, and vulva, using a light source and a binocular microscope | Used to facilitate detailed evaluation of a suspect malignancy and to assist in directed biopsies of suspicious areas. It can also be used to detect inflammatory or infectious changes, and traumatic injuries to the cervix, vagina, and vulva | Minimal risk | Can be performed in the office and rarely requires any anesthesia |
| Computed axial tomography (CT) | It is a form of imaging that uses x-ray information to generate detailed cross-sectional images of internal structures | Can help evaluate for pelvic masses, signs of adenopathy, and plan for radiation therapy CT heavily relies on the use of IV contrast and this contrast can cause kidney damage. Should not be used in patients with advanced renal failure | Superior contrast resolution which provides a significant amount of information. However, it is considered as a moderate to high radiation diagnostic technique | CT is best suited to study bone and calcifications in the body, or vessels and bowel which have been enhanced with contrast |

(*Continued*)

### Common Gynecologic Procedures (*Continued*)

| Procedure | Description | Indications/Contraindications | Benefits/Risks | Comments |
|---|---|---|---|---|
| Cryotherapy | It is a technique to destroy tissue by freezing with liquid nitrogen or liquid carbon dioxide | Most frequently used to destroy dysplastic sections of the cervix and other benign lesions (i.e., condyloma) | Minimal risk. Inexpensive and generally effective, although not as precise as laser ablation | Not as useful for treating changes in the upper cervix; a cone biopsy is recommended instead |
| Culdocentesis | It is the passage of a needle into the cul-de-sac to obtain fluid from the pouch of Douglas | It is a diagnostic procedure to check for abnormal fluid. Blood fluid may indicate a ruptured ectopic pregnancy; pus-filled fluid indicates acute infection; ascetic fluid may indicate cancer | There is a slight risk of puncturing any mass or uterine wall | Not as commonly performed today with advances in ultrasound technology |
| Dilation and curettage (D&C) | It is a process of opening and dilating the cervix using a series of graduated dilators followed by curettage, or scraping of the uterine lining | It may be used to take an endometrial biopsy, remove polyps, other tumors, or excess endometrial lining, or to treat cases of incomplete spontaneous abortion | If done roughly, uterine perforation may occur or scarring could develop leading to infertility | It is generally performed under local or general anesthetic in the operating room |
| Dilation and evacuation (D&E) | It is a procedure used in the second semester to remove the products of conception by | It is used in pregnancy termination | Mild bleeding, cramping. There is also slight risk of uterine perforation and scarring | D&E is the most common and safest |

| | | | | |
|---|---|---|---|---|
| | first dilating the cervix and then using destructive grasping forceps. Vacuum aspiration may also be used to facilitate the removal | | | procedure used (95% of the time) for an abortion in the second trimester |
| Fern test for ovulation | Cervical mucus is spread on a clean, dry slide and allowed to dry in the air. A fern-frond pattern is seen under the microscope when ovulation has failed to occur. A non-frond-like pattern is seen when ovulation has occurred | To determine the presence or absence of ovulation at the ovulatory time of cycle | | A fern-frond pattern is induced by unopposed estrogen. Progesterone inhibits the effects of estrogen on ferning and makes the mucus thick and cellular (seen in ovulation). See Figure 2-2, page 22 |
| Genital tract biopsy | It is the removal of tissue from lesions of the vulva, vagina, cervix, and endometrial cavity | Allows for histopathologic assessment of the specimen to evaluate any malignancy and may also serve to fully excise small lesions | Minimal risk | Usually performed in the office and requires only local anesthetic |

(*Continued*)

Common Gynecologic Procedures (*Continued*)

| Procedure | Description | Indications/Contraindications | Benefits/Risks | Comments |
|---|---|---|---|---|
| Hysterectomy | It is the removal of the uterus. It can be performed by entering the abdomen (abdominal hysterectomy) or extracting the uterus through the vagina (vaginal hysterectomy) | It may be indicated for patients with benign or malignant changes in the uterine wall or cavity, for menstrual disturbances or abnormal bleeding, endometriosis, uterine prolapse, or chronic pelvic pain<br>It is not recommended for the sole purpose of sterilization | Advantages include the elimination of future pregnancies, cessation of menses, and possibility of uterine and cervical cancer | There are different types of hysterectomy:<br>*Total*: removal of all of the uterus and not the fallopian tubes or ovaries<br>*Subtotal or supracervical*: body of the uterus is removed near the level of the internal cervical os, leaving the cervix in place<br>*Radical*: is a cancer surgery procedure where the uterus is removed with wide margins of surrounding tissues |

| | | | | |
|---|---|---|---|---|
| Hysterosalpingography | It is an x-ray of the uterus, fallopian tubes, and abdominopelvic cavity that involves the injection of dye through the cervix | It is useful to assess the size, shape, and anatomy of the uterine cavity for evaluation of infertility or genital anomalies | There is a risk of infection of the uterus or pelvis, bleeding, pain, and allergic reaction to the dye | Can be performed with hysteroscopy and hysterosonography |
| Hysteroscopy | It is a small endoscope which has a built-in viewing camera that allows direct visualization of the endocervix and endometrial cavity | It is used for evaluation of bleeding or structural abnormalities which may cause infertility, or location of missing intrauterine devices; it is also used for therapeutic reasons (i.e., polypectomy, endometrial ablation, removal of the uterine septum) | Mild bleeding, cramping | Fluid may be used to distend the uterine cavity. Usually performed as an outpatient procedure under local or general anesthesia |
| Hysterosonography | It is a new minimally invasive technique used to visualize the uterine cavity by use of ultrasound and slow infusion of sterile saline | It is used to evaluate abnormal growths inside the uterus; abnormalities of the tissue lining the uterus (the endometrium); or disorders affecting deeper tissue layers | Does not use ionizing radiation, contrast media, or invasive surgical techniques. Mild bleeding and cramping may occur postprocedure | It is useful as a screening test to minimize the use of more invasive diagnostic procedures, such as tissue biopsies and D&C |

*(Continued)*

## Common Gynecologic Procedures (*Continued*)

| Procedure | Description | Indications/Contraindications | Benefits/Risks | Comments |
|---|---|---|---|---|
| Laparoscopically assisted vaginal hysterectomy (LAVH) | It is a procedure using laparoscopic surgical techniques and instruments to remove the uterus and/or tubes and ovaries through the vagina | Indications are similar to that of a hysterectomy | Advantages include avoiding a large abdominal incision, less postoperative pain and recovery time.<br>Disadvantages include technical difficulty leading to increased operative time and increased anesthesia exposure | Recently, laparoscopic supercervical hysterectomy (LSH) has been advocated by some. This preserves the cervix and its supporting structures, and allows for lubrication and maintenance of sexual response |
| Laparoscopy | It is the inspection and manipulation of tissue within the abdominal cavity using endoscopic instruments (camera) | It is used for diagnostic and therapeutic purposes. It can help in diagnosis of the source of pelvic pain, pelvic masses, infertility, and congenital abnormalities. It can treat endometriosis, lyse adhesions, and be used to perform minimally invasive surgeries (eg, bilateral salpingo-oophorectomy [BSO]) | Less morbidity than laparotomy, but injury to the bowel and vessels can occur. Postsurgical infection and bleeding is possible | The abdominal cavity is usually distended with carbon dioxide or nitrous oxide gas to facilitate viewing and prevent bowel injury |

| | | | | |
|---|---|---|---|---|
| Laparotomy | It is a surgical maneuver involving an incision through the abdominal wall to gain access into the abdominal cavity | It is for both diagnostic and therapeutic purposes. Exploratory laparotomy is used to identify the cause of disease; whereas, in therapeutic laparotomy, the nature of disease is known | The operative procedure time may be less time consuming compared to laparoscopic technique, but there is more postoperative pain and recovery time | The Pfannenstiel's incision is a transverse incision below the umbilicus and just above the pubic symphysis. It is the incision of choice for cesarean delivery and abdominal hysterectomy for benign disease |
| Laser vaporization | High-energy light waves are used to destroy abnormal cells and dysplastic tissue | Can be used to treat cervical dysplasia. Also used to make incisions | Painless can replace cryotherapy. However, due to its sophistication it is expensive | Infrared and $CO_2$ lasers are commonly used in the office, and can be coupled to colposcopes |
| Loop electro-surgical excision procedure (LEEP) | It is an instrument that consists of a thin wire loop electrode and an electrosurgical generator, and uses electrical currrent to cut away cervical tissue in the immediate area of the loop wire | It has both diagnostic and therapeutic uses. It is most commonly used to excise vulvar condylomas and cervical dysplasias. It is also used for cone biopsies of the cervix | Minimal pain, minimal damage to the surrounding tissue, and low morbidity | It is an office procedure and requires only local anesthetic |

(*Continued*)

Common Gynecologic Procedures (*Continued*)

| Procedure | Description | Indications/Contraindications | Benefits/Risks | Comments |
|---|---|---|---|---|
| Magnetic resonance imaging (MRI) | It is a form of imaging that is based on the magnetic characteristics of various atoms and molecules in the body. It uses nonionizing radiofrequency signals | Used to evaluate any soft tissue mass but emerging clinical applications include assessment of breast lesions and staging of cervical cancer | There are no harmful effects to the fetus | MRI is best suited to evaluate soft tissue or non calcified tissue |
| Mammography | It is an x-ray examination of the breasts. The breasts are placed between two plates and pressed flat. An x-ray is taken of each | It is used as a diagnostic and screening modality for breast masses | Lower dose radiation exposure makes this exam safe | Women should receive screening mammograms every 1–2 years when they reach age 40 |

| | | | | |
|---|---|---|---|---|
| Pap smear | It is a microscopic examination of cells scraped from the ectocervix and endocervix | Mainly used as a screening modality, it can detect cancerous or precancerous conditions of the cervix | | ACOG recommends annual Pap smear screenings from 3 years after the start of sexual intercourse but not later than age 21 years. Women at risk should have annual Pap smears; women who have had three consecutive negative tests can be screened every 2–3 years |
| Schiller's test for neoplasia | Iodine solution is placed on areas of the cervix and vagina that are suspect for dysplasia.Any portion of the tissue that does not absorb the dye is biopsied for signs of cancer | It is performed on areas of the cervical or vaginal mucosa where malignant changes are suspected | | Colposcopy is a more accurate diagnostic tool. |
| Suction and curettage (S&C) | It is a procedure used in the first trimester to remove the products of conception by first dilating the cervix, followed by suction and scraping inside the uterus | It is used in pregnancy termination | Suction curettes are preferred because they are less likely to cause damage to the uterus. Other risks may include bleeding and cramping | This is an outpatient procedure and may be done in the office using local anesthetics |

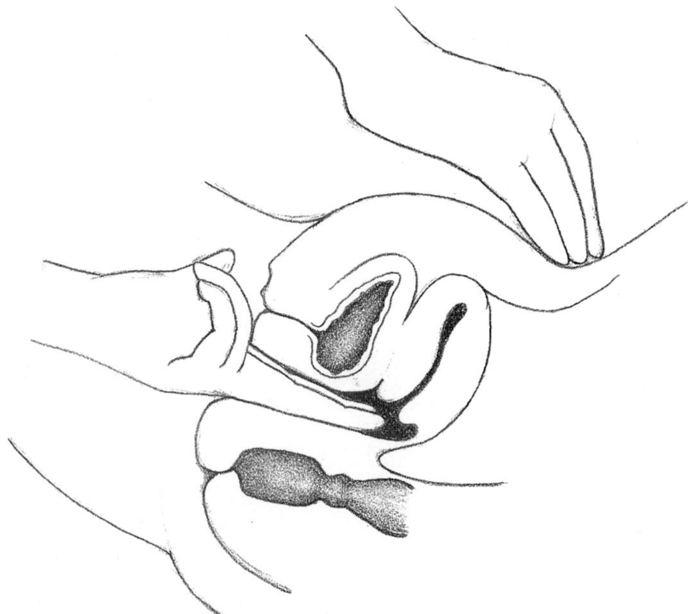

**Figure 2-1** Bimanual examination of the uterus and adnexa.

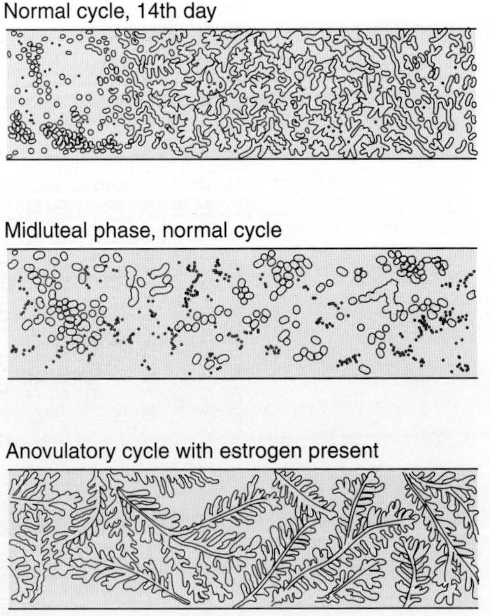


**Figure 2-2** Fern test for ovulation.

CHAPTER 3

# Female Anatomy

## BONY PELVIS

**What forms the bony pelvis?**

Sacrum

Coccyx

Paired hip bones (ilium, ischium, and pubis)

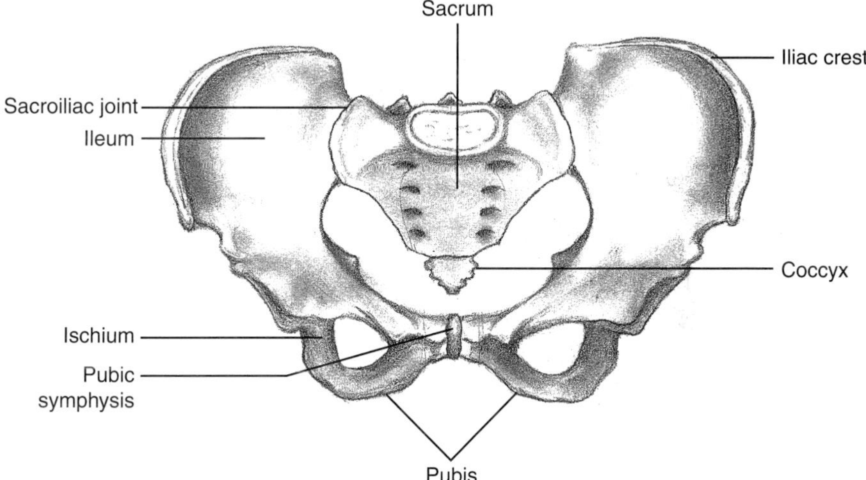


**Figure 3-1** The bony pelvis.

**What is the sacral promontory and what is its significance?**

The most anterior projection of the sacrum, it is a landmark for the insertion of a laparoscope as it demarcates the point of bifurcation of the common iliac arteries

**What is the arcuate line and what is its significance?**

Also called the linea semicircularis, it is the line that marks the pelvic brim. It lies between the first two segments of the pelvis and demarcates the site of entry of the inferior epigastric artery into the rectus sheath

**What is the ischial spine and what is its significance?**

It is the medial protrusion of the ischium and an important landmark for giving a pudendal nerve block. It also provides a good landmark by which to assess progression of fetal descent during labor

**What are the four pelvic configurations found in females and how common are each?**

Gynecoid (50%); anthropoid (25–50%); android (16–33%); platypelloid (3%)

**Describe the shape of a gynecoid pelvis.**

It is **wider** and **lower** than the male pelvis. The pubic arch is wide and round, the iliac bone is flatter, and the ischial spines are not prominent. The anterior-posterior and transverse diameters are roughly equal. All of this makes the pelvic basin more spacious

**Describe the shape of an anthropoid pelvis.**

It is **heart-shaped** with a wider anterior-posterior diameter than a transverse diameter

**Describe the shape of an android pelvis.**

It is **narrower** and **taller** than the gynecoid pelvis

**Describe the shape of a platypelloid pelvis.**

It has a wider transverse diameter than an anterior-posterior diameter

**What is the pelvic inlet?**

The superior circumference of the lesser pelvis. Its boundaries include the sacral promontory, the pubic ramus and symphysis pubis, and the linea terminalis

**Describe the following:**

**Obstetric conjugate**

The shortest pelvic diameter through which the fetal head passes; it can only be measured radiographically; the distance from the sacral promontory to the symphysis pubis; the normal diameter is >10 cm

**True conjugate**

The AP diameter that lies between the sacral promontory and the superior symphysis pubis

**Diagonal conjugate**

Only one measured clinically; the distance between the sacral promontory and the inferior margin of the symphysis pubis

## PELVIC ORGANS

**What is the major blood supply to the pelvic organs?**

Internal iliac artery (aka hypogastric artery)

**Describe the branches of the internal iliac artery.**

Coming off the common iliac artery, the internal iliac typically but not always divides into anterior and posterior trunks

Anterior trunk: Superior vesical
Middle vesical
Inferior vesical
Middle hemorrhoidal
Obturator
Internal pudendal
Inferior gluteal
Uterine
Vaginal

Posterior truck: Iliolumbar
Lateral sacral
Superior gluteal

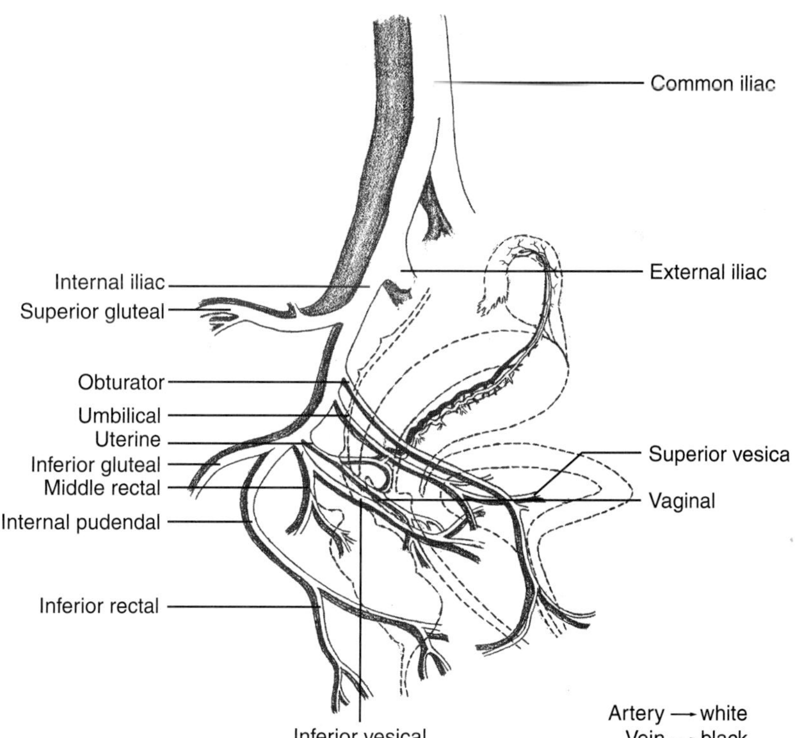


**Figure 3-2** Arteries and veins of the female reproductive system.

**Describe the position of the vagina in the pelvis.**

It extends from the vulva to the cervix. The bladder lies anterior, separated from the vagina by the vesicovaginal septum. The rectum lies posterior, separated from the vagina by the rectovaginal septum

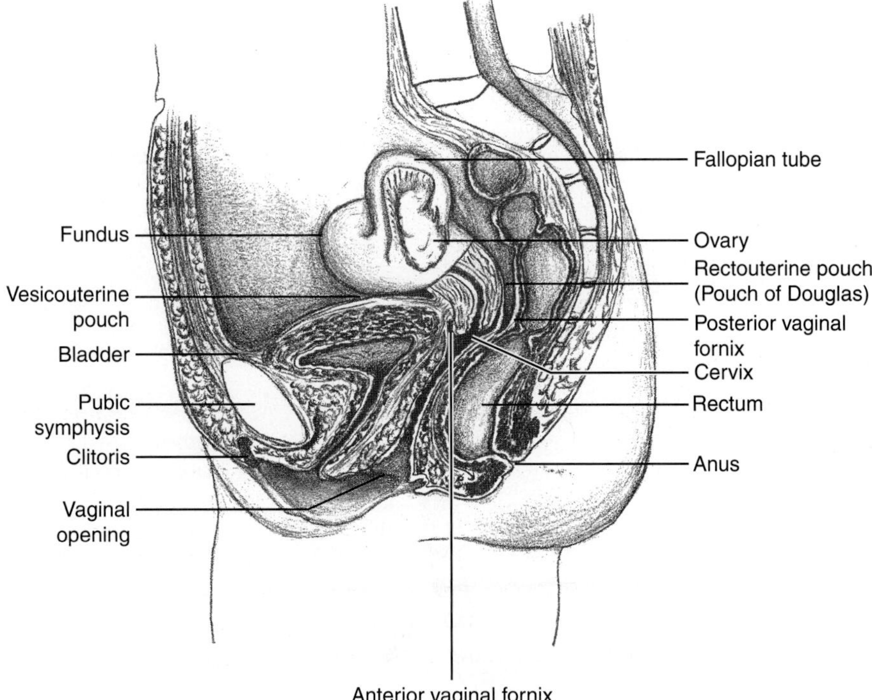


**Figure 3-3** Midsagittal view of pelvic viscera.

**What is the major blood supply to the vagina?**

The vaginal artery (can also arise from hypogastric artery or the uterine artery)

**What is the innervation to the vagina?**

Parasympathetics via S2-S4 for the upper two-thirds and general somatic efferent to the lower one-third via the pudendal nerve; there are no other specific nerve endings

**What is the lymphatic drainage of the vagina?**

The upper two-thirds drain into the internal and external iliac nodes. The lower one-third drains into the inguinal nodes

**Describe the layers of the vaginal wall (from interior to exterior).**

It is composed of a smooth muscle layer (arranged in an outer longitudinal layer, circumferential layer, and a poorly differentiated inner longitudinal layer) followed by a mucosal layer. The mucosa of the vagina is lined by stratified squamous epithelium

**Describe the vaginal fornices.**

The area of the vagina surrounding the cervix; divided into anterior, posterior, and two lateral fornices

**Describe the position of the uterus in the pelvis.**

It is covered by the peritoneum (vesicouterine peritoneum anteriorly and the peritoneal reflection called the pouch of Douglas posteriorly) and is between the bladder and rectum, directly touching the bladder

**What ligaments support the uterine position in the pelvis?**

Uterosacral, cardinal, round, and broad

**What are the anatomic portions of the uterus?**

Fundus (most superior portion of the uterus [above the entrance of the fallopian tubes]); Corpus (the uterine body); Isthmus (area where the uterus begins to constrict); Cervix (inferior portion of the uterus that extends into the vagina)

**What is meant by flexion of the uterus?**

The angle between the long axis of the uterine body and the cervix; can be anteflexed or retroflexed

**What is meant by the terms anteversion and retroversion?**

The angle between the cervix and the vagina

**What are the histological layers of the uterine wall (from interior to exterior)?**

Endometrium (ciliated columnar epithelium, glands, and spiral arteries); Myometrium (smooth muscle and connective tissue); Serosa

**What are the major blood supplies to the uterus?**

Uterine and ovarian arteries (there are extensive anastomoses which allow for ligation of the uterine or internal iliac during hemorrhage to control bleeding without compromising blood supply to the uterus)

**Describe the course of the uterine artery in the pelvis.**

Arises from the internal iliac → divides into cervicovaginal and uterine branches → uterine branch divides into the fundal, ovarian, and tubal arteries and provides radial arteries that perforate into the uterus

**What is the relationship of the uterine artery with the ureter?**

The ureter crosses under the artery ("water under the bridge") 2 cm lateral to the cervix

**What is the lymphatic drainage of the uterus?**

Internal and external iliac nodes (although the fundus can drain into the para-aortic lymph nodes)

**Describe the following portions of the cervix:**

**Portio**

The portion of the cervix that is visible from the vagina

**Cervical canal**

Area in between the internal and external os

**External os**

Inferior opening of the cervix into the vagina

**Internal os**

Superior opening of the cervix into the uterine cavity

**What is the major blood supply to the cervix?**

Cervical branch of the uterine artery

**What is the innervation to the cervix?**

Autonomics, sympathetics (T12–L3), and parasympathetics from S2, S3, S4

**What is the lymphatic drainage of the cervix?**

Internal and external iliacs to the common iliacs

**What are the fallopian tubes?**

These are 8–10 cm tubes that extend laterally from the body of the uterus

**What are the histological layers of the fallopian tubes (from interior to exterior)?**

Mucosal layer (ciliated columnar epithelium covered in cilia); Muscular layer (external longitudinal layer and internal circular layer); Serosa

**What are the segments of the fallopian tubes (from medial to lateral)?**

Interstitial, isthmic, ampullary, infundibular, and fimbrial

**What is the major blood supply to the fallopian tubes?**

Uterine and ovarian arteries

**What is the lymphatic drainage of the fallopian tubes?**

Aortic nodes

**Describe the position of the ovaries in the pelvis.**

They lie in the ovarian fossae, which are lateral to the uterus in the pelvic sidewall where the common iliac artery bifurcates

**What are the histological layers of the ovary (from interior to exterior)?**

Medulla (connective tissue and blood supply); cortex (ova and tunica albuginea); germinal epithelium

**What is the major blood supply to the ovaries?**

Branches of the uterine artery and the ovarian arteries

**Where do the right and left ovarian veins drain?**

The right ovarian vein drains through the inferior vena cava (IVC) and the left drains through the left renal vein

**Describe the position of the bladder in the pelvis.**

It sits between the abdominal wall/pelvic bones (anteriorly) and the vagina/cervix (posteriorly)

**What are the major blood supplies to the bladder?**

Superior vesical artery, inferior vesical artery, and middle hemorrhoidal artery

**What is the innervation to the bladder?**

Parasympathetics, sympathetics, and the pudendal nerve (innervates the external urethral sphincter)

**What is the lymphatic drainage of the bladder?**

Internal iliac nodes

**Describe the course of the ureter through the abdomen and pelvis.**

In the abdomen, it is retroperitoneal on the anterior surface of the psoas muscle. It then crosses the common iliac artery (the right at the bifurcation and the left 1–2 cm above the bifurcation) and then follows the pelvic wall laterally to the medial broad ligament. It then crosses under the uterine artery and courses medially to enter the cardinal ligaments. It enters the bladder at the trigone

**How is the ureter distinguished during surgery?**

(1) Ureteral peristalsis
(2) Auerbach's plexus (only on the ureteral anterior surface)

**What are the most common sites of ureteral injury?**

(1) Pelvic brim
(2) Where the ureter crosses the uterine artery
(3) Bladder trigone

**How can the rectum be differentiated from the rest of the bowel?**

It begins after the sigmoid colon where the mesentery ends and it does not have teniae coli or appendices epiploicae

**Why is the rectum sometimes injured during vaginal surgery?**
Because of its proximity to the posterior vaginal wall

**What is the blood supply to the rectum?**
Hemorrhoidal arteries (superior, middle, and inferior)

**What is the lymphatic drainage of the rectum?**
Iliac nodes

**Name the ligamentous structures in the pelvis. Describe each.**

**Broad ligaments**
Reflections of peritoneum from the lateral margin of the uterus to the pelvic sidewall; contain the uterine vessels and ureters in their base

**Round ligaments**
Homologue of the male gubernaculums; also contain an artery of the round ligament, connects lateral uterine fundus to the upper labia majora

**Uterosacral ligaments**
Extend from posterior-inferior uterus to the presacral fascia

**Cardinal ligaments**
Support the uterus; at base of broad ligament, contain uterine artery

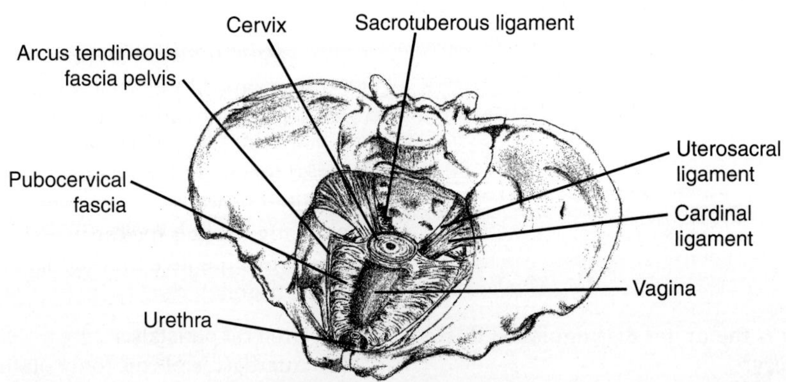


**Figure 3-4** Ligaments of the female pelvis.

**Describe the clinical manifestations of damage to each of the following nerves:**

**Femoral nerve**
Problems with hip flexion

**Obturator nerve**
Problems with adduction of thigh/ hip; loss of sensation in medial thigh

| | |
|---|---|
| **Genitofemoral nerve** | Loss of sensation in perineum |
| **Peroneal nerve** | Foot drop; loss of sensation in lateral lower leg and dorsum of the foot |

**During which types of surgeries can each of the following nerves be injured?**

| | |
|---|---|
| **Femoral nerve** | Abdominal surgery or inguinal node dissection |
| **Obturator nerve** | Radical hysterectomy or node dissection |
| **Genitofemoral nerve** | Radical hysterectomy or node dissection |
| **Peroneal nerve** | Improper placement of legs in stirrups |

## PERINEUM

| | |
|---|---|
| **What is the perineum?** | Area between the mons pubis and the buttocks |

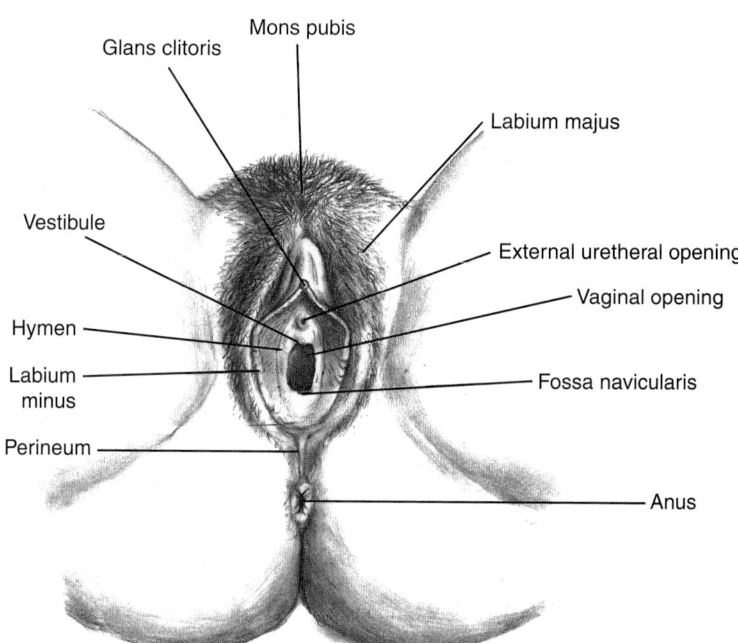


**Figure 3-5** External genitalia of the adult female.

**What is the major blood supply to the perineum?**
Internal pudendal artery

**What is the major innervation to the perineum?**
Pudendal nerve

**What is the lymphatic drainage of the perineum?**
Inguinal nodes

**Name the muscles of the perineum**
Superficial and deep transverse perineal
Bulbocavernosus
Ischiocavernosus
External anal sphincter
Urethral sphincter

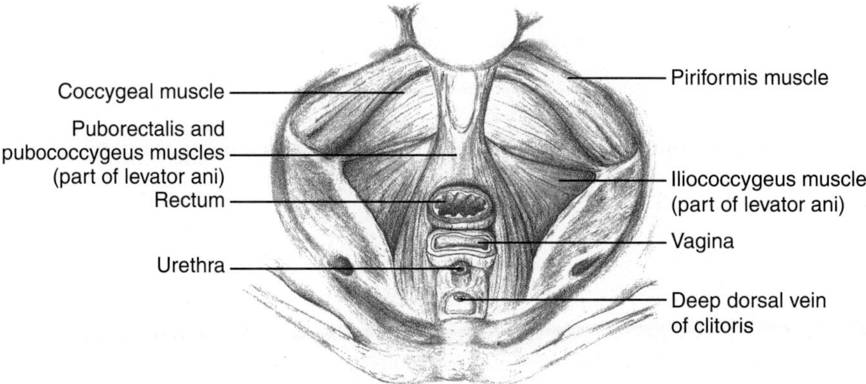


**Figure 3-6** Pelvic diaphragm—superior view.

**What is the urogenital diaphragm?**
Muscles between the pubis symphysis and the ischial tuberosities that support the perineum

**Name the muscles of the urogenital diaphragm.**
Urethral sphincter and deep transverse perineal

**What is the pelvic diaphragm?**
Muscles from the upper pubis and ischium to the rectum that support the perineum

**What muscles comprise the pelvic diaphragm?**
Levator ani; coccygeal

**What structures comprise the external genitalia of the female?**
Mons pubis, labia majora, labia minora, clitoris, vestibule, urethral opening, vagina, perineum, and perineal body

**What are the muscles of the vulva?**

Superior transverse perineal

Bulbocavernosus

Ischiocavernosus

(All lie superficial to the urogenital fascia [perineal membrane])

**What is the difference between the labia minora and the labia majora?**

Labia majora are skin folds with adipose tissue that connect with the mons anteriorly and the perineum posteriorly. They contain hair follicles, sweat glands, and sebaceous glands. Labia minora are narrower skinfolds medial to the labia majora that contain sweat and sebaceous glands but no hair follicles or adipose tissue. They connect with the prepuce and frenulum of the clitoris anteriorly and the labia majora and perineum posteriorly

**What is the frenulum?**

The anterior junction of the labia minora; ventral to the clitoris

**What is the vestibule?**

The area between the labia minora, clitoris, and perineum where the vaginal and urethral openings are located

**What are Bartholin's glands?**

Glands found deep to the vestibule, lateral to the vagina that open into the vestibule

**Where is the urethral opening in relation to other perineal structures?**

It is located in the anterior aspect of the vestibule

**What are Skene's glands?**

Also called paraurethral glands; they are homologues of the prostate that surround the urethral opening and empty into the vestibule

**What are the embryologically homogenous male structures for the labia majora and the clitoris?**

Scrotum for the labia majora and glans penis for the clitoris

## ABDOMINAL WALL

**What are the layers of the abdominal wall?**

Skin → subcutaneous fat → outer fatty layer (Camper) of superficial fascia → inner membranous layer (Scarpa) of superficial fascia →

anterior rectus sheath → rectus abdominus muscle → posterior rectus sheath → preperitoneal fat subserous or extraperitoneal fascia → parietal peritoneum

**Describe the blood supply to the lower abdomen.**

Deep circumflex iliac (off of the external iliac) and external pudendal artery

**What is the arcuate line?**

Also called the linea semicircularis; above it the posterior aponeurosis of the internal oblique and the aponeurosis of the transversus abdominus comprise the posterior portion of the rectus sheath. Below the arcuate line they contribute to the anterior leaflet of the rectus sheath

**What is the linea alba?**

The medial aspect of the rectus abdominus; formed by the fusion of the aponeuroses of the anterior abdominal muscles

**What are the linea semilunara?**

The lateral borders of the rectum abdominus muscles

**What structures pass through the inguinal canal in the female?**

Round ligament

An artery and vein passing to the uterus

Extraperitoneal fat

SECTION II

# Topics in Gynecology

CHAPTER 4

# General Gynecology

## Menstrual Cycle Physiology

**What is the average duration of the menstrual cycle, duration of menses, and amount of blood loss during menses?**

The average duration of the menstrual cycle is **28 days**. The average duration of menstrual flow is **4 days**. On an average, women lose less than **60 mL of blood** during each menses

**What are the two phases of the menstrual cycle and how long does each last?**

**Follicular** (or **proliferative**) phase and the **luteal** (or **secretory**) phase, separated by **ovulation**. (Follicular/luteal describe the ovarian changes, proliferative/secretory describe the endometrial changes)

By convention, day 1 marks the onset of menses. The follicular phase begins on day 1 and lasts approximately **14** days (days 1–14) in a 28-day cycle, until ovulation occurs. The luteal phase then commences and lasts until approximately day **28** (days 14–28)

**What causes the variability in the length of the menstrual cycle?**

The duration of the follicular phase (the luteal phase is constant)

**Describe the hormone pathway involved in the menstrual cycle (see Fig. 4-1) and name which structures produce each hormone**

The cycle begins in the arcuate nucleus of the **hypothalamus** where **gonadotrophin-releasing hormone (GnRH)** is released in a pulsatile fashion. GnRH stilmulates the **anterior pituitary** to release **follicle-stimulating hormone (FSH)** and **luteinizing hormone (LH)**. These gonadotropins then cause the ovaries to release the sex steroid hormones **estradiol** and **progesterone**. Estrogen

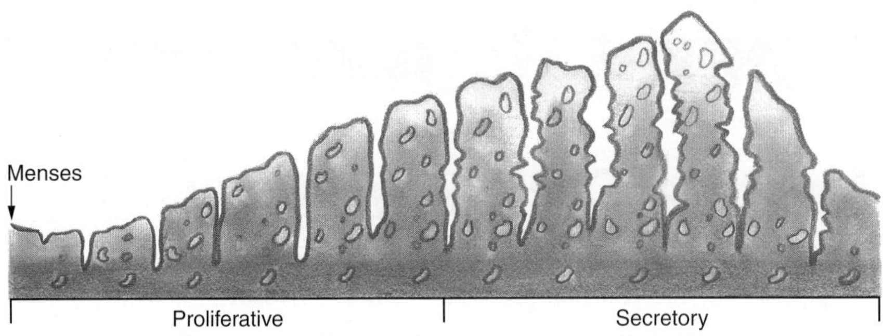


Endometrial histology

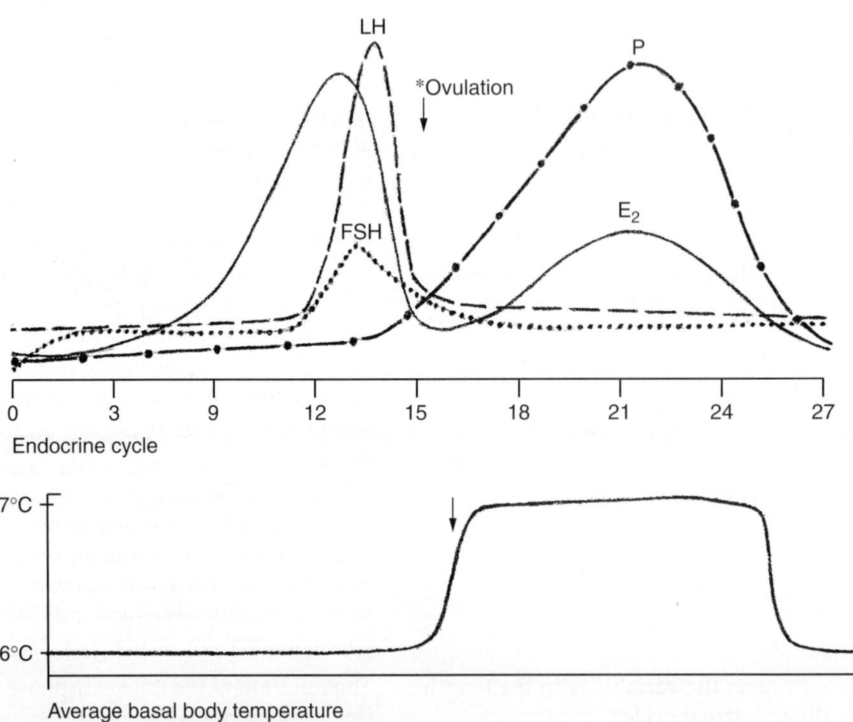


**Figure 4-1** The menstrual cycle.

and progesterone feedback negatively on both the hypothalamus and the pituitary gland

**What is happening in the ovary during the menstrual cycle?**

The ovary beings with approximately one million **primordial follicles at birth (20 million at week**

**20 in utero)**. Each follicle contains an oocyte arrested in **prophase of meiosis**. The oocyte is surrounded by pre-granulosa cells and these are surrounded by pre-theca cells. In the follicular phase, FSH stimulates the pre-granulosa cells to become granulosa cells. The **granulosa cells** secrete **estradiol**. The pre-theca cells in turn become **theca cells** and secrete **androgens**, which are aromatized by the granulosa cells into estradiol.

One follicle with the highest number of granulosa cells, FSH receptors, and estradiol production becomes the **dominant follicle** and all other follicles become atretic. This follicle is released during ovulation and becomes the **corpus luteum**. The corpus luteum secretes progesterone and a smaller amount of estrogen during the follicular phase of the cycle. If fertilization does not occur, it degenerates into the **corpus albicans**

**What is the function of the corpus luteum?**

Secretion of **progesterone** and **estradiol**. It is the only structure that produces progesterone in significant quantities which sustains the pregnancy until the placenta is developed

**What is happening to hormone levels in the follicular phase?**

At menstruation, concentrations of **estradiol**, **progesterone**, and **LH** are at their **lowest** point. **FSH and LH levels begin to rise** in response to the low estrogen and progesterone.

**Estradiol** levels, secreted from the dominant ovarian follicle, begin to rise by day 4. Just before ovulation, estradiol levels peak. This peak causes a positive feedback on LH secretion, leading to the **LH surge** and a **smaller FSH surge**, which results in **ovulation** 30–38 hours later. **Progesterone** levels remain **low** throughout the follicular phase

**What is happening to hormone levels in the luteal phase?**

The LH surge causes granulosa and theca cells to secrete **progesterone** and smaller amounts of **estrogen. Progesterone peaks** 3–4 days after ovulation.

Estrogen levels decrease immediately after ovulation but slowly rise with the growth of the corpus luteum. Progesterone and estrogen (at low to moderate levels) both act via negative feedback to **suppress LH** and **FSH**. If fertilization and implantation do not occur, progesterone and estradiol levels diminish after 11 days. FSH increases as the corpus luteum regresses

**What is happening to the endometrium in the proliferative phase?**

At menses, the **endometrium sloughs off** until it becomes a thin line. During the proliferative phase estradiol levels rise, resulting in the proliferation of the uterine endometrium. The endometrium becomes **thicker** and **more glandular** and the **spiral arteries elongate**. On ultrasound, it appears as a "**triple stripe**" pattern

**What is happening to the endometrium in the secretory phase?**

The progesterone released from the corpus luteum leads to **slowing of endometrial proliferation**, reorganization of the glands (resulting in a more **edematous stroma**), and further **coiling of the spiral arteries**. This results in the loss of the "triple stripe" pattern and its replacement with a **uniformly bright** endometrium. If pregnancy does not occur, the endometrium degenerates

**What are the primary clinical manifestations of estradiol and progesterone during the menstrual cycle?**

**Estradiol**
Endometrium: thickens stroma and elongates glands (creates **proliferative endometrium**); Endocervix: stimulates secretion of thin, **watery mucus**. Produces "**ferning**" pattern when spread on a glass slide;
Vagina: promotes **vaginal thickening**

**Progesterone**
Endometrium: causes tissue to become edematous and blood vessels to thicken and twist (creates **secretory endometrium**);
Endocervix: **thickens** endocervical

**mucus, causing it to become stringy**; Breast: stimulates acinar glands, causing breasts to round; Other: **raises basal body temperature** by 0.6–1°F. Causes some women to have the emotional, physical, and behavioral changes of premenstrual syndrome (PMS)

**What layer of the endometrium sloughs off during menses?**

The **functionalis layer (inner layer)** sloughs off after glandular and stromal degeneration

**What hormone mediates menstrual cramps and how is it synthesized?**

**Prostaglandins**, especially $PGF_{2\alpha}$. It is released by the secretory endometrium in response to progesterone and causes uterine contractions

# Family Planning

## CONTRACEPTION OVERVIEW

**How many American women use contraception and what are the rates of unintended or mistimed pregnancy in the United States?**

Between **89% and 93%**; yet **53%** of births are either unintended or mistimed

**What are some of the reasons for contraception failure?**

Failure of the method; Incorrect use; Nonadherence

**What are the two measures for effectiveness of a contraceptive method?**

1. **Theoretical effectiveness (perfect use)**—the pregnancy rate among women who use the method correctly every time
2. **Actual effectiveness (typical use)**—includes the chances of inconsistent or incorrect use

**What factors about each method must be considered when counseling about contraception?**

Coital dependence, convenience, cost, duration of action, protection against sexually transmitted infections (STIs), effect on menses, religion, reversibility, acceptability, and side effects

**What are the five main classes of contraception?**

1. Rhythm method
2. Barrier methods

3. Hormonal contraceptives
4. Intrauterine devices (IUDs)
5. Sterilization

**Rank the following contraceptives from the highest to the lowest with respect to actual effectiveness. What is the failure rate associated with each?**

**Condom, diaphragm/cervical cap, injectable/implantable hormonal contraception, oral contraception, periodic abstinence (fertility awareness method), spermicide, sterilization, withdrawal**

IUDs (0.1–2%)

Sterilization (0.4–4%)

Injectable hormonal contraception (<1%)

Oral contraceptives (5%)

Male condom (14%)

Diaphragm or cervical cap (20%)

Female condom (21%)

Periodic abstinence (25%)

Withdrawal (19%)

Spermicide (26%)

**What is the fertility awareness method?**

Predicting the time of month when a woman is **most fertile** and **abstaining** during that time. Also known as the rhythm method

**What three methods can be used to predict fertility and which days are women presumed to be fertile?**

1. **Date of the last menstrual period:** days 8–19 of the cycle (peri-ovulation)
2. **Changes in body temperature:** after menstruation until 3 days after an increase in basal body temperature by 0.5–1°F
3. **Changes in cervical mucus:** when the mucus becomes clear and stretchy (peri-ovulation) known as spinbarkeit

**Why are fertility awareness methods unreliable?**

Because people **do not always abstain** during this time and because there is always **some chance of fertility** on the "non-fertile" days. Body temperature and cervical mucus (especially if used together) are more effective than the calendar method because of irregular cycle lengths

**What is the withdrawal method?**

The withdrawal method is when the male **withdraws** from the vagina **before ejaculation**. It is ineffective when not timed correctly or when the pre-ejaculatory fluid contains sperm

**Is lactation an effective means of birth control?**

Lactation is somewhat effective as a means of birth control because of the **prolactin-induced inhibition of GnRH**, which leads to a delay in return to ovulation. Additional contraception should be used by breast- feeding women to prevent pregnancy

**What factors affect the effectiveness of lactation as a means of birth control?**

The number of times a woman breast feeds each day; How effective breast feeding is (i.e., how much milk she is producing); If the child is getting any supplemental feeding

## STERILIZATION METHODS

**What methods are available for surgical sterilization?**

**Male: vasectomy**—ligation of vas deferens preventing passage of sperm into seminal fluid

**Female:**

1. **Ligation/removal** of a section of the fallopian tube—involves laparotomy or laparoscopy
2. **Mechanical blockage**—using rings, coils, clips, or plugs
3. **Coagulation-induced blockage**—usually through cauterization methods

**What are the overall risks and benefits of female sterilization?**

Risks:

1. Anesthesia/surgical complications
2. Ectopic pregnancy—failed procedures can result in an increased risk of ectopic pregnancies
3. Regret of the procedure (especially in younger people)

4. Does not stop the spread of HIV or other STIs

Benefits: 1. Not coitally dependent
2. Decreased risk of ovarian cancer
3. No evidence of menstrual irregularity or dysmenorrhea

**What are the risks and benefits of each of the female sterilization procedures?**

**Ligation** is one of the **oldest methods** of sterilization with the **lowest failure rate (0.8%)** but it is not easily reversed

**Mechanical blockage** with a clip is the **most readily reversed method** but it also has the **highest failure rate (3.7%)**

**Coagulation-induced blockage** with electrocautery is the **fastest procedure** with a **low failure rate (2.5%)**, but there is increased risk of electrical damage to surrounding structures

**What are some advantages and disadvantages of a vasectomy?**

Advantages: effectiveness is very high—typical first-year failure rate 0.15%; simpler, surgically safer, more cost-effective than female sterilization; Males share contraception responsibility with females

Disadvantages: does not protect against STIs

**Is reversibility after a female sterilization procedure and vasectomy possible?**

Reversibility after a female sterilization procedure is generally very difficult and has been reported as only **60%** effective.

**As for vasectomy**, men are generally counseled that it is permanent. About **50–70%** of men who have a reversal become fertile. The chance of becoming fertile decreases with increasing time after the procedure

**If a woman in her early twenties with two children requests tubal sterilization, what is the next appropriate recommendation?**

Considering the woman's age, you must inform her of the risk for regret of the procedure and of the permanence of tubal sterilization/ difficulty of reversal

## Hormonal Contraceptives

**What types of hormonal contraceptives are available?**

Oral contraceptives; Injectable contraceptives; Contraceptive patch; Implants; Vaginal ring

**What is the general mechanism of action of hormonal methods of contraception?**

Hormonal contraceptive methods act primarily by **inhibiting** the midcycle surge of **gonadotropin secretion** and thereby **inhibiting ovulation**. They also **alter the endometrium and cervical mucus** to **decrease sperm transport and implantation**, and **decrease tubal motility**

**Do hormonal contraceptives protect against STIs?**

No. Condoms must be used to prevent transmission of STIs

## Oral Contraceptive Pills

**What are the types of oral contraceptive pills (OCPs) available and which is the most effective?**

**Combined estrogen-progesterone pills** are the most effective (2–3% actual failure rate). **Progestin-only pills** are indicated for women who have contraindications to estrogen-containing pills

**How are OCPs dosed?**

**Cyclic**—OCPs are taken for 21 consecutive days, followed by 7 days of placebo

**Extended cycle**—OCPs are taken for 84 consecutive days, followed by 7 days of placebo

**When should OCPs be started?**

On the **first day of menstruation**

**Sunday starter schedule**: take the pill on the Sunday after the beginning of menses. This method requires **another nonhormonal form of contraception** for the first **7 days of OCP use**

**Quick-start regimen:** begin taking the pill ASAP, even in the doctor's office/clinic; increases adherence, decreases failures, side effects the same

**What type of OCP should be started first?**

Low-estrogen OCPs (20–35 μg of ethinyl estradiol [EE]) or very low estrogen OCPs (20 μg of EE) should be started in the average patient

**In addition to contraception, what other advantages are conferred by taking OCPs?**

Decreases menorrhagia, dysmenorrhea, and ovulation pain

(mittelschmerz); regulates menses; Lessens anemia; Improves acne (with estrogen-containing pills); protects against benign breast disease, formation of new corpus luteum cysts, osteoporosis, hirsutism; may reduce fibroids (controversial); decreases risk for ovarian cancer, endometrial cancer, pelvic inflammatory disease (PID), colorectal cancer, ectopic pregnancy

**What are the risks of taking OCPs?**

Increased risk of **thromboembolic disease/stroke; hepatocellular adenoma**; adenocarcinoma of the cervix; myocardial infarction (MI) (especially in high estrogen formulations); subarachnoid hemorrhage; hypertension; insulin dependence in diabetics

**Is there a risk of developing breast cancer when using OCPs?**

Experts agree there is most likely **no** risk between birth control pills and breast cancer

**What are the absolute contraindications to the use of estrogen-progesterone OCPs?**

History of thromboembolic disease/thrombophlebitis; smokers >age 35; cerebrovascular disease/coronary artery disease; congenital hyperlipidemia; history of an estrogen-dependent tumor; liver disease; pregnancy

**What are the relative contraindications to the use of estrogen-progesterone OCPs?**

Diabetes mellitus (may need to change insulin dose)

Epilepsy (can use the higher dose E2 pills if their medicines stimulate the $P_{450}$ system; if their medicines do not, there is no contraindication)

Gallbladder disease (although benign disease is not a contraindication)

Hypertension (requires close monitoring)

Use of some antibiotics

Postpartum state (women may be susceptible to clots following delivery)

Migraines/vascular headaches with aura

Obesity

**What are the possible side effects of OCPs?**

Breakthrough bleeding (especially first 3 months)

Amenorrhea

Depression/mood changes

Nausea

Bloating

Breast tenderness

Headaches

Acne (with some progestin-only pills)

**Do OCPs cause weight gain?**

OCPs have not been proven to cause weight gain

**How do OCPs affect acne?**

**Progestins worsen acne** by increasing sebum production whereas **estrogen relieves acne**. Combined OCPs are used to treat acne. Use of a less androgenic progesterone-only pill will lower the risk of acne

**What mediates the increased risk of thromboembolic disease with OCPs?**

**Estrogen**. It **increases** the levels of **clotting factors VII** and **X** and **decreases** levels of **antithrombin III**

**What is a hepatocellular adenoma?**

A rare **benign liver tumor** associated with long-term OCP use, diagnosed by a **right upper quadrant pain** or a palpable **mass** on physical examination. Rupture of the adenoma can lead to hemodynamic instability

**How is hepatocellular adenoma treated?**

**Discontinuation of OCPs is the treatment for hepatocellular adenoma.** Pregnancy should be avoided in patients with this diagnosis unless the tumor is surgically removed

**What is breakthrough bleeding?**

**Intermenstrual bleeding** that occurs because of an **imbalance of estrogen and progesterone**. Occurs in 10–30% of women on low-dose OCPs.

Early occurrences usually **resolve spontaneously**, but if bleeding does not resolve within 4 months, the patient can be switched to a pill with **increased estrogen** or a **lower dose** progesterone. Pathologic causes of abnormal bleeding should also be considered.

**What is post-pill amenorrhea?**

The **failure to menstruate by 6 months after cessation of OCPs.** Most cases **resolve spontaneously**

**How is post-pill amenorrhea managed?**

An endocrine workup is necessary after 6 months to rule out pregnancy and functional causes of amenorrhea (anorexia, excessive exercise). It should also include a **progestin challenge test** to rule out hypothalamic-pituitary dysfunction

**What is a progestin challenge test?**

100 mg of progesterone is administered. Withdrawal bleeding should occur within a few days if ovulation is occurring

**What drugs interfere with OCP metabolism?**

OCPs are metabolized by the **cytochrome $P_{450}$**. Drugs including **anticonvulsants** (phenytoin), **antibiotics** (isoniazid, rifampin, penicillin, tetracycline), and some **anti-retrovirals** decrease their effectiveness by increasing their metabolism

**What should be done if the patient must take these drugs: for a short duration, for a long duration?**

**Back-up contraception** should be used if the drugs are used for a short duration; however, one must seek an **alternative contraceptive modality if the drugs are used for long duration**

**What should a patient do if she forgot to take pills in following cases?**

**One pill:** take the missed dose as soon as possible and take the following dose at her regular time

**Two pills:** take two pills immediately and then continue the following day

**Three or more pills:** stop taking the pills in order to have menses and then restart the cycle

**Note: In all of the above cases, an additional contraceptive measure for the rest of that cycle is required. A pregnancy test is recommended if menstruation does not occur**

## Injectable Contraceptives

| | |
|---|---|
| **What injectable contraceptive is available in the United States?** | **Depot medroxyprogesterone acetate** (DMPA or Depo-Provera)—a progestin-only injectable |
| **What is its typical use failure rate in the first year?** | Less than 1%—similar (if not lower) to that of a tubal ligation |
| **How is DMPA administered?** | An **intramuscular (IM) injection** of 150 mg **every 3 months** |
| **When should DMPA be started?** | DMPA should be begun **within 5 days of the onset of menses**. If received after this time window, another nonhormonal method must be used for the first 7 days |
| **What are the contraindications to the use of DMPA?** | Undiagnosed abnormal uterine bleeding; cerebrovascular disease/ coronary artery disease; liver disease; pregnancy; thromboembolic disease/ thrombophlebitis (relative contraindication) |
| **In addition to contraception, what other advantages are conferred by DMPA?** | Decreased risk of **endometrial cancer and pelvic inflammatory disease (PID); decreased volume of menstrual bleeding; decreased pain associated with endometriosis;** can be used while breast-feeding and in cases where estrogen is contraindicated |
| **What are the potential side effects of taking DMPA?** | **Amenorrhea** (eventually occurs in most women within 1 year of consistent use); **irregular bleeding** (spotting); decreased bone density **(fully reversed once DMPA is stopped)**; acne; headache; depression<br><br>There is **no evidence** to date that DMPA leads to **weight gain** |
| **How long does it take to restore fertility after DMPA is stopped?** | Most women return to fertility in **9–12 months** after their last injection; however fertility can be delayed for up to 18 months after cessation |

## Hormonal Implants, Patches, and Rings

| | |
|---|---|
| **What are contraceptive implants?** | Small **rods placed surgically** in the inner part of the upper arm **subdermally**. They **release progestin** in a controlled manner and can be left in place for **3–5 years**, depending on the implant |
| **What is the typical use failure rate in the first year?** | 0.05% |
| **What are the absolute contraindications to hormonal implants?** | Pregnancy, undiagnosed vaginal bleeding, liver disease, breast cancer, thrombophlebitis/embolism |
| **What are the main side effects of contraceptive implants?** | **Irregular bleeding** (common), amenorrhea, headache, acne, weight gain |
| **What is the contraceptive patch ?** | A **transdermal patch** that delivers **estrogen** and **progestin** in a controlled manner daily |
| **How is the contraceptive patch administered?** | It is placed on the buttock, abdomen, upper arm, or upper torso (but not breast). It is **changed once per week** for 3 weeks, followed by a patch-free week<br><br>Note: If detached for more than 24 hours, it must be replaced and an additional method of contraception should be used for 7 days |
| **What is the overall failure rate for the contraceptive patch?** | 0.3–1% |
| **What is the main advantage of the patch over OCPs?** | Better compliance by avoiding daily pill taking |
| **What are the side effects of the contraceptive patch?** | **Skin reactions at site of placement; breakthrough bleeding; breast discomfort;** dysmenorrhea; headache; abdominal pain; nausea |
| **Is there an increased risk of blood clots with the contraceptive patch?** | Theoretically, yes. The patch delivers a higher dose of estrogen (area under the curve) than typical OCPs and so it may increase the risk for blood clot development. However, no studies to date have documented this effect. |
| **What is the contraceptive vaginal ring?** | An **intravaginal ring** that releases **estrogen** and **progestin** daily |
| **How is the vaginal ring administered?** | It is inserted within 5 days of the onset of menses and requires an |

additional form of contraception for the first 7 days. The ring is taken out after **3 weeks** to allow 1 week of withdrawal bleeding

Note: If the ring is displaced for more than 3 hours, an additional contraceptive method must be used for 7 days

**What are the potential side effects of the vaginal ring?**

**Device-related discomfort; irregular bleeding;** headache; vaginal discharge/irritation; nausea; breast tenderness; mood changes

## Emergency Contraception ("Morning-After Pill")

**What is emergency contraception (EC)?**

A postcoital method of contraception

**How does EC work?**

EC works by preventing ovulation and fertilization. **EC will not terminate a pregnancy** if implantation has already occurred

**Which methods are recommended in the United States?**

High-dose progestin-only contraceptive pills **(Plan B)**

High-dose estrogen and progesterone pills **(Yuzpe method)**

Plan B is routinely recommended over the Yuzpe method

**How is EC administered?**

It can be taken up to 3 days after unprotected intercourse, but is more effective if taken sooner. It is now recommended that both doses of Plan B be taken together ASAP!

**How effective are the Yuzpe method and Plan B at preventing pregnancy?**

The Yuzpe method **reduces the risk of pregnancy by approximately 75% whereas** Plan B **reduces the risk of pregnancy by up to 89%**. Both methods are more effective the closer they are taken to the unprotected act of coitus

**How effective is Plan B at preventing pregnancy if started:**

**Within 24 hours of unprotected intercourse?**

95% effective

**Within 72 hours of unprotected intercourse?**

58% effective

**Who should be prescribed EC?**

**Every sexually active woman** at risk of pregnancy should be prescribed EC as a backup in the event of primary contraceptive failure

**What are the major side effects of EC?**

**Nausea** and **vomiting. Both are seen more commonly with the Yuzpe method**. Antiemetics may be used prophylactically prior to EC use

**Can EC prevent against future pregnancies?**

No. Barrier or hormonal contraceptives should be used to prevent future pregnancy

**Is EC teratogenic to the fetus if pregnancy occurs?**

No. There is no evidence that emergency contraceptive pills (ECPs) increase the risk of fetal anomalies or miscarriages

**Are there any nonhormonal methods of emergency contraception?**

Yes—an IUD can also be used. It is 92–98% effective in preventing pregnancy if placed within 120 hours of unprotected intercourse

## BARRIER METHODS OF CONTRACEPTION

**What are the types of barrier methods available?**

Male condom; female condom; diaphragm; cervical cap; Lea's shield; contraceptive sponge; spermicide

**What are the advantages of barrier contraception over other methods?**

Many **prevent STI transmission** and they have **no hormonal side effects**

**What are the disadvantages of barrier contraception over other methods?**

Coital dependence (less reliable); Risk of breakage

**Which barrier method is the most effective at preventing STI transmission?**

**Male condoms** are the most **effective**. The **diaphragm, cervical cap, and sponge** have more **limited protection** against STIs because they do not cover the entire genital tract

**What are the two types of male condoms and what are the disadvantages of each?**

1. **Latex**—the most common type of condom; Disadvantages: risk of latex sensitivity, breaks with oil-based lubricants
2. **Synthetic**—such as polyurethane; Disadvantages: less effective, more likely to break

Male condoms have a typical use failure rate of 15% in the first year

**Do spermicidal condoms offer more protection compared to non-spermicidal condoms?**

No. They have no added protection against STIs or pregnancy. Many manufacturers have stopped producing spermicidal condoms

**What is the female condom and how it is used?**

The female condom is a **lubricated polyurethane sheath** with a flexible ring on each end. One ring covers the cervix and the other remains external, partly covering the labia. It should be **left in place for 6–8 hours after intercourse**

*Female condoms have a typical use failure rate of 21% in the first year

**What is a diaphragm, what is a cervical cap, and how are they used?**

Cup-shaped rubber barriers that, when **used with spermicide**, are effective contraceptive modalities

**How are the diaphragm and cervical cap used?**

Both require initial fitting by a clinician and are inserted to cover the cervix. They should be inserted no more than 6 hours before coitus. Both must be **left in the vagina 6–8 hours after intercourse**. The diaphragm can be left in place for up to 24 hours and the cervical cap can be left in place for up to 48 hours

**What are the side effects of the diaphragm and cervical cap?**

Increased risk of **UTI** (with diaphragm)

Possible increased risk of **toxic shock syndrome**

Increased risk of **vaginal irritation**/discharge

**For which women are diaphragms and caps not recommended and why?**

Women who are at risk for HIV or who are infected with HIV. The nanoxynol-9 placed on the device may induce vaginal irritation and destroy normal vaginal flora thereby increasing the risk for HIV infection

**What is Lea's shield?**

A dome-shaped silicone bowl placed over the cervix. It has a one-way valve that allows egress of secretions but keeps sperm out. It does not protect against STDs

**How is Lea's shield used?**

It does not need to be fitted by a physician. It is inserted before sexual intercourse and must be taken out 8–48 hours after intercourse

**What is the contraceptive sponge?**

A circular polyurethane foam sponge containing **nonoxynol-9** attached to a loop for removal

**How is the contraceptive sponge used?**

It is moistened and placed **intravaginally** up to 24 hours before coitus. The sponge can be left in place for **up to 24 hours** after intercourse

**What are the side effects of the cervical sponge?**

Increased risk of **toxic shock syndrome**

**What type of spermicide is available over the counter in the United States?**

Nonoxynol-9. It is available as a vaginal cream, film, foam, and gel

**How is spermicide used?**

It is placed intravaginally at least 15 minutes prior to intercourse and remains effective for up to 1 hour

**What are the disadvantages of spermicide?**

Relative **high failure rate** (29% typical use failure rate in first year)

It is not an effective vaginal microbicide and does not protect against HIV, gonococcus, or chlamydia transmission

## INTRAUTERINE DEVICES

**What are IUDs and how are they administered?**

**T-shaped devices** placed by a clinician through the cervix and **into the uterus**. They have a small string that hangs down from the external cervical os into the vagina for removal (see Fig. 4-2). They can be **left in place for 1–10 years** (depending on specific device)

**What are the two types of IUDs available and how do they work?**

**Copper IUDs** (*Paragard*)—prevent sperm from reaching the fallopian tubes by inducing a **sterile inflammatory reaction in the endometrium**. They can be left in place for up to 10 years

**Levonorgestrel-releasing IUDs** (*Mirena*)—**prevent sperm from reaching the ovum** by causing the cervical mucus to become thicker. Also can cause **anovulation** after 1 year as well as decreased menstrual flow and amenorrhea. They can be left in place for up to **5 years**

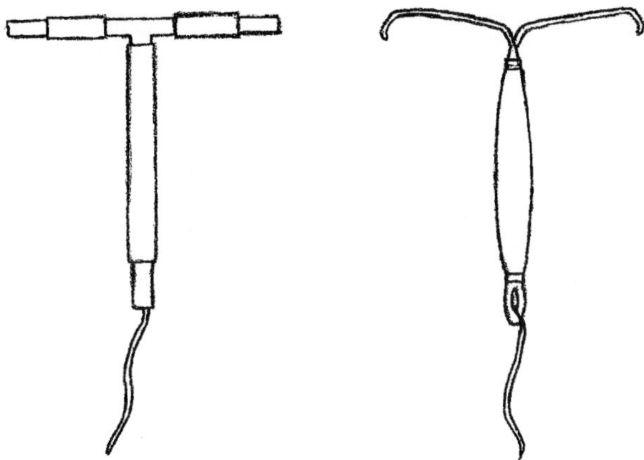

**Figure 4-2** Examples of commonly used intrauterine devices.

**What are the benefits of IUDs?**

Very effective (typical use failure rate in first year <0.1%); Decreased risk for ectopic pregnancy (compared to non-contraception users); possible protective effect against endometrial and cervical cancer; highly cost-effective over a 5-year period; immediate return to baseline fertility after removal; menorrhagia and dysmenorrhea improvement (with Mirena*). Mirena may help reduce the risk of pelvic inflammatory disease (PID) because of its cervical mucus effects

***It has the highest level of user satisfaction of any contraception being used by women**

**What are the risks of IUD placement?**

Uterine perforation; infection (risk of PID highest in first 20 days after placement); expulsion (patients should be encouraged to look/feel for string monthly); potential complications if pregnancy does occur

**What are the side effects of IUD use?**

Menorrhagia and dysmenorrhea (with Paraguard); can be relieved with NSAIDs; amenorrhea (with Mirena); no protection from STIs or HIV

**What are the contraindications to IUD placement?**

**Absolute contraindications:** pregnancy, endometrial cavity distortion, undiagnosed uterine bleeding, active, recent, or recurrent pelvic infection, copper allergy/Wilson disease (for Paraguard only), pelvic malignancy

**Relative contraindications:** multiple sexual partners, dysmenorrhea/menorrhagia (for Paraguard only)

**What is the relationship between IUD use and PID?**

PID development risk is greatest in the **first 20 days** after IUD insertion and rare thereafter. If a woman develops a gonococcal or chlamydial infection, she is **much more likely to develop PID** if she has an IUD in place. IUD use is related to the development of PID with **actinomycosis** infection

**Should the IUD be removed if a woman is found to have a positive gonorrheal or chlamydial culture?**

**Yes**, and the patient must be treated promptly

**What are the four signs of IUD expulsion and what should be done?**

1. Cramping
2. Vaginal discharge
3. Irregular spotting
4. Dyspareunia

However, expulsion may be asymptomatic and so it is important to check monthly for **elongation or absence of the vaginal string** to ensure continued placement

**What should be done if expulsion occurs?**

The patient should immediately begin to **use another form of contraception** until she sees her physician

## ELECTIVE ABORTION

**How common is elective abortion?**

Very common; in the United States 50% of all pregnancies are unintended and half of these are terminated

**Is there an impact of elective abortion on future pregnancies?**

No—there is no evidence to prove that a single termination has any impact on future fertility or the risk of spontaneous abortion. However there is an increased risk of Asherman syndrome (intrauterine synechiae) if the dilation and curettage (D&C) is done in the presence of infection or if multiple procedures are done

**What examinations/tests need to be done before an elective termination of pregnancy?**

**Pelvic examination** (to assess uterine size and position); **β-hCG** or ultrasound (to confirm pregnancy); **ultrasound** (to assess dates and confirm intrauterine pregnancy); **hematocrit** and **Rh(D)** status.

Some providers screen and treat for STIs prior to the procedure

**What are the surgical procedure options for evacuation of products of conception (POC)?**

Manual vacuum aspiration (**MVA**); suction dilation and curettage (suction **D&C**); dilation and evacuation (**D&E**); dilation and extraction (**D&X**)

**What are the risks of these procedures?**

- Risks of anesthesia
- Infection
- Hemorrhage
- Embolus (pulmonary or other)
- Cervical laceration
- Uterine perforation with/ without pelvic
- Organ damage
- Potential for adhesion development

**Does an abortion increase the risk of breast cancer?**

No

**What are the mortality rates associated with elective terminations?**

In the United States, mortality rates for first trimester abortions are 0.1–0.4 per 100,000 and 1.7–8.9 per 100,000 in the second trimester. However, internationally, where many abortions are done illegally, one in eight maternal deaths is because of abortion-related complications

**What should be done if uterine perforation is suspected?**

Immediate **laparoscopy** or **laparotomy** to examine the abdominal contents to assess bowel injury

**How and when is an MVA performed?**

Anytime before 12 weeks. The cervix is dilated using cervical dilators and the uterine contents are evacuated using a cannula that is attached to a handheld syringe which has the vacuum source

**How is a suction D&C performed?**

The cervix is dilated using cervical dilators and the uterine contents are evacuated using an electrically powered vacuum device

**When can a D&C be performed?**

Anytime before 14 weeks

**How is a D&E performed?**

The cervix is dilated using osmotic dilators placed intracervically 1–2 days prior to the procedure to slowly soften and dilate the cervix and thus minimize mechanical damage to the cervix. At the time of the procedure, these are removed and mechanical dilators are used for further dilation as needed. The uterine contents are evacuated using specialized forceps (sophers and bierers). Many people confirm completion by performing a curettage and feeling a good "cri" (gritty texture) throughout the cavity. Vacuum can also be used to remove any remaining blood or tissue

**When can a D&E be performed?**

Anytime before 24 weeks, depending on the legal limit in the state

**How is a D&X performed?**

It is similar to a D&E except that the fetus is delivered in breech presentation through the dilated cervix and the cranial contents are suctioned before delivery of the fetal head

**When can a D&X be performed?**

From approximately 18–24 weeks

**What is the advantage of a D&X procedure over a D&E?**

It potentially minimizes uterine and cervical injury from the fetal bones and from instrumentation

**Are prophylactic antibiotics indicated to prevent infection?**

Yes. Women given antibiotics peri-abortion have a lower risk of postoperative infection

| | |
|---|---|
| **What types of antibiotics can be used prophylactically?** | Doxycycline, ofloxacin, or ceftriaxone |
| **What is a medical abortion?** | Termination of pregnancy or evacuation of POCs using medications only |
| **How effective is medical abortion?** | Very effective—it is successful in 90–98% of women |
| **What are the various modalities for medical abortion?** | Intravaginal **misoprostol** alone<br>Oral or IM **methotrexate** followed by intravaginal, oral, or buccal misoprostol 3–7 days later<br>Oral mifepristone followed by intravaginal, oral, or buccal **misoprostol** 6–72 hours later (up to 49–63 days) |
| **How do each of the following agents work?** | **Misoprostol:** a prostaglandin analogue; increases contractility by directly stimulating the myometrium<br>**Methotrexate:** blocks dihydrofolate reductase, an enzyme necessary for the production of thymidine during DNA synthesis, thus affecting the rapidly growing cytotrophoblast<br>**Mifepristone:** binds to the progesterone receptor with a greater affinity than progesterone itself, and therefore blocks the "pro-gestation" action of progesterone |
| **What are the side effects of a medical abortion?** | Cramping, bleeding (often heavier than a menstrual period)<br>Gastrointestinal (GI) distress (nausea, vomiting, diarrhea) |
| **What are the contraindications to a medical abortion?** | Allergies to any of the medications<br>An in situ IUD<br>Severe anemia<br>Coagulopathy/use of an anticoagulant<br>Active liver disease<br>Cardiovascular disease<br>Uncontrolled seizure disorder<br>Adrenal disease |
| **Is there any effect of medical termination on subsequent pregnancies?** | No |

**What is a septic abortion?**

Evidence of localized infection and systemic infection after a spontaneous or elective abortion

**How is a septic abortion managed?**

Stabilize the patient

Take blood and endometrial cultures

Administer parenteral broad-spectrum antibiotics

Surgically evacuate the uterine contents

Administer anti-D immunoglobulin if it is warranted

**What antibiotic combinations can be used to treat septic abortion?**

Clindamycin and gentamicin with or without ampicillin

Ampicillin and gentamicin and metronidazole

Ticarcillin-clavulanate or piperacillin-tazobactam or imipenem alone

**What are the indications for laparotomy in the management of a septic abortion?**

Failure to respond to evacuation/antibiotics

Pelvic abscess

Gas gangrene or other fulminant disease (i.e., *Clostridium sordelii*)

**Who should be given Rh(D)-immune globulin postabortion?**

All Rh(D)-negative women who are unsensitized

**When does ovulation resume postabortion?**

As early as 2 weeks after an abortion. Therefore if pregnancy is undesired, contraception must be started immediately

**When do menses resume postabortion?**

Usually within 6 weeks (average 4 weeks)

**What conditions need to be considered if menses do not resume within 6 weeks?**

Pregnancy and gestational trophoblastic disease; less likely are Asherman syndrome or other systemic diseases (e.g., thyroid disorder)

**What instructions should be given postabortion?**

Women should be advised to have **nothing per vagina** for 2 weeks after the procedure/passage of POC. Some recommend deferment of pregnancy (if desired) for 2–3 months, although there is no data to support this recommendation

**When should a woman return to clinic postabortion?**

If she experiences heavy bleeding, fever, or abdominal pain

# Sexually Transmitted Diseases and Pelvic Infections

## SEXUALLY TRANSMITTED INFECTIONS OF THE LOWER GENITAL TRACT

### Condyloma Accuminata

**What is condyloma accuminata?**
**Genital warts**. It is the most common sexually transmitted infection

**How is condyloma accuminata transmitted?**
Through skin-to-skin contact; it is primarily transmitted through sexual activity

**What is the pathogen and which subtypes are associated more commonly with genital warts?**
A DNA virus called human papillomavirus (**HPV**); subtypes **6 and 11**

**What are the clinical manifestations of condyloma accuminata?**
**Warts** located on the external genitalia, perineum, anus, cervix, mouth, inside the vagina, and urethra; These are generally raised, pedunculated/**cauliflower-shaped** lesions but they can vary in number, size, and color (flesh-colored, pinkish-white, grayish-white)

**What other disease should be excluded?**
**Condyloma lata** of secondary syphilis

**How is condyloma accuminata diagnosed?**
Visualization by colposcopic examination and cytologic smear. Biopsy can be performed if the diagnosis is uncertain

**What would a biopsy of the specimen reveal?**
**Koilocytosis** (vacuolated keratinocyte with peri-nuclear halo). It is often also associated with atypia and dysplasia

**What is the treatment?**
Cryotherapy, laser excision, trichloroacetic acid, podophyllum, or imiquimod cream. If left untreated, visible lesions may resolve on their own, remain unchanged, or increase in size or number

| | |
|---|---|
| | **The virus cannot be eradicated once present in the genital tract; therefore, warts can recur** |
| **What are Buschke-Lowenstein tumors?** | **Giant condylomas** caused by HPV that are found in **immunocompromised patients** |
| **What else can HPV cause?** | **Preinvasive and invasive cervical cancer**. Dysplasia is more commonly caused by **subtypes 16 and 18** |
| **How can HPV infection be prevented?** | A quadrivalent recombinant vaccine against HPV serotypes 6, 11, 16, 18 (Gardasil) can be given to females between the ages of 9 and 26 |

## Molluscum Contagiosum

| | |
|---|---|
| **What is genital molluscum contagiosum?** | A benign, usually asymptomatic, infection of the vulva caused by poxvirus |
| **How is genital molluscum transmitted?** | Through sexual contact, casual skin-skin contact, fomites (substances that absorb and transport infectious disease particles, i.e., underwear), or auto-inoculation |
| **What is the typical clinical presentation?** | Single or multiple (<30) small, white, pink, or flesh-colored **dome-shaped papules** with **central umbilication** in the genital/inguinal area. It is usually asymptomatic but **eczema** may surround the lesion and **pruritus** may occur |
| **How does genital molluscum contagiosum present in an immunocompromised person?** | Large lesions (>1 cm) or a clustering of numerous small lesions; intra-oral or peri-oral lesions can arise |
| **What are the differential diagnoses?** | Multiple small lesions: condyloma accuminata<br>Large, solitary lesions: basal or squamous cell carcinoma |
| **How is the diagnosis made?** | Usually based on clinical manifestations. Biopsy can be performed for definitive diagnosis and will reveal **intracytoplasmic inclusions** |
| **What are the treatment options?** | It is usually self-limiting; cosmetic options include curettage or |

cryotherapy of lesions with liquid nitrogen; topical imiquimod is also used

**Sexual partners do not need to be treated**

## Pediculosis Pubis (Crabs) and Scabies

**What are pediculosis pubis and scabies?**
Parasitic infections of the pubic area

**What causes pediculosis pubis?**
The crab louse *Phthirus pubis*—a blood-sucking parasite that lives on hair shafts and lays eggs (nits)

**What causes scabies?**
The itch mite *Sarcoptes scabiei*—a parasite that burrows underneath the skin and lays eggs

**How are pediculosis pubis and scabies transmitted?**
Primarily through sexual contact. Can also be through fomites (clothing, sheets)

**What is the typical presentation of these infestations?**
Intense pruritus over the genital area, especially at night. Polymorphic papules may be seen in scabies.

**How are pediculosis pubis and scabies diagnosed?**
Visualization of the parasites or eggs (nits) under a microscope (skin scrapings) or magnifying glass

**What is the treatment?**
**Permethrin** 1% cream (first line)

Lindane 1% shampoo (second line) (contraindicated in pregnant/ lactating women)

**All clothing and sheets should be washed in hot water and isolated for at least 3 days after treatment. All contacts must be treated**

**What other tests should be ordered?**
Screening tests for other sexually transmitted diseases (HIV, syphilis, gonorrhea, *chlamydia*)

# SEXUALLY TRANSMITTED INFECTIONS CAUSING GENITAL ULCERATIONS

**What are the most common infectious causes of genital ulcers in the United States?**
Herpes simplex virus (HSV) > syphilis > chancroid >>> lymphogranuloma venereum and granuloma inguinale

**Is coinfection with multiple organisms common?**

Yes. Making a diagnosis based on the history and physical can be very difficult and requires a thorough workup and knowledge of the most likely causal organism in the specific patient population

**What are some of the most common noninfectious causes of genital ulcers?**

Behcet disease, drug reactions, trauma, neoplasma

**What are the tests used to diagnose a genital ulcer?**

**Darkfield microscopy** (syphilis)

**Serologic tests** (syphilis and lymphogranuloma venereum [LGV])

**Gram stain** and **viral culture** on selective media (*Haemophilus ducreyi*)

**Tzanck preparation**, direct fluorescence antibody (DFA), viral culture, or polymerase chain reaction (PCR) for HSV

**Tissue biopsy** (syphilis, granuloma inguinale)

**With what other disease are these genital ulcer diseases associated?**

HIV

**Which of these diseases must be reported?**

Syphilis (and HIV)

## Genital Herpes

**What is genital HSV?**

A DNA virus **transmitted through infectious secretions** that causes recurrent, **lifelong disease**

**What is the difference between HSV-1 and HSV-2?**

Both are implicated in genital herpes and have the same clinical presentation. However, **HSV-2** more commonly infects the **genitalia** whereas **HSV-1** more commonly affects the **oral mucosa**

**What is the natural history of the HSV infection?**

**Primary episode**: mucocutaneous infection occurs via direct sexual contact with an infected person. After a 4-day incubation period, ulcerating pustular lesions erupt, often associated with local pain, lymphadenopathy, and systemic symptoms

**Viral latency**: after primary infection, there is a period of **viral latency** as the virus ascends along the sensory nerve roots and becomes latent in the dorsal root ganglion

**Reactivation**: can occur at any interval when the virus travels back down the sensory nerve. This can either cause a mucocutaneous outbreak (**recurrence**) or sometimes no symptoms may be detected

**What is the strongest risk factor for genital HSV infection?**

A large number of lifetime sex partners

**What clinical presentation is suggestive of primary genital herpes?**

A **prodrome** of 2–24 hours characterized by **localized/regional burning and pain**

Systemic symptoms including **fever, malaise, and bilateral inguinal lymphadenopathy**

**Grouped vesicles, uniform in size, mixed with multiple, shallow, severely tender ulcers** around the vulva, perineum, and perianal area are pathognomonic

**Cervical lesions** are also common and cause intermittent bleeding and vaginal discharge

**Dysuria and urinary retention syndromes** may occur because of contact with urethral and vulvar ulcers

**Are all primary outbreaks clinically symptomatic?**

No. 70–80% of infected persons have unrecognized symptoms or completely asymptomatic infections; therefore, transmission of this virus can be high and unrecognized

**What laboratory tests help make a diagnosis of HSV?**

**Type-specific viral cultures** (highest sensitivity and specificity; highest yield if done early when you can attain more vesicle fluid)

Direct fluorescence antibody test

Type-specific serologic testing (best for those with a questionable hx, subclinical infection, or suspicion of a false-negative viral culture)

Tzanck smears

Polymerase chain reaction (PCR)

**What is the presentation of a secondary outbreak?**

They vary widely in their frequency, are **milder** and **shorter in duration**, and may not have prodromal symptoms of pain, burning, and itching. Viral shedding can occur for weeks after the appearance of lesions.

**What are some precipitating factors of a recurrent outbreak?**

Immunodeficiency, trauma, fever, nerve damage, concurrent infection, and sexual intercourse

**What are the treatment options for genital herpes?**

**Oral acyclovir** for primary and recurrent episodes. It reduces viral shedding and shortens the clinical course. Can also be used prophylactically for patients with frequently recurring episodes, decreasing the recurrence rates by 70–80%

**Intravenous (IV) acyclovir** should be considered for severe/disseminated disease or in immunocompromised patients

Other therapies include keeping the affected area clean and dry, wearing loose clothing and undergarments, washing hands after contact with affected areas, and using an ice pack or sitz bath for soothing sores

**All sexual partners should be evaluated for infection**

**Screening tests should be considered for what other diseases?**

**Syphilis and HIV**

**What is the most common cause of urogenital complaints in the emergency room setting?**

Genital herpes

**If a pregnant woman carries HSV, what is the risk of transmission to the neonate?**

The risk of transmission by an infected mother is 30–50% among women with a primary outbreak during the third trimester, and <1% in those with recurrent infection or a primary infection during the first half of the pregnancy

**What precautions should be considered to decrease neonatal transmission from an affected mother?**

In the presence of a genital lesion or prodrome, delivery should be via cesarean delivery

Prophylactic antivirals may be administered in the third trimester to reduce the incidence of HSV recurrence

## Syphilis

**What organism causes syphilis?**
*Treponema pallidum*

**How is it transmitted?**
Usually via sexual transmission. It enters the body by penetrating intact mucous membranes or by invading epithelial abrasions

**Is it *always* sexually transmitted?**
No. Skin contact between any skin abrasions and an ulcer infected with *T. pallidum* can result in infection

**Which population is highest at risk?**
Black heterosexual women and homosexual men in urban areas

**What are the clinical manifestations for the three stages of syphilis?**
Primary, secondary, and tertiary syphilis

**Describe primary syphilis**
Symptoms occur approximately 3 weeks after infection and include a **painless chancre** (a single, clean-based ulcer usually on labia/vaginal wall/cervix) and **painless lymphadenopathy**

**Describe secondary syphilis**
**Systemic disease** results from hematogenous dissemination that occurs 6–8 weeks after infection. Symptoms include a **maculopapular rash on the palms and soles, condyloma latum** (moist, grayish papules-like warts), malaise, fever, arthralgias, pharyngitis, and generalized lymphadenopathy

**Describe tertiary syphilis**
Occurs 3–10 years after initial infection. Symptoms include **gummas** (noninfectious granulomatous lesions found in skin and bones), cardiovascular syphilis (**aortitis** or an **aortic aneurysm**), and neurosyphilis (**general paresis, tabes dorsalis,** or an **Argyll-Robertson pupil**)

**What is the latent period?**
A period of anywhere from 2–20 years that occurs **between the second and third stages** of syphilis. Most patients are asymptomatic (some have recurrences) and are considered noninfectious, although their serologic tests remain positive

**What is the gold standard for diagnosis of syphilis and when can it be used?**
**Dark field microscopy** of a specimen from the primary chancre,

condyloma latum, or the maculopapular rash reveals **spirochetes**. It is only useful during the active stages of primary and secondary syphilis

**What other tests are available to help with diagnosis?**

Nonspecific and specific serological screening tests:

**Nonspecific**: venereal Disease Research Laboratory **(VDRL)** and rapid plasma reagin **(RPR). A positive result must be confirmed with a specific treponemal antibody test given high rate of false positives!**

**Specific**: Fluorescent treponemal antibody absorption **(FTA-ABS),** microhemagglutination assay **(MHA-TP),** and treponemal hemagglutination tests for syphillis **(HATTS)**

**How would you interpret the following laboratory results:**

**Positive nonspecific test and positive specific test**

Active treponemal infection

**Positive nonspecific test and negative specific test**

False positive

**Negative nonspecific test and positive specific test**

Successfully treated syphilis

**Negative nonspecific test and negative specific test**

Syphilis unlikely

**What other common conditions may cause a false positive nonspecific test result?**

Systemic lupus erythematosus (SLE), rheumatic heart disease, pregnancy, infectious mononucleosis, intravenous drug use, viral hepatitis, recent immunization

**What is the treatment for syphilis?**

Penicillin or tetracycline (for nonpregnant penicillin allergic patients) for primary, secondary, and early latent syphilis are first-line drugs. Erythromycin is second-line but is contraindicated in pregnant patients

**What is Jarisch-Herxheimer phenomenon?**

A self-limiting, **acute worsening of symptoms after antibiotics are started**. Symptoms include headache, fever, chills, muscle aches, and other flu-like symptoms

**What diagnosis should be considered for unexplained rashes, arthralgias, neurologic or systemic complaints?**

Syphilis

## Chancroid

**What is chancroid?**

An **acute, curable, sexually transmitted disease** caused by ***H. ducreyi.*** It is uncommon in the United States but is a predominant cause of genital ulcer disease in sub-Saharan Africa

**What clinical presentation highly suggests chancroid?**

**One to three extremely painful ulcers** around the perilabial area that are deep, purulent, and have ragged edges. These are associated with **unilateral, suppurative, painful swollen inguinal lymph nodes** that, in 25% of cases, will rupture, releasing a heavy, foul discharge that is contagious **(suppurative adenopathy = bubo)**. Systemic symptoms (fevers, myalgias) are typically **not** present

**What other infections must be ruled out before a diagnosis of chancroid can be made?**

Syphilis, HSV, lymphogranuloma venereum (LGV), and granuloma inguinale

**What laboratory tests help make a diagnosis of chancroid?**

Culture on selective media isolates *H. ducreyi*

Gram stain of a specimen from the ulcer base or bubo aspirate: reveals gram-negative rods in a chain; referred to as a "**school of fish**" pattern

PCR

**What is the treatment for chancroid?**

**Azithromycin** (oral) or **ceftriaone** (IM)

Treat sexual partners

## Lymphogranuloma Venereum

**What is LGV?**

A **sexually transmitted ulcerative disease** that occurs in **three stages** and involves **infection of the lymphatic tissue** in the genital region

**What is the causal agent?**

*Chlamydia trachomatis;* serotypes L1, L2, and L3 are most common

**What are key risk factors one should be aware of in the history and physical (H&P)?**

Travel and unprotected sex in tropical regions or regions where LGV is endemic (Africa, Southeast Asia, India); anal sex

**What are the key physical findings at each stage of this disease?**

Stage 1: **small, painless papules/ shallow ulcerations** typically on the vaginal wall that often go unnoticed

Stage 2: **painful unilateral inguinal lymphadenopathy** (typically in men); women may complain of lower back/ abdominal pain because of deep pelvic node involvement; **bubo** (matted nodes that adhere to the overlying skin); systemic symptoms; **groove sign** (enlargement of the nodes above and below the inguinal ligament)

Stage 3: **rupture of the bubo** leads to **genitoanorectal syndrome** (strictures and fistulas in the anogenital tract); constitutional symptoms; **proctocolitis**; abscesses

**At what stage do most women present?**

Stage 3

**Which finding is pathognomic for LGV?**

**Groove sign** (inguinal buboes with nonsignificant ulcers = LGV)

**What other diseases may present with similar cutaneous lesions?**

Granuloma inguinale, tuberculosis (TB), early syphilis, and chancroid

**What are the most common laboratory tests used to diagnose LGV?**

**Complement fixation tests** (used most often)

Serologic tests for IgG antibodies

Immunofluorescence on aspirates from bubo for the presence of inclusion bodies

PCR for *C. trachomatis* or DNA swab from lesion

Genital or lymph node specimen tested by culture

**How is LGV treated?**

Oral **doxycycline** or erythromycin for 3 weeks

Lymph node aspiration if needed

**What are some complications of LGV?**

Fistulas, strictures, tissue ischemia and necrosis; elephantiasis of the female genitalia (esthiomene)

## Granuloma Inguinale (Donovanosis)

**What is granuloma inguinale?**

A slow, progressive genital ulcerative disease that is primarily sexually transmitted. It is most common in the developing world; it is rare in the United States

**What is the cause?**

***Klebsiella granulomatis (previously known as Calymmatobacterium granulomatis)***, a gram-negative pleomorphic bacillus

**What are the typical manifestations of granuloma inguinale?**

Large, **painless**, and **spreading ulcers** typically in the vulva area; the lesions are clean but have **friable bases with raised, rolled margins that bleed easily**. They are typically **beefy red** in appearance and exude a malodorous discharge. **Inguinal lymphadenopathy is rare**

**What is the classic finding for establishing a diagnosis of granuloma inguinale?**

**Donovan bodies** (intracytoplasmic safety pin shaped organisms seen after Giemsa or Wright staining of tissue specimens)

**What is the treatment?**

**Doxycycline or trimethoprim-sulfamethoxazole**. (Tetracycline is no longer recommended because of bacterial resistance)

# CERVICITIS

## *Chlamydia*, Gonorrhea, and Other Causes of Cervicitis

**What cell types make up the cervix and where are they located?**

Columnar epithelium—endocervix

Non-keratinizing squamous epithelium—ectocervix

**What is mucopurulent cervicitis (MPC)?**

Inflammation of the **endocervix** most commonly caused by sexually transmitted organisms. It is characterized by a **yellow-greenish mucopurulent discharge** on visual inspection or on an endocervical swab specimen.

**What are the two most common infectious etiologies of MPC and what kind of organisms are they?**

1. *C. trachomatis*: gram-negative, obligate intracellular bacterium

2. *Neisseria gonorrhoeae*: gram-negative diplococci

**What is ectocervicitis?**

Inflammation of the ectocervical epithelium. This squamous epithelium is an extension of the vaginal epithelium and can be infected by the same organisms that cause vaginal infections

**What are some infectious causes of ectocervicitis and what are some key clues, if any, that lead you to that etiology?**

Trichomonas: strawberry cervix (small petechiae to large punctuate hemorrhages on the ectocervix)

HSV: ulcerative and hemorrhagic lesions/vesicles during the primary infection

HPV: genital warts, cervical dysplasia on Pap smear

**What age group is most frequently affected with cervicitis?**

15–25 year olds

**What are the typical symptoms of MPC?**

Vaginal discharge, dysuria, urinary frequency, dyspareunia, postcoital bleeding

**What findings are found on clinical examination?**

A tender, friable cervix that may also be erythematous and/or edematous

**Patients infected with *C. trachomatis* or *N. gonorrhoeae* are frequently asymptomatic!**

**What laboratory test supports a diagnosis of MPC?**

>30 polymorphonuclear (PMN) leukocytes on a Gram-stained specimen from the endocervix

**How is the diagnosis of each of the following organisms made?**

*C. trachomatis:* **cell culture** (gold standard, but difficult), nucleic acid amplification tests (NAAT) from urine, DNA probe, enzyme immunosassay

*N. gonorrhoea:* **Thayer-Martin agar culture** (gold-standard), DNA probe, enzyme immunoassay

*T. vaginalis:* visualization of motile trichomonads on **wet mount**

**HSV:** Tzanck smear test, serologic testing, viral culture

**HPV:** clinical appearance, cytology

**What is the treatment for each of these causes of cervicitis?**

*C. trachomatis:* doxycycline × 7 days or azithromycin (single dose)

*N. gonorrhoeae:* ceftriaxone (IM), ciprofloxacin plus doxycycline, azithromycin (single dose)

*T. vaginalis:* metronidazole (PO)

**HSV:** acyclovir (PO)

**For all of the above infections, sexual partners also must be treated**

**What is the treatment for *C. trachomatis* in a pregnant patient or a noncompliant patient?**

Azithromycin (single dose PO)

**What other organism should be treated in a patient diagnosed with *N. gonorrhoeae*?**

*C. trachomatis*

**What are some serious complications of cervicitis?**

**Pelvic inflammatory disease** (PID), pregnancy and neonatal complications, cervical cancer, increased risk of HIV transmission

**What are the guidelines for STI screening?**

Annual screening of *C. trachomatis* and *N. gonorrhoeae* for all sexually active women ”25 years of age, or those at high risk >25 (new sex partner or multiple sex partners)

**What other necessary steps should be taken with a patient diagnosed with an STD-induced cervicitis?**

Treat all partners and test for HIV, syphilis, hepatitis B and C

## INFECTIONS OF THE UPPER GENITAL TRACT

### Pelvic Inflammatory Disease

**What is PID?**

An **acute infection** that may involve parts or all of the female genital tract, including the **cervix, endometrial cavity (endometritis), fallopian tubes (salpingitis), ovaries (oophoritis), parametrial tissues/ligaments (parametritis), and/or peritoneal cavity (peritonitis)**. It is *typically* initiated by **sexually transmitted agents**

**What are the usual presentation/symptoms/signs of this disease?**

The patient is typically a **13–35-year-old sexually active female** who presents with **lower abdominal pain** (not more than of 2 weeks' duration), **adnexal tenderness** (usually bilateral), or **cervical motion tenderness** on physical examination (PE) (only one must be present). While not required to establish the diagnosis of PID, **the presence of one or more of the following enhances the specificity of the minimum criteria: fever (>101°F); purulent cervical discharge; elevated erythrocyte sedimentation rate (ESR)/C-reactive protein level; leukocytosis**

**What are other immediate differential diagnoses of a patient who presents with lower abdominal pain?**

Appendicitis, endometriosis, (ruptured) ectopic pregnancy, irritable bowel syndrome, inflammatory bowel disease, ruptured/hemorrhagic ovarian cyst, abortion, gastroenteritis, ovarian torsion, renal colic, tubo-ovarian abscess (TOA), UTI, somatization, mesenteric adenitis

**For each of the following differential diagnosis related to Ob-Gyn, list the main symptoms/signs that would differentiate between that diagnosis and PID**

**Endometriosis**: medical history of chronic pelvic pain, dysmenorrhea, deep dyspareunia, low sacral backache, dischezia, perimenstrual bleeding, cystic ovarian enlargement, tender adnexae, uterosacral tenderness and nodularity, retroflexed uterus

**(Ruptured) ectopic pregnancy**: history of amenorrhea, crampy abdominal pain, abnormal uterine bleeding, nausea/vomiting (N/V), dizziness/light-headedness, palpable tender adnexal mass; other signs depend on extent of rupture and hemorrhage (peritoneal signs, tachycardia, tachypnea, and orthostatic changes)

**Ruptured/hemorrhagic ovarian cyst**: sudden-onset bi/unilateral lower abdominal pain, rebound tenderness, guarding, N/V

**Ovarian torsion**: intense, progressive unilateral pain combined with tense, tender, and enlarged ovarian mass. History of repetitive, transitory pain. "Wave-like" episodes of N/V may also be experienced

**TOA**: usually associated with PID. Symptoms can be consistent with sepsis: high fever, N/V, tachycardia, abdominal rigidity and guarding, rebound tenderness

**Abortion**: amenorrhea, vaginal spotting, crampy abdominal pain

**What are the risk factors for PID and what pathogens (if any) are associated with these risk factors?**

<35 years old (recent reports state <25 years old); multiple sexual partners; sexual partners with *Chlamydia,* gonorrhea, or other urethritis, nonbarrier protection

-common pathogens: ***C. trachomatis and N. gonorrhoeae***

Instrumentation of the cervix

-common pathogen: ***Actinomyces israelii***

Bacterial vaginosis (BV)

-common pathogens: ***Bacteroides, Peptostreptococcus, Escherichia coli***

Alterations in vaginal flora (i.e., douching, changes in vaginal pH, necrotic tissue, foreign body reaction

-common pathogens: ***Bacteroides, Clostridia***

**What is Fitz-Hugh–Curtis (FHC) syndrome?**

Focal perihepatitis, causing right upper quadrant tenderness in 15–30% of patients with PID. **Right upper quadrant pain does *not* rule out PID!**

**Name the diagnostic tests and the expected results that help you make a diagnosis of PID**

***β*-hCG pregnancy test** (rule out ectopic pregnancy or complications of an intrauterine pregnancy)

Microscopic examination of vaginal discharge in saline (78% for ≥3 WBC/hpf)

Gram stain tests for *Chlamydia* and gonococcus

Urinary analysis (UA) (rule out UTI)

Complete blood count (CBC) (leukocytosis)

Fecal occult blood tests (r/o acute abdomen)

C-reactive protein (CRP) (elevated in PID)

ESR (elevated in PID)

**What other methods of evaluation could you consider?**

Culdocentesis, ultrasound, endometrial biopsy, laparoscopy

**How is the diagnosis of PID for empiric treatment made?**

The **minimum criteria** include **cervical motion tenderness or adnexal tenderness**. No other causes of these symptoms/signs should be present

**Additional criteria that increase the suspicion for PID include:**

Oral temperature of >101°F (>38.3°C)

Abnormal cervical or vaginal mucopurulent discharge

Presence of white blood cells on saline

**What is the gold standard for diagnosis of PID?**

**Laparoscopy (**usually used in severe cases, patients who have tubo-ovarian drainage, or when the diagnosis is in question)

**What are important points to remember regarding treatment?**

***Always* rule out pregnancy!**

**Always use multiple antimicrobial agents** to provide coverage for *N. gonorrheae*, *C. trachomatis*, gram-negative facultative bacteria, streptococci, and anaerobes

**Better to "over diagnose"** to prevent sequelae such as scarring, infertility

**Reassess** in 48–72 hours after initiating treatment! If no improvement, change treatment or diagnosis

**Always treat sexual partners** (asymptomatic or symptomatic)

**When should you consider inpatient management?**

Pregnancy

Inability to exclude surgical emergency (i.e., appendicitis) or uncertain diagnosis

Failure to respond to outpatient oral therapy within 72 hours, requiring IV medicines

Inability to tolerate oral therapy (e.g., severe N/V)

Severe illness (e.g., high fever, peritonitis)

Presence of a TOA

Noncompliance, +IUD, +peritoneal signs, +pelvic mass

Nulliparity with initial infection will also be a case for hospitalization to avoid sequelae (i.e., scarring and infertility)

**What are the first-line regimens for inpatient therapy of PID?**

**Cefotetan** and **doxycycline**

**Clindamycin** and **gentamicin**

**What are the first-line regimens for outpatient therapy of PID?**

**Ofloxacin**; or levofloxacin ± metronidazole

**Ceftriaxone** (or cefoxitin with probenecid) plus doxycycline ± metronidazole

**What are complications of PID?**

**Tubal factor infertility** (tubes are scarred), ectopic pregnancy, chronic pelvic pain, TOA, perihepatitis (FHC syndrome), adhesions

**What is the most likely cause of infertility in a normally menstruating woman <30 years old?**

Pelvic inflammatory disease

**How can PID be prevented?**

**Education** of young women and teenagers-at-risk (primary prevention)

**Annual screening** for *Chlamydia* in all sexually active women <25 and women >25 if they have new or multiple partners (secondary prevention)

**Consistent use of barrier contraception**

**Oral contraception**

**Treatment of sexual partners**

## Fitz-Hugh–Curtis Syndrome

**What is FHC syndrome?**

Inflammation of the liver capsule and diaphragm most often associated as an extrapelvic manifestation of PID

**What organisms are typically cultured from the infection?**

*C. trachomatis* > *N. gonorrhoeae*

**What are the typical presenting symptoms?**

Acute phase: **right upper quadrant pain** that may radiate to the right shoulder

Chronic phase: **chronic abdominal pain** (commonly over the right upper quadrant)

**How is the diagnosis of FHC syndrome made?**

Clinical presentation

Elevated WBC count and ESR

Positive cervical and/or abdominal cultures of *C. trachomatis* and/or *N. gonorrhoeae*

**What is the gold standard for diagnosis and what are the expected findings?**

Diagnostic laparoscopy

Acute phase: inflammation (gray and flaky exudates) of the peritoneum and liver capsule

Chronic phase:"**violin-string" adhesions** of the anterior liver capsule to the anterior abdominal wall or diaphragm

**What is the treatment for FHC syndrome?**

Medical (same as for PID: doxycycline plus ceftriaxone or ofloxacin plus metronidazole) or surgical (lysis of adhesions)

## Tubo-Ovarian Abscess

**What is a TOA?**

An abscess of the ovary and fallopian tube that almost always arises as a complication of PID in premenopausal women

**In what settings does a TOA develop?**

Most commonly, it occurs in the setting of a history of **chronically damaged adnexal tissue** with a **superimposed recurrent infection.** Secondary TOA results from intraperitoneal spread of infection by bowel perforation (appendicitis or diverticulitis) or in association with a pelvic malignancy

**What are the most common pathogens associated with TOA?**

Mixed polymicrobial infection with a high prevalence of **anaerobes** (*Bacteroides* and *Peptostreptococcus*)

and **gram-negative organisms** (*E. coli* and streptococcal species)

**What is the typical presentation of a patient with TOA?**

The patient is usually young and of low parity with a **history of PID**. Typical symptoms and signs include **severe abdominal** and/or **pelvic pain**, **fever**, leukocytosis, **N/V**, **rebound tenderness** in lower quadrants, diminished bowel sounds, distension, and tympany

**How does a ruptured TOA present?**

As **septic shock**: fever, chills, tachycardia, hypotension, disorientation, tachypnea, and oliguria

**What is on the list of differential diagnoses for an unruptured TOA?**

Unruptured ectopic pregnancy, ovarian torsion, pelvic neoplasm, cul-de-sac (pelvic) abscess, acute appendicitis, septic incomplete abortion, perforation of a diverticular abscess or a diverticulum, perforation of a peptic ulcer

**What tests are used to diagnose TOA?**

**Pelvic ultrasound (first choice)**

CT (used if ultrasound is uninformative)

Exploratory laparoscopy (gold standard)

Culdocentesis

**What are the findings on culdocentesis?**

Unruptured TOA: "cloudy reaction" fluid

Ruptured TOA: grossly purulent material

**What is the difference between a TOA and a tubo-ovarian complex (TOC)?**

TOC is an inflammatory pelvic mass consisting of living tissue from adherent, infected pelvic structures in PID. Unlike TOA, there is no abscess wall or pus contained within a cavity. It can be distinguished from TOA by ultrasound and it is responsive to medical treatment

**What are the appropriate steps in management of TOA?**

Admit the patient

Begin IV fluids followed by IV antibiotics (ampicillin plus gentamicin plus metronidazole *or* imipenem-cilastin)

| | |
|---|---|
| | Monitor for signs of sepsis (vital signs, CBC, chest x-ray/EKG, urine output) |
| | If there is no response to antibiotics, drain transvaginally or perform exploratory laparotomy |

## Pelvic Actinomycosis

| | |
|---|---|
| **What is pelvic actinomycosis?** | It is a very rare infection of the upper genital tract caused by ***Actinomyces israelii*, a gram-positive anaerobic organism**. It is usually part of a polymicrobial infection |
| **Is it normally part of the female genital tract?** | Yes—the presence of *Actinomyces* in the vagina or cervix is neither diagnostic nor predictive of disease |
| **With which gynecologic diseases has *Actinomyces* been associated?** | PID, TOA, chronic endometritis, retroperitoneal fibrosis |
| **With what gynecologic procedure has *Actinomyces* been associated?** | IUD placement—*Actinomyces* has been identified in 8–20% of women with an IUD |
| **How is the diagnosis of actinomycosis infection made in a symptomatic patient?** | Microscopically. A hematoxylin and eosin (H&E) stain reveals sulfur granules and a Gram stain reveals gram-positive filaments |
| **If a Pap smear returns positive for *Actinomyces* on an asymptomatic patient with an IUD, what are the next steps in management?** | IUD removal or antibiotic treatment. Repeat the Pap in 1 year |
| **When are both removal of the IUD and treatment with antibiotics necessary?** | In a patient showing symptoms/signs of a pelvic infection |

## Pelvic Tuberculosis

| | |
|---|---|
| **Which bacteria commonly cause pelvic TB?** | *Mycobacterium tuberculosis* or *Mycobacterium bovis* |
| **How does TB reach the pelvic organs?** | Via hematogenous dissemination from either the lung or the GI tract |
| **What parts of the upper genital tract does TB usually affect?** | Oviducts and endometrium |
| **Which population is most affected?** | Premenopausal women; immigrants from Asia, the Middle East, and Latin America |

**What are the most common presenting complaints of patients with a chronic infection of pelvic TB?**
**Infertility**, abnormal uterine bleeding, pelvic pain, and abdominal distension (ascites)

**What are some findings on the PE?**
Pelvic examination is normal 50% of the time; however, patients may have mild adnexal tenderness and/or bilateral adnexal masses

**How is the diagnosis of pelvic TB made?**
Positive chest x-ray and lung scan, positive purified protein derivative (PPD), and positive sputum smears/cultures are suggestive. A **positive acid-fast stain and culture from menstrual discharge or biopsy of the endometrium** is diagnostic

***Suspect TB if a patient is not responding to conventional antibiotics for bacterial PID**

**What are the histologic findings of the endometrial biopsy?**
Classic giant cells, granulomas, and caseous necrosis

**What are the next steps in management?**
Chest x-ray, intravenous pyelogram, serial gastric washings, and urine cultures (for urinary tract TB)

**What is the treatment?**
A multidrug regimen consisting of isonicotinyl hydrazine (INH), rifampicin, pyrazinamide, and ethambutol

**What are some complications of pelvic TB?**
Infertility and chronic endometritis

## VAGINITIS

### Introduction

**What are the characteristics of normal vaginal discharge?**
White or transparent in color, thick, and odorless

**What is the normal vaginal pH?**
<4.5

**What is the microbiology of normal vaginal flora?**
There is an average of six different species of bacteria, which are predominantly aerobic. The most common is the **hydrogen peroxide-producing lactobacilli**

**What does microscopy of normal vaginal secretions reveal?**
Predominantly squamous epithelial cells, few white blood cells (<1 per epithelial cells), and possibly a few clue cells

**What are the typical symptoms of vaginitis?**

Increased vaginal discharge, pruritus, irritation, soreness, odor, dyspareunia, bleeding, dysuria, and mucosal erythema

**What are some of the most important etiologies to consider in your differential diagnoses?**

Most common infectious causes (bacterial vaginosis > vulvovaginal candidiasis > trichomoniasis)

Less common "infectious" causes (desquamative inflammatory vaginitis, foreign body with secondary infection)

Noninfectious causes (atrophic vaginitis, contact dermatitis, allergens, irritants, hypersensitivity)

**What laboratory tests are typically ordered to diagnose the etiology of vaginitis?**

pH, amine test (whiff test), saline microscopy

## Bacterial Vaginosis (Nonspecific Vaginitis)

**What is BV?**

The most common cause of infectious vaginitis and results from an **alteration of the normal vaginal bacteria flora**. Loss of the normal hydrogen peroxide-producing lactobacilli results in an **overgrowth of anaerobes** such as ***Gardnerella vaginalis*** and ***Mycoplasma hominis***

**What are the key distinguishing symptoms?**

"**Musty**" or "**fishy**" vaginal odor; **thin, homogenous, gray-white discharge;** less inflammatory symptoms; dyspareunia absent

**What are risk factors for BV?**

Multiple sex partners

A new sex partner

Douching

Lack of vaginal lactobacilli

**What are the three major diagnostic findings in BV?**

**Vaginal pH >4.5**

**Positive amine/whiff test** (release of fishy, amine-like odor when vaginal fluid is alkalinized with KOH)

**Saline microscopy reveals >20% of clue cells** (vaginal epithelial cells with adherent bacterial clusters)

**What are some important complications of BV?**

Cervicitis, increased risk of PID, increased risk of HIV infection, preterm delivery, intrapartum and postpartum infections, first trimester miscarriages

**What is the treatment for BV?**

Oral or intravaginal metronidazole or clindamycin

*Pregnant patients should not receive topical clindamycin

**Do sexual partners need to be treated?**

No. BV is not a sexually transmitted disease

## Vulvovaginal Candidiasis

**What is vulvovaginal candidiasis (VVC)?**

It is a **yeast infection** of the vagina primarily caused by ***Candida albicans*** because of a change in the vaginal flora

**What are the major risk factors for VVC?**

Immunosuppression (**corticosteroids**, AIDS)

Changes in normal vaginal flora (**antibiotics**)

Hormonal changes (**pregnancy**, menstruation, higher dose estrogen OCP)

Intrauterine devices and vaginal sponges

**Diabetes mellitus**

**What key symptoms and signs distinguish candidiasis from other causes of *infectious* vaginitis?**

Intense vulvovaginal pruritis, soreness, vulvar mucosal erythema and edema, and vaginal discharge that resembles **white "cottage cheese"**

**What are other conditions that must be considered in the differential diagnosis?**

Hypersensitivity, allergic or chemical reactions, and contact dermatitis

**What is the pH of the vagina in patients with VVC?**

Normal pH (4–4.5)

**How would you definitively diagnose vaginal candidiasis?**

Microscopic evaluation of a wet saline or KOH prep of vaginal fluid reveals **hyphae, pseudohyphae, or budding yeast ("spaghetti and meatballs")**

**What is the treatment?**

Either **oral fluconazole** (single dose in nonpregnant women) or **topical or intravaginal antifungal drugs**

(3–7 days). About 1% hydrocortisone may be used to relieve external irritative symptoms

**When is oral fluconazole contraindicated?**

**During pregnancy**. A 7-day course of topical antifungal therapy is recommended for pregnant patients

**Does the patient's sexual partner need to be treated as well?**

No. Candidiasis is not typically a sexually transmitted disease

## Trichomonas Vaginalis

**What is trichomoniasis?**

A sexually transmitted vaginal infection caused by the flagellated protozoan, *T. vaginalis*. There is a strong association with BV

**What are the key presenting characteristics of trichomoniasis?**

**Malodorous, purulent, greenish, frothy, profuse watery discharge**; vulvovaginal erythema and irritation, dyspareunia, dysuria; punctate hemorrhages on the cervix ("**strawberry cervix**")

**How is the diagnosis usually made?**

**pH of vaginal secretions >5.0**

Microscopic examination of a wet saline prep of vaginal fluid reveals **motile trichomonads**

**What are some complications of trichomoniasis?**

Increased HIV transmission; increased risk of PID; preterm delivery; premature rupture of membranes; low birth weight infants

**What is the treatment?**

Oral metronidazole

Pregnant patients should receive oral metronidazole (category B drug)

**All sexual partners should be treated**

**What other tests should be considered?**

Tests for *N. gonorrhoeae*, *C. trachomatis*, syphilis, HIV

## Desquamative Inflammatory Vaginitis

**What are the three characteristics of desquamative inflammatory vaginitis?**

Diffuse, exudative vaginitis

Vaginal-epithelial cell exfoliation

Profuse and purulent vaginal discharge

**What causes inflammatory vaginitis?**
Replacement of normal lactobacilli with gram-positive cocci (usually streptococci)

**What type of patients present with desquamative inflammatory vaginitis?**
Premenopausal women with normal estrogen levels

**How do these patients typically present?**
With a purulent vaginal discharge, vulvovaginal burning, dyspareunia, vaginal erythema, and a vulvovaginal-cervical spotted rash

**What are some laboratory findings?**
Vaginal secretion pH >4.5

Increased number of parabasal cells

Gram-positive cocci (usually streptococci) on Gram-staining

**What is the treatment?**
2% clindamycin cream intravaginally × 7 days

## Atrophic Vaginitis

**Which women are more likely to be affected by atrophic vaginitis?**
Postmenopausal women

**What causes atrophic vaginitis?**
Thinning of the vaginal epithelium because of a reduction of endogenous estrogen. Reduction of lactobacilli and lactic acid increases the vaginal pH and leads to an overgrowth of non-acidophilic organisms

**What are some common symptoms?**
Mild vaginal atrophy is usually asymptomatic. Advanced vaginal atrophy can present with vaginal soreness, purulent vaginal discharge, dysparenuia, and postcoital irritation and bleeding

**What does a physical examination reveal?**
Atrophy of external genitalia, loss of vaginal folds, thin and diffusely erythematous vulvovaginal mucosa with some ecchymoses, and watery or serosanguineous discharge

**What do laboratory tests of the vaginal secretions reveal?**
pH >5.0–7.0

Increased number of leukocytes and parabasal epithelial cells

Increased gram-negative rods

**What is the treatment?**
Topical estrogen vaginal cream

## Noninfectious Causes of Vaginitis

**What are some causes of noninfectious vaginitis?**

Topical antimycotic drugs

Spermicides

Mini-pads/pantyliners and other feminine products

Soaps

Povidone-iodine

Latex condoms

Seminal fluid

**What are the symptoms of noninfectious vaginitis?**

Pruritus, irritation, burning, soreness, and variable discharge (similar to infectious vaginitis)

**With what disease can noninfectious vaginitis be confused?**

Acute *Candida* vaginitis

**How is the diagnosis made?**

Based upon symptoms and exclusion of all infectious etiologies

**What is the treatment?**

Removal of causative agent

Local relief by sodium bicarbonate, sitz baths, and topical vegetable oils

# OTHER GYNECOLOGIC INFECTIONS

## Postoperative Pelvic Infection

**What are some gynecologic postoperative infections?**

Cuff and pelvic cellulitis

Salpingitis

Suppurative pelvic thrombophlebitis

TOA with and without rupture

**What are the five major causes of fever in the postoperative gynecology patient?**

The five "W"s:
Wind = pulmonary atelectasis or pneumonia

Water = urinary tract infection

Walk = deep vein thrombosis (DVT) or superficial phlebitis

Wound = infection from the abdominal incision or from a pelvic source

Weird drugs = drug-causing fevers

**On what postoperative day does fever because of pelvic infection commonly occur?**

Between postoperative day (POD) 2–4

**What should one think of if fevers continue and there is no clinical response to antibiotics?**

Pelvic abscess

## Toxic Shock Syndrome

**What is toxic shock syndrome (TSS)?**

An **acute** illness characterized by **high fevers** which may quickly lead to **hypotensive shock** and **multisystem failure**

**What is the cause of toxic shock syndrome?**

Preformed exotoxins produced by ***Staphylococcus aureus***

**In which patients has this syndrome been associated?**

**Menstruating women** between ages 12–24 who use **superabsorbent tampons**

Postpartum women

Women who use a diaphragm

In both men and women following surgical procedures

**What are the major clinical findings in TSS?**

Abrupt onset of **high fevers**, **vomiting**, and **diarrhea**. Within 48 hours, **signs of shock** occur (temperature ≥102.2°F, dehydration, tachycardia, hypotension) and a **diffuse "sunburn-like" rash** appears over the face, trunk, and proximal extremities. **Desquamation (particularly affecting the palms and soles)** may occur 1–2 weeks after the onset of illness

**Involvement of three or more organ systems (GI, CNS, renal, mucous membrane, skin, cardiac, hepatic) is essential for diagnosis**

**What information should be sought during the H&P that is pertinent to this diagnosis?**

Ask the patient if she is **menstruating or using tampons!!!** You must perform a vaginal examination and remove the tampon immediately if one is present

**What laboratory should be ordered?**

Complete panel of blood tests

Cultures from blood, sputum, CSF, and the **vagina**

**What will the vaginal culture yield in TSS?**

Penicillinase-producing *S. aureus*

**What is the management and treatment for a patient with TSS?**

Assess hemodynamics

Replace fluid volume and electrolytes (may require dopamine infusion)

Monitor urine output

IV antibiotics: β-lactamase-resistant antibiotic (nafcillin or oxacillin)

Vancomycin (for penicillin-allergic patients)

**What are the three most common causes of death from TSS?**

Acute respiratory distress syndrome

Intractable hypotension

Hemorrhage secondary to DIC

## HIV/AIDS

**What is HIV?**

A single-stranded **RNA retrovirus** that infects **CD4 receptor lymphocytes** and other target cells and causes a progressive **decrease in cellular immunity** leading to AIDS

**What are the three means of HIV transmission?**

Sexual contact

Parenteral exposure to blood or bodily fluids (i.e., IV drugs, occupational exposure)

Vertical transmission (from an infected mother to her fetus)

**How do HIV-infected patients initially present?**

With mononucleosis-like symptoms such as **fever, weight loss, night sweats**, pharyngitis, lymphadenopathy, erythematous maculopapular rash. This is followed by a long asymptomatic period lasting from months to years

**What percent of those diagnosed with AIDS in the United States are women?**

25%

**What are some symptoms of HIV infection in females?**

Difficult-to-treat vaginal infections (**candidiasis**, BV, and common STDs)

Increase in frequency, severity, and recurrence of HSV ulcers, HPV infections, and cervical dysplasia

Presence of idiopathic genital ulcers

**How is it diagnosed?**

Screening test: **ELISA** (detects antibodies to HIV)

Confirmation test: **Western blot**

**When can the ELISA test give a false-negative result?**

In early infection (<**12 weeks**). All patients with recent exposure need to be tested again after this window period

**What vaccinations should be offered to HIV-infected patients?**

Hepatitis B, influenza, and pneumococcus

**What organism commonly causes pneumonia in HIV-infected patients?**

*Streptococcus pneumoniae*

**What is the most common opportunistic pneumonia in HIV-infected patients? How is it detected and treated?**

*Pneumocystis carinii* (PCP)

Diagnosis: bronchoalveolar lavage with silver stain (Giemsa)

Treatment: trimethoprim-sulfamethoxazole or pentamidine

**What is the current treatment regimen for HIV infection?**

Two anti-retrovirals and one protease inhibitor

# Pelvic Pain

## CHRONIC PELVIC PAIN

### Etiologies

**How is chronic pelvic pain (CPP) defined?**

It is **noncyclic pain** of nonmenstrual origin that **lasts ≥6 months duration** and is located **below the umbilicus**. The pain is severe enough to **cause functional disability or require medical treatment**

**What is the prevalence of chronic pelvic pain?**

Approximately 15–20% of women aged 18–50 years have chronic pelvic pain of greater than 1 year duration

**What are the most common gynecologic conditions that cause chronic pelvic pain?**

**Pelvic inflammatory disease (18–35%); endometriosis;** adenomyosis; gynecologic malignancies (late stages); tuberculous salpingitis

**How often is endometriosis diagnosed by laparoscopy in women with chronic pelvic pain?**

Diagnosis of endometriosis by laparoscopy is made in 33% of women with chronic pelvic pain

**What are the most significant non-gynecological causes of chronic pelvic pain?**

Consistent scientific evidence has shown that interstitial cystitis, irritable bowel syndrome, chronic coccygeal or back pain, and depression may cause or exacerbate chronic pelvic pain

**What is the relationship between chronic pelvic pain and involvement of more than one organ system?**

Pain is more severe when more than one organ system is involved. Women with chronic pain are more often found to have dysmenorrhea and dyspareunia compared to the general population. The severity of pain is greater in women who have gastrointestinal or urologic symptoms in addition to the chronic pelvic pain

**What is the association between physical or sexual abuse, and chronic pelvic pain?**

About 40–50% of women with chronic pelvic pain have a history of some form of abuse. A direct causal relationship and mechanism to chronic pelvic pain has not been established

**What other mental disorders should be considered in a patient with chronic pelvic pain?**

Somatization, opiate abuse, depression

**What type of obstetrical history may lead to chronic pelvic pain?**

Known as "peripartum pelvic pain syndrome," this is a musculoskeletal source of pain that manifests in women with lumbar lordosis, delivery of a large infant, muscle weakness and poor physical conditioning, a difficult delivery, vacuum or forceps delivery, and use of gynecologic stirrups for delivery

## Workup

**What information should be gathered when taking the history of the patient's pain?**

A thorough review of systems should be performed with emphasis on urinary tract disease, bowel disease, reproductive tract disease, musculoskeletal disorders, and psychoneurologic disorders

**What characteristics of the pain should be investigated as part of the detailed history?**

Location, intensity, quality, duration, temporal pattern, precipitating patterns (exertion, sexual activity, menses, pregnancy), radiation, and relationship to urination and defecation

**How do the nature and the quality of pain give a clue to the source of the pain?**

**Somatic pain** is usually localized and sharp, indicating a musculoskeletal origin

**Visceral pain** is usually vague, aching, and difficult to localize; this may indicate an intraperitoneal or upper reproductive tract etiology

**What should be looked for on physical examination?**

The physical exammination should concentrate on looking for points of localized or generalized tenderness, surgical scars, masses, and hernias. The pelvic examination should focus on identifying physical findings consistent with pelvic floor dysfunction, painful bladder syndrome, endometriosis, adenomyosis, or leiomyomat

**What are the physical findings that suggest the following etiologies of chronic pelvic pain?**

**Endometriosis**: uterosacral ligament nodularity or thickness, cervical stenosis, lateral displacement of the cervix because of shortening of one of the ligaments

**Adenomyosis**: slightly enlarged, globular, tender uterus on examination

**Leiomyomat**: enlarged, mobile uterus with an irregular contour on bimanual or abdominal examination

**Pelvic inflammatory disease (PID)**: uterine tenderness or cervical motion tenderness on examination

**Neuropathy**: burning, shock-like, paresthesia, and dysesthesia

**Neoplasm**: adnexal mass, ascites

**What is Carnett's sign?**

It refers to **increased local tenderness during muscle tensing by raising both legs straight up while lying supine**. This maneuver tightens the rectus abdominis muscles, increasing pain if there is **myofascial pain** (e.g., trigger points, entrapped nerve, hernia, myositis), while true visceral sources of pain are associated with less tenderness when abdominal muscles are tensed

**Which laboratory and imaging tests should be ordered in a patient with chronic pelvic pain?**

Complete blood count (CBC) with differential and ESR

Pregnancy test

Urinalysis

Occult blood test

Pelvic ultrasound

*Chlamydia* and gonorrhea infection

CA-125

**When should MRI or CT scan be used?**

Only when abnormalities are found on ultrasound examination

**What is the role of laparoscopy in evaluation of women with chronic pelvic pain?**

It is indicated in women who have symptoms and signs of endometriosis and/or adhesions. It is also indicated in women with **chronic pelvic pain** who have not had relief of symptoms with nonsteroidal anti-inflammatory drugs (NSAIDs) or estrogen-progestin treatment and have no strong contraindications to laparoscopic surgery

**What is conscious laparoscopic pain mapping?**

It refers to laparoscopy performed under local anesthesia in which the tissues are probed and pulled with surgical instruments while the patient is asked about the severity and nature of any pain she perceives. It can lead to the treatment of subtle or atypical areas of disease that might have been previously overlooked. It may also help prevent surgical treatment when no painful lesions are identified

## Treatment

**How is endometriosis-associated chronic pelvic pain treated?**

Empirical sequential treatment with nonsteroidal anti-inflammatory drugs, oral contraceptives administered in monthly or longer cycles, GnRH agonist analogues (nafarelin, goserelin, and leuprolide), progestins (medroxy-progesterone acetate)

**In what other sources of chronic pelvic pain are GnRH agonists effective?**

Irritable bowel syndrome, pelvic congestion syndrome, and interstitial cystitis also respond to GnRH agonists

**When are oral contraceptives indicated for treatment of chronic pelvic pain?**

To decrease pain from primary dysmenorrhea

**What is the role of antidepressants in treatment of chronic pelvic pain?**

Currently, evidence is insufficient to substantiate efficacy of antidepressants for the treatment of chronic pelvic pain. However, adding psychotherapy to medical treatment of chronic pelvic pain appears to improve response over that of medical treatment alone and should be considered

**What is the role of surgery in treatment of chronic pelvic pain?**

Excision or destruction of endometriotic tissue, lysis of adhesions, and hysterectomy (in women who have finished childbearing) have been proposed to relieve chronic pelvic pain

**What is presacral neurectomy and is it effective for treatment of chronic pelvic pain?**

It is the surgical resection of the superior hypogastric plexus which innervates the cervix, uterus, and proximal fallopian tubes with afferent nociception. It may be used to treat centrally located dysmenorrhea but has limited efficacy for chronic pelvic pain or pain that is not central in its location

**What is the main take-home point of treatment for chronic pelvic pain?**

Multimodal therapy (medical therapy, surgical therapy, and behavioral/mental health treatment, along with pain consultation) is superior to treatments that emphasize a single approach

# ACUTE PELVIC PAIN

## Etiologies

**What are the obstetric and gynecologic differential diagnoses for acute pelvic pain?**

Pelvic inflammatory disease

Adnexal cysts/masses/abscesses with bleeding, torsion, or rupture

Ectopic pregnancy

Spontaneous abortion

Endometritis

Degeneration, infarction, or torsion of leiomyomas (fibroids)

**What are non-gynecologic differential diagnoses for acute pelvic pain?**

Appendicitis

Diverticulitis

Urinary tract infection or obstruction

Renal colic

**Which of these diagnoses are life threatening and must be ruled out quickly?**

Ectopic pregnancy

Tubo-ovarian abscess

Ruptured ovarian cyst

Appendicitis

**On what additional points should the history taking focus to determine a pelvic etiology?**

The regularity and timing of menstrual periods, possibility of pregnancy, presence of vaginal discharge or bleeding, and a recent history of dyspareunia or dysmenorrhea

**What findings on physical examination may lead you to the appropriate gynecologic/obstetric etiology for acute pelvic pain?**

**Ectopic pregnancy:** unruptured pregnancy leads to localized unilateral pain because of fallopian tube dilatation. If it ruptures, the pain becomes generalized because of peritoneal irritation. A pelvic examination may reveal cervical motion tenderness that is exaggerated on the side of the tubal pregnancy

**Tubo-ovarian abscess**: patients present with generalized abdominal pain and rebound tenderness caused by peritoneal inflammation. Bilateral, palpable, fixed, and tender masses are commonly found on examination

**Acute PID**: lower abdominal tenderness, cervical motion tenderness, adnexal tenderness

**Ovarian torsion/rupture**: severe unilateral, lower abdominal pain, adnexal mass, nausea and vomiting

**Uterine infection or pathology (torsion, degeneration, infarction)**: irregular enlargement and painful uterus on palpation

**Endometriosis**: localized pain in the cul-de-sac or uterosacral ligaments, palpable tender nodules in the cul-de-sac, uterosacral ligaments, or rectovaginal septum, possible fixation of adnexa or uterus in a retroverted position

**What labs or tests should be considered in the workup of acute pelvic pain?**

CBC; urinary analysis (UA); pregnancy test; tests for *Chlamydia* and gonorrhea in women with suspected PID; microscopic examination of (wet mount) of any abnormal vaginal discharge; culdocentesis; vaginal ultrasound; laparoscopy

**How do differences in the clinical and laboratory findings help point out the etiology of acute gynecologic pelvic pain?**

See Table 4.1

**What is mittelschmerz?**

It is recurrent acute midcycle abdominal pain because of leakage of prostaglandin-containing follicular fluid at the time of ovulation. The pain associated is typically mild, unilateral, midway between menstrual periods, and lasts for a few hours to a couple of days

# Endometriosis

**What is endometriosis?**

A benign yet very debilitating gynecologic disease where **endometrial glands and stroma** are present in an **extrauterine location**

**Table 4-1** Differential Diagnosis of Acute Gynecologic Pelvic Pain

| | Clinical and Laboratory Findings | | | | | |
|---|---|---|---|---|---|---|
| Disease | CBC | UA | Pregnancy Test | Culdocentesis | Fever | Nausea and Vomiting |
| Ruptured ectopic pregnancy | Hematocrit low after treatment of hypovolemia | Red blood cells rare | Positive, beta-hCG low for gestational age | High hematocrit<br>Defibrinated, nonclotting sample with no platelets<br>Crenated red blood cells | No | Unusual |
| Salpingitis/PID | Rising white blood cell count | White blood cells occasionally present | Generally negative | Yellow, turbid fluid with many white blood cells and some bacteria | Progressively worsening; spiking | Gradual onset with ileus |
| Hemorrhagic ovarian cyst | Hematocrit may be low after treatment of hypovolemia | Normal | Usually negative | Hematocrit generally <10% | No | Rare |
| Torsion of adnexa | Normal | Normal | Generally negative | Minimal clear fluid if obtained early | No | Rare |
| Degenerating leiomyoma | Normal or elevated white blood cell count | Normal | Generally negative | Normal clear fluid | Possibly | Rare |

Reprinted, with permission, from Pearlman MD, Tintinalli JE, eds. *Emergency Care of the Woman*. New York, NY: McGraw-Hill; 1998: 508.

**To which hormone does ectopic endometrial tissue respond? What is the significance of this?**

**Estrogen**. It **changes in a cyclic manner** according to menstrual changes in estrogen levels. The ectopic tissue can release a small amount of blood into the surrounding tissues leading to repeated **tissue inflammation, pelvic pain, scarring, and eventually adhesions in the reproductive organs, pelvis, and other intestines**

**Who develops endometriosis?**

**Reproductive-age women** and postmenopausal women on estrogen-replacement therapy

**What is the prevalence of endometriosis in the United States?**

7% of reproductive-age women are diagnosed with endometriosis

**What are the two most common symptoms associated with endometriosis and what percentage of women with these complaints are found to have endometriosis?**

**Chronic pelvic pain** (71–87%); **Infertility** (38%)

**How does endometriosis lead to infertility?**

1. It causes the **formation of adhesions** that distort the normal uterine/tubal/ovary anatomy, inhibit tubo-ovarian motility, and block ovum release
2. The release of other substances (such as **cytokines**) may be "toxic" to normal ovarian function/fertilization/implantation

**What other common complication can endometrial adhesions cause?**

Small bowel obstruction

**For what other disease is endometriosis a risk factor?**

**Epithelial ovarian cancer** (EOC)

Since both are estrogen-dependent diseases, the presence of endometriosis may indicate a risk for developing EOC

**Do genetic factors increase the risk for endometriosis?**

Yes. There is a seven- to tenfold increased risk of developing endometriosis if a first-degree relative has been affected by endometriosis. The mode of inheritance is polygenic and multifactorial

**What three leading theories explain the etiology of endometriosis?**

1. **Retrograde menstruation:** a reverse flow of endometrial tissue through the fallopian tubes

during menses leads to the seeding of endometrial cells in the peritoneal cavity

2. **Lymphatic and vascular spread:** spread of endometrial cells through lymphatic and vascular channels
3. **Coelomic metaplasia:** transformation of coelomic epithelium or undifferentiated peritoneal cells into endometrial tissue by an endogenous undefined biochemical factor

**In what sites are endometrial implants found?**

Most common: **ovaries**, anterior and posterior cul-de-sac, uterosacral ligaments, posterior uterus, posterior broad ligaments, sigmoid colon, appendix, round ligaments

Less common: vagina, cervix, rectovaginal septum, cecum, ileum, inguinal canals, abdominal or perineal scars, ureters, urinary bladder, and umbilicus

Rare: breast, pancreas, liver, gallbladder, kidney, urethra, extremities, vertebrae, bone, peripheral nerves, lung, diaphragm, and central nervous system

**What are the common presenting symptoms of endometriosis and how do ectopic lesions explain these symptoms?**

**Chronic pelvic pain**: local peritoneal inflammation secondary to formation of adhesions and fibrosis

**Acute exacerbations of pelvic pain**: peritoneal inflammation secondary to the release of hemolyzed blood and other contents of ruptured endometriomas

**Secondary dysmenorrhea**: cyclical changes in ectopic lesions secondary to changes in estrogen levels

**Dyspareunia**: deep infiltration and scarring of the uterosacral ligaments and rectovaginal septum by endometriotic lesions. Can also be caused by a retroverted uterus secondary to adhesions (leads to deep dyspareunia)

**Infertility**: invasive endometriosis and the formation of adhesions distorts the normal uterine/tubal/ovary anatomy, inhibits tubo-ovarian motility, and blocks ovum release

**Many women are asymptomatic**

**What symptom is pathognomonic for endometriosis?**

Cyclical rectal bleeding

**What are endometriomas?**

Invasive endometriotic lesions found inside the ovary. Often described as a **"chocolate cyst"** because it contains old blood that has undergone hemolysis

**What are the complications of endometriomas?**

Rupture of endometriomas can cause periteonal inflammation, scarring, and pelvic adhesions

**What findings are typically found on physical examination?**

**Tenderness upon pelvic examination during menses** (most common finding)

Uterosacral or cul-de-sac nodularity

**Retroverted uterus** and limited motion of ovaries and fallopian tubes

Tender, enlarged adnexal mass (unilateral)

There are often no abnormal findings on physical examination

**What is the differential diagnosis for the presentation of endometriosis?**

Pelvic inflammatory disease (PID)

Acute or chronic inflammation

Ectopic pregnancy

Kidney stones

Cystitis

Pelvic tumors

**What laboratory tests would help you rule out the diseases on your differential diagnoses list?**

Complete blood count (CBC) and erythrocyte sedimentation rate (ESR); cervical Cx; urine β-hCG; urinalysis and urine culture

**How do the following tests help you in your diagnostic decision making?**

**CBC and ESR**

Positive findings are nonspecific; leukocytosis may be seen in infection

**Cervical Cx**

Positive cultures for guanylyl cyclase c (GC/C) may indicate PID

**Urine β-hCG**

Positive test indicates pregnancy, ruling out ectopic pregnancy is necessary

**Urinalysis and urine culture**

Ruling out UTI

**What value does CA125 have in the clinical management of endometriosis?**

CA125 is not a sensitive diagnostic test for endometriosis (especially in minimal to mild disease). However, it may be used as a **marker to follow medical treatment response** for endometriosis. CA125 levels may decrease during treatment compared to pretreatment values; however, normal posttreatment values do not confirm the absence of endometriosis nor are they useful markers for predicting disease recurrence

**Are imaging tests a sensitive modality for diagnosing endometriosis?**

No. However, ultrasound, CT, and MRI are useful for detecting pelvic or adnexal masses (i.e., endometriomas) or ruling out other causes of pelvic pain. Deeply infiltrating endometriosis that involve the uterosacral ligaments and the cul-de-sac may be detected by MRI

**How is the diagnosis of endometriosis made?**

Direct visualization by laparoscopy/ laparotomy with histologic confirmation

**What are the characteristic findings of endometriosis found during laparoscopy/ laparotomy?**

**Classic lesions**: brown/black/ blue **"powder burn," "gun shot"** lesions, nodules or small cysts containing old hemorrhage surrounded by fibrosis on the serosal surfaces of the peritoneum

Atypical/subtle lesions: clear vesicles, white opacifications, red, white, yellow/ brown plaques, excrescences, scars or lesions of varying sizes

**Note: Normal appearing peritoneum may have microscopic evidence of endometriosis**

**What histologic findings confirm the diagnosis of endometriosis?**

The **presence of two or more** of the following histologic features: endometrial epithelium, endometrial glands, endometrial stroma, hemosiderin-laden macrophages

**What is the current classification system for endometriosis staging?**

One created by the American Society for Reproductive Medicine. It uses point scores for disease staging and is used primarily for the uniform recording of operative findings

**What are the limitations of this system?**

It is not good for correlating disease stage with pain and/or dyspareunia. It also does not predict the chance of pregnancy following treatment

**What is the typical clinical outcome of endometriosis and what is the goal of treatment?**

Endometriosis is a progressively deteriorating disease that rarely improves. Elimination of endometriotic implants by medical or surgical intervention provides only temporary relief. However, **the goal of treatment should be to eradicate the lesions, treat endometriosis-related pelvic pain and infertility, and prevent bowel and extra-pelvic complications**

**What factors must be considered when choosing the appropriate treatment regimen?**

Patient's desire for future fertility, side effects of medication, cost, and patient's tolerance

**What type of medical therapy is most effective for endometriosis?**

Hormonal therapy that **suppresses estrogen synthesis** (induces atrophy of ectopic lesions) and/or **disrupts the menstrual cycle** (abrogates or diminishes retrograde bleeding)

**What are the most commonly used hormonal medications for the treatment of endometriosis?**

**Oral contraceptive pills (OCPs)**: best for minimal to mild pain, reduces menstrual flow

**Progestins**: good for moderate to severe disease, excellent pain relief, induces atrophy of endometrial implants, few side effects, inexpensive

**Danazol**: effective for mild to moderate disease, relieves dysmenorrhea, inhibits midcycle

LH/FSH surge, induces endometrial atrophy within uterus and ectopically ultimately leads to amenorrhea

**GnRH agonists**: inhibit pituitary gonadotropin secretion which suppresses ovarian estrogen production, induces amenorrhea, relieves pain

**What other nonhormonal medication treats endometriosis-related pain?**

Nonsteroidal anti-inflammatory drugs

**When is surgery indicated for the treatment of endometriosis?**

1. When symptoms have not improved or worsened with medical management
2. When symptoms of endometriosis are severe and incapacitating
3. For advanced disease
4. To treat endometriomas, bowel or urogenital tract obstruction, or anatomically distorted pelvic structures because of adhesions/ invasive endometriotic lesions

**What are the indications for conservative surgery (preserves uterus and ovarian tissue)?**

Less severe disease or for those who want to preserve fertility

**What are the indications for definitive surgery (hysterectomy with or without removal of the fallopian tubes and ovaries)?**

For patients with advanced disease and for those who no longer want/ need fertility conservation

**What is the impact of medical management versus surgical management on recurrence and infertility?**

Similar or higher rates of recurrence have been reported with medical management versus surgical management. Surgery has been reported to improve rates of fertility compared to expectant management

**What is the most likely cause of infertility in a menstruating woman without a history of PID?**

Endometriosis

**What is the management of endometriosis-related infertility?**

Assisted reproduction technologies (ART) such as IVF

**What is adenomyosis?**

The presence of **ectopic endometrial glands and stroma within the uterine musculature**

**What is the prevalence of adenomyosis?**

It is thought to affect 20% of all women

**What is the classic presentation of a patient with adenomyosis?**

A **parous, middle-aged** woman with **menorrhagia** and **dysmenorrhea** with a **symmetrically enlarged, tender, and "boggy" uterus**

**How is the diagnosis of adenomyosis made?**

A presumptive diagnosis is based on the clinical presentation in the absence of endometriosis or leiomyomas. A definitive diagnosis requires histologic assessment of the uterine tissue

**What is the differential diagnosis for adenomyosis?**

Leiomyoma

Intra-abdominal neoplasia

Endometriosis

PID

**Is adenomyosis related to endometriosis?**

Although they are both disorders of the ectopic endometrium, they are unrelated

**What is the definitive treatment for adenomyosis?**

Hysterectomy

**What is the prognosis for adenomyosis?**

Good—it is a self-limited process that often becomes asymptomatic after menopause

# Benign Pelvic Masses

## BENIGN CERVICAL MASSES

### Cervical Cysts

**What four types of cervical cysts are there?**

1. Nabothian
2. Mesonephric
3. Endometrial
4. Adenosis

**What are the symptoms of a cervical cyst?**

Usually **asymptomatic** but can cause dyspareunia

**What is a nabothian cyst and how does it develop?**

A discrete mucus-filled cyst that appears grossly as a small translucent or yellow elevation on the cervix. Nabothian cysts are often discovered on pelvic examination. They occur via metaplasia, a process by which cervical cells convert from glandular cells that secrete mucus to squamous cells. Sometimes a cleft of **columnar endocervical** epithelium becomes covered by **squamous** epithelium, trapping the mucus secretions and forming cysts.

**How are nabothian cysts treated?**

- Most are asymptomatic and therapy is not needed
- If symptomatic, treatment can be via excision, electrocautery or cryotherapy

**Which other cervical cyst may be confused with a nabothian cyst? How can it be distinguished from a nabothian cyst?**

The mesonephric (Wolffian) cysts are found deep in the stroma of the **ectocervix** and are lined by **Wolffian-type cells**

**What conditions are most associated with cervical cysts?**

Pregnancy, menopause, and cervicitis

## Cervical Polyps

**What are cervical polyps?**

Small, pedunculated, benign neoplasms of the cervix composed of a vascular connective tissue stroma covered by epithelium. They commonly arise via focal hyperplasia of the endocervix and protrude from the cervical canal out of the external os.

**How common are they and in whom do they develop?**

Relatively common—especially in multigravidas over 20 years of age. They are rare before menarche but may develop after menopause

**How are cervical polyps diagnosed and managed?**

- Asymptomatic polyps often are discovered on routine pelvic examination. Otherwise they usually present with **intermenstrual** or **postcoital bleeding** or discharge
- Although carcinoma developing in a polyp is rare, polyps should be **removed** close to their attachment and **pathologically reviewed**

# BENIGN UTERINE MASSES

## Leiomyomas

**What are uterine leiomyomas?**

**Benign** tumors of the **smooth muscle** cells (myometrium) of the uterus; Also known as **fibroids, fibromyomas**, or **myomas**

**What are the three types of leiomyomas? (see Fig. 4-3)?**

1. **Intramural**—located **within the wall of the myometrium** and may distort the shape of the uterine cavity and surface
2. **Submucosal**—originate in the myometrium and **grow toward the endometrial cavity**, protruding into the uterine lumen
3. **Subserosal**—originate in the myometrium and grow out toward **the serosal surface** of the uterus; extend from the uterine surface into the peritoneum and abdominal cavity

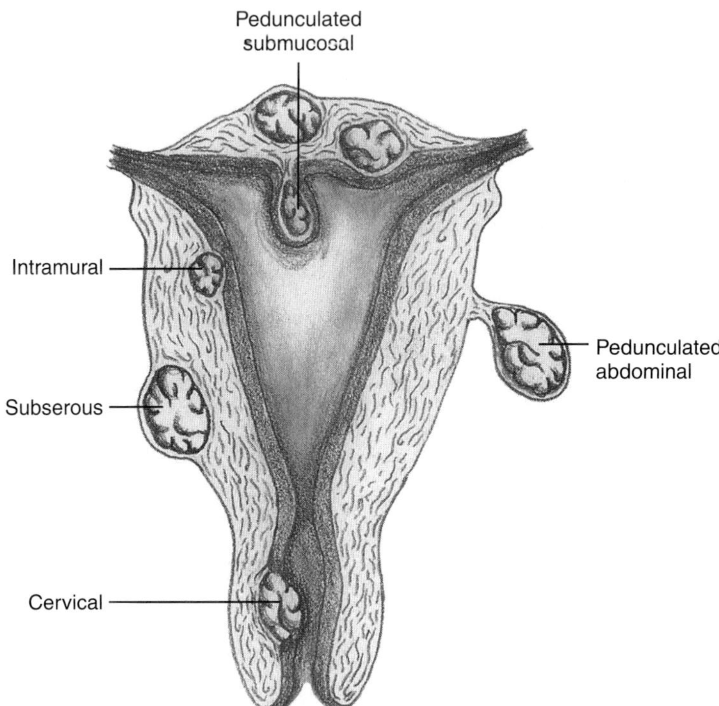


**Figure 4-3** Types of leiomyomas.

**What is the prevalence of leiomyomas and in whom do they occur?**

Leiomyomas are **hormonally responsive** and are found in **20–30% of reproductive-age women.** Most women diagnosed with leiomyomas are **between 30 and 50 years old**. **Black women** are 2–3 times more likely to develop fibroids than white women.

**What are the risk factors for leiomyomas?**

**Black race**

**Nulliparity**

**Oral contraceptives (OCPs)** are mostly **protective**

Diet—a diet high in red meat and low in green vegetables has been suggested to increase the risk for fibroids

Genetics

Alcohol

**What are the usual presentation/symptoms/signs of fibroids?**

Most are **asymptomatic** and so are diagnosed based on the finding of an **irregularly enlarged, mobile uterus** on gynecologic examination

If symptoms do occur, the most common are:

**Abnormal uterine bleeding** (menorrhagia or metrorrhagia)

**Pelvic pressure/pain** (dysmenorrhea, urinary frequency, constipation, or dyspareunia)

**Infertility**

**Aside from leiomyomas, what are other differential diagnoses of a patient who presents with menorrhagia and pelvic pressure/pain?**

Adenomyosis; primary dysmenorrhea; endometriosis; tubo-ovarian abscess; malignancy (cervical, endometrial, or ovarian)

**How is the diagnosis of fibroids usually made?**

Via ultrasonography

**Describe the theoretical mechanisms for increased bleeding associated with leiomyomas.**

1. An **alteration in myometrial cells contractile ability** leading to lack of control of bleeding from the endometrial arterioles
2. The endometrium is **unable to respond to hormonal changes** in the menstrual cycle, leading to sloughing off of excess tissue

3. Increased pressure causes **necrosis of the endometrium**, which leads to exposure of the vasculature surfaces and increased bleeding

**What other methods of evaluation could you consider for the diagnosis of fibroids?**

**Hysterosalpingography** allows for visualization of submucosal fibroids

**MRI** or **CT**

**Hysteroscopy and/or dilation and curettage (D&C)**

**What causes the development and growth of leiomyomas?**

It is unknown what causes their development. Their growth is responsive to both **estrogen** and **progesterone**. Estrogen may increase the production of extracellular matrix. Progesterone increases the mitotic activity of myomas and inhibits apoptosis

**What is the molecular pathogenesis of leiomyomas?**

First, **normal myocytes transform into abnormal myocytes** either via somatic mutation or in response to injury

Second, the abnormal myocytes **grow via clonal expansion** into clinically significant tumors

Molecular alterations that lead to **increased or abnormal vasculature** are also involved in fibroid formation

**What is degeneration of a leiomyoma and what types can occur?**

Various histologic and gross changes occur in leiomyomas when they outgrow their blood supply. The types are as follows:

**Red degeneration**—hemorrhagic changes that occur as a result of rapid growth. Can cause acute pain, low-grade fever, and an elevation in white blood cell (WBC) count; most common during pregnancy

**Hyaline degeneration**—mildest form of degeneration: hyalization of the smooth muscle of the leiomyoma represented by loss of the whorled pattern and an overall homogenous appearance

**Calcification**—occurs especially in inactive smooth muscle elements after menopause

**When do fibroids need to be treated?**

Most women **do not need surgical or medical treatment**. Expectant management with annual pelvic examinations to monitor growth is warranted. Intervention is indicated with worsening symptom or with a rapidly enlarging uterus

**What are the treatment options for symptomatic leiomyomas?**

**Progestin supplementation**

**Prostaglandin synthetase inhibitors**—reduce bleeding

**Other NSAIDs**

**GnRH analogs** → inhibit estrogen which reduces the size of the leiomyoma

**Myomectomy** → indicated in symptomatic women desiring future fertility

**Hysterectomy** → indicated in symptomatic women not desiring future fertility

**Embolization of the uterine arteries** → indicated in symptomatic premenopausal women not desiring fertility and who want to preserve their uterus and avoid surgical intervention

**What are the risks of myomectomy?**

**Intraoperative blood loss;** postoperative **hemorrhage; postsurgical adhesions; risk of recurrence**. These risks are higher with myomectomy than with hysterectomy

**What types of complications can occur which are secondary to leiomyomas?**

Iron-deficiency anemia

Acute blood loss

Hydroureter or hydronephrosis

**Can leiomyomas ever metastasize?**

Rarely. In those cases, leiomyomas can grow beyond the uterus or even invade intravascularly to spread to the peritoneum or lung

**What types of metastatic disease can develop from a leiomyoma?**

Intravenous leiomyomatosis

Benign metastasizing leiomyoma

Leiomyomatosis peritonealis disseminate

Leiomyosarcoma

**Who is most likely to develop a malignancy from a leiomyoma?**

Postmenopausal women, especially those presenting with rapid tumor growth, vaginal bleeding, and/or pain

**What is a leiomyosarcoma?**

A **malignant neoplasm of the uterine smooth** muscle. It occurs most commonly in postmenopausal women, is rapidly expanding, and carries a poor prognosis

## Benign Ovarian Masses

**What is the differential diagnosis of an ovarian mass?**

Functional ovarian cysts; dermoid cyst; PCOS; endometriomas; ectopic pregnancy; tubo-ovarian complex; malignancy

## Functional Ovarian Cysts

**What are functional ovarian cysts?**

Benign anatomic variations resulting from irregularities in normal ovarian function

**What are the three types of functional ovarian cysts and how do they form?**

1. **Follicular cysts**: ovulation fails to occur and the remaining fluid does not become reabsorbed but gets accumulated into a cystic structure
2. **Corpus luteum cysts**: the corpus luteum formed after ovulation persists and grows larger than 3 cm
3. **Theca lutein cysts**: most frequently occur iatrogenically following ovulation induction or in young girls with hypothyroidism. Also may be seen with high levels of hCG (e.g., in patients with hydatidiform mole or choriocarcinoma)

**What are the typical symptoms (if any) of each of the following types of ovarian cysts?**

**Follicular** — Typically asymptomatic; can cause midcycle pelvic pain, dyspareunia, and abnormal uterine bleeding

**Corpus luteum** — Localized tenderness, amenorrhea, and delayed menstruation (often confused with ectopic pregnancy)

**Theca lutein** — Pelvic heaviness/aching, hyperemesis, and breast paresthesias

**What is the appearance of each of the following types of cyst?**

**Follicular** — Smooth, thin walled, unilocular

**Corpus luteum** — More complex, usually yellowish-orange lining consisting of luteinized granulose and theca cells

**Theca lutein** — Usually bilateral, multicystic, filled with clear, straw-colored fluid.

All are usually <10 cm

**What is the diagnostic workup for a patient with a suspected functional ovarian cyst?**

Pelvic exam; ultrasound; repeat examination and sonography at 6–8 weeks; laparoscopy if symptomatic, concern for torsion or persistence after 3–6 months

**What findings raise your suspicion that a cyst may be neoplastic?**

- Patient is prepubescent or postmenopausal
- Patient has history of another malignancy (especially breast or gastric)
- Patient has ascites
- Ultrasound findings are significant for: large size, loculations, septa, papillae, or increased blood flow
- Continued presence of cyst at 3–6 months follow-up

**How are asymptomatic functional ovarian cysts treated?**

**Expectant management** with analgesics as needed (usually resolve within weeks); OCPs are often used—they do not promote faster resolution of the cyst, but reduce the risk of future cyst development

**When do functional ovarian cysts need to be treated?**

When there is severe pain or when there is suspicion of malignancy, rupture, or torsion

## Benign Ovarian Neoplams

**How are ovarian neoplasms categorized?**

Epithelial; germ cell; stromal cell

**How are benign ovarian neoplasms treated?**

Laparoscopy with unilateral cystectomy or oophorectomy (if the patient wishes to preserve fertility). Conversion to laparotomy and staging if malignancy is found

## Benign Fallopian Tube Masses

**What are the types of benign fallopian tube neoplasms?**

Paraovarian cysts; paratubal cysts

**What is another name for paratubal cysts? Describe them.**

Hydatid cysts of Morgagni. They are located near the fimbriated end of the tube, filled with clear fluid, and ~1 cm in diameter

**How do these masses usually present?**

Usually asymptomatic and the diagnosis is usually made as an incidental finding in the OR

# Sexual Dysfunction

**Describe what happens during the four phases of sexual response described by Masters and Johnson**

1. **Excitement: internal or external stimuli** → activation of the central nervous system (CNS) → deep breathing, increase in heart rate, blood pressure, and sexual tension; generalized vasocongestion → skin flush, breast engorgement, nipple erection, engorgement of labia and clitoris, vaginal transudation, and uterine tenting
2. **Plateau: marked degree of vasocongestion throughout the body** → further engorgement of the labia, lower third of vagina, breast, and areolae. Secretion from

the Bartholin glands, retraction of the clitoris, vagina lengthens with dilation of the upper two-thirds, muscle tension begins to build up
3. **Orgasm**: release of sexual tension, generalized myotonic contractions, perivaginal muscles and anal sphincter contract at precise intervals, vaginal and uterine contractions
4. **Resolution:** a gradual diminution of sexual tension and response

**What is the biopsychosocial model of female sexual response?**

The biopsychosocial nature of female sexual response is influenced by the dynamic interaction of four components: **biologic**, **psychologic**, **sociocultural influences**, and **interpersonal relationships**. All of these components must be addressed in order to achieve sexual satisfaction

**What are the possible etiologies of sexual dysfunction?**

1. Change in vascularity (atherosclerosis, pudendal artery insufficiency affecting vaginal vasocongestion)
2. Neurogenic causes (spinal cord dysfunction or injuries)
3. Depression or anxiety disorders
4. Medications (selective serotonin reuptake inhibitor [SSRI], tricyclic antidepressants, $H_2$ blocker, and some antihypertensive medication)
5. Psychosocial factors (prior history of sexual abuse, religious or cultural expectation, fear of rejection or intimacy, and distorted body image)
6. Hormonal changes (premature ovarian failure and menopause)

**What is the prevalence of sexual dysfunction?**

**Studies show a range of 10–60%; the average is 43%**

**What are the types of female sexual dysfunction and what is the main symptom of each?**

1. **Sexual desire disorders:** decreased sexual fantasy and/or desire, sexual aversion
2. **Sexual arousal disorders: decreased genital vasocongestion** and lubrication

3. **Orgasmic disorders:** anorgasmia
4. **Sexual pain disorders**: vaginismus, dyspareunia, noncoital sexual pain

**How should the question of sexual dysfunction be addressed?**

The evaluation should involve an interview of the couple and each partner separately. A complete assessment should include past medical, psychological, sexual history and physical examination including gynecologic examination. Each patient should be asked if she has any questions or concerns about her sexual activity. The most important aspect of taking a sexual history is to make the patient feel comfortable

**What hormones influence vaginal blood flow?**

**Estrogen** and **testosterone** increase vaginal blood flow; **Progesterone** diminishes vaginal blood flow

**What types of therapies are available for the treatment of sexual dysfunction?**

1. **Nonpharmacologic therapy: Patient education, lifestyle** and **behavioral changes**—should be tried first
2. **Pharmacologic therapy**: Hormones: **estrogen**—increases genital blood flow and enhanced lubrication

**Testosterone**—may improve libido, data nonconclusive

Herbal therapy: (e.g., St. John's wort, ginseng, yohimbine) generally ineffective

L-Arginine: increases nitric oxide (NO) leading to genital vasocongestion; needs further study

Tibolone: used for osteoporosis; has androgenic activity that may improve sexual function

Sildenafil: a vasodilator; data inconclusive on its benefit for women, not FDA approved

**Describe what changes occur with aging that affect sexual function**

1. **Decreased libido**
2. **Hormonal changes**—estrogen levels gradually drop leading to vaginal atrophy and dryness. Testosterone levels decrease,

leading to a decrease in arousal and intensity and frequency of orgasm

3. **Medical issues**—increase in medical problems and use of medications that may affect sexual function
4. **Past experiences**—for example, recurrent dyspareunia can lead to introital spasm, which can further impede sexual function
5. **Relationship issues**
6. **Self-esteem changes**

**What types of medication or substances can lead to sexual dysfunction?**

Alcohol; antihypertensives; illicit drugs; SSRIs

Psychotropic

Antihistaminic

**What are the adverse effects of SSRI use on sexual function?**

SSRIs have been reported to reduce libido in women and men, to cause anorgasmia in women, and to increase ejaculation latency in men

**What types of changes occur under the following circumstances that may affect female sexual function?**

**During pregnancy**: breast tenderness, mild cervical bleeding during intercourse, and uterine contractions with orgasm

**Postpartum**: fatigue, vaginal dryness, bleeding, vaginal discomfort

**What is hypoactive sexual desire disorder (HSDD)?**

**Recurrent and persistent lack of sexual fantasies or desires** or receptivity to sexual activity that causes personal distress

**How should HSDD be evaluated?**

Take a careful history including medications, medical illness, depression, substance abuse, and stress. Thyroid test and prolactin levels may be indicated if there is any suggestion of hyperprolactinemia. Androgen levels are not useful in the majority of cases

**How should HSDD be treated?**

Physiologic causes should be assessed and managed. Further treatment may require individual therapy or relationship therapy

**What is sexual aversion disorder?**

It is characterized by a phobia with **avoidance of sexual contact** and severe anxiety associated with contemplation of sexual activity

**What are sexual arousal disorders and how are they treated?**

When women experience desire and orgasm, but **lack signs of sexual stimulation**, such as lubrication and genital vasocongestion. Treatment includes masturbation, vaginal lubricants, vibrator to increase stimulation, foreplay, distraction technique to alleviate anxiety, and/or estrogen replacement therapy for postmenopausal women

**What is orgasmic dysfunction and how is it treated?**

A **persistent delay in or absence of orgasm** after sufficient stimulation and arousal resulting in distress or interpersonal difficulty. Treatment involves orgasm goal directed sexual counseling

**What types of orgasmic dysfunction exists?**

**Primary anorgasmia** is found in 5–10% of women and is lifelong

**Secondary anorgasmia** is often related to relationship problems, medications, medical illness, depression, substance abuse, and self-monitoring/anxiety during arousal

**What types of sexual pain disorders exist and what are they?**

**Vaginismus (recurrent involuntary contraction of the vaginal musculature** during vaginal penetration)

**Dyspareunia** (**general pain** that occurs before, during, or after intercourse)

**What organic disorders must be ruled out when vaginismus is diagnosed?**

Endometriosis; PID; partial imperforate hymen; vaginal stenosis

**How is vaginismus treated?**

Education; relaxation techniques; kegel exercises; progressive vaginal dilatation

**What organic disorders must be ruled out when dyspareunia is diagnosed?**

Bartholin cysts; vulvitis; vestibulitis; vaginitis; clitoral irritation/hypersensitivity; rigid hymenal ring/introital scar tissue; vaginal atrophy and dryness; pelvic adhesion; fibroid; endometriosis

**How is dyspareunia treated?**

The treatment depends on the etiology

# Benign Conditions of the Vulvavagina

## DYSTROPHIES

**What are vulvar dystrophies?**

A group of disorders characterized by lesions that are **white, intensely pruritic** with or without pain, and may occur with **vulvar epithelial changes. Lesions should be biopsied to rule out malignancy**

**What is vulvar lichen sclerosis?**

A **benign, progressive, and chronic dermatologic condition** more common in older women and characterized by **intense pruritus and pain**, which may be so severe that it leads to **sleep disturbances**

**What are other sequelae of lichen sclerosis?**

Painful defecation, anal pruritus, dyspareunia, and dysuria. **They may also develop into invasive squamous cell cancer of the vulva**

**How does lichen sclerosis appear on clinical examination?**

Thin, white, wrinkled skin often resembling **"parchment paper" or "cigarette paper"** that is localized to the labia minora and/or labia majora. It may extend toward the anus

**What is the treatment for lichen sclerosis?**

Super potent topical corticosteroids (Clobetasol)

**What other additional steps should be considered in management of these patients?**

Strong encouragement of vulvar hygiene. Given the risk of malignant vulvar cancer, the skin should be examined yearly and suspicious lesions should be biopsied

**What is vulvar lichen planus?**

An inflammatory dermatologic condition with unknown etiology that mainly affects the skin and mucous membranes of the oral cavity and genital area

**How does lichen planus clinically present on the vulva?**

With either **violaceous papules**, hyperkeratosis, or bright erythematous erosions with a white border or white striae along the margins

**How does lichen planus clinically present on the skin and oral mucous membranes?**

**Skin**—eruption of multiple, shiny, polygonal, flat-topped, purple papules with white striae

**Oral mucous membranes**—white plaques

**How is lichen planus different from lichen sclerosis?**

The vagina is involved 70% of the time in lichen planus

**What is vulvovaginal-gingival syndrome?**

A variant of lichen planus that involves lesions on the vulva, vestibule, vagina, gingival epithelium, and/or skin. These affected areas may or may not occur concurrently

**What is the treatment of lichen planus?**

Ultra-potent topical corticosteroids

**What is vulvar dermatitis?**

Also known as vulvar eczema, it is the most common inflammatory skin disease characterized by intense pruritus and irritation, leading to chronic scratching and eventual changes in the dermis. It can have a familial predisposition (atopic dermatitis) or occur with allergens (contact dermatitis)

**What is the end result of constant irritation and scratching in vulvar dermatitis?**

**Lichen simplex chronicus**. It appears as a raised, hyperkeratotic white lesion. Biopsy reveals hyperkeratosis and acanthosis

**What is the difference between lichen simplex chronicus, and lichen sclerosis and lichen planus?**

Lichen simplex chronicus is a reactive change whereas lichen sclerosis and lichen planus are primary dystrophies

**What is the treatment?**

Medium-to-high-potency topical steroids

**What other vulvar dystrophy has the same histologic appearance as lichen simplex chronicus?**

Squamous cell hyperplasia

**In what setting does lichen simplex chronicus arise?**

In patients who have chronic vulvovaginal infections or other causes of chronic irritation

**What is the treatment for squamous cell hyperplasia?**

The goal is symptomatic relief. Sitz baths and lubricants are recommended to restore moisture to cells. Medium potency topical steroids are used to decrease inflammation and pruritus

**What is the gold standard for diagnosis of any of these dystrophies?**

Biopsy of the lesion

**How does psoriasis appear on physical examination of the vulva?**

Red moist plaques covered by silver scales. Topical corticosteroids are the treatment of choice

**What are the most common differential diagnoses among all of the vulvar dystrophies?**

Lichen sclerosis, squamous cell hyperplasia, lichen planus, lichen chronicus, vulvar eczema, psoriasis, vulvovaginal candidiasis, vitiligo, desquamative inflammatory vaginitis, pemphigus, Behcet disease

## BENIGN CYSTS

**What are the most common benign vulvovaginal cysts?**

Bartholin ducts cysts, epidermal, sebaceous, and apocrine sweat gland cysts

**Where are Bartholin glands and ducts located?**

Deep in the labia majora at about four and eight o'clock positions. They are not palpable in healthy women

**What is the role of Bartholin glands?**

As a homologue to the male bulbourethral glands, they secrete mucus to provide moisture for the vagina

**How do Bartholin gland cysts develop?**

Infection can cause inflammation and obstruction of the main duct of Bartholin glands leading to cystic dilation. They may enlarge up to 1–3 cm and are usually asymptomatic

**What may Bartholin gland cysts develop into?**

Bartholin gland abscesses

**When symptomatic, what are the acute symptoms and signs of Bartholin gland cysts and abscesses?**

Pain, dyspareunia, and difficulty ambulating or sitting. Physical examination may reveal swelling, erythema, edema, and a large fluctuant mass in the medial labia majora. This is usually because of infection or swelling

**How are Bartholin gland cysts treated?**

Asymptomatic cysts need no intervention or antibiotic treatment

Symptomatic cysts are incised and drained, and **a catheter is placed to form a tract for the drainage of glandular secretions (Word catheter).** If this procedure fails, then a marsupialization can be done (the creation of a new ductal orifice). The most definitive procedure for a Bartholin cyst after failure of all previous methods is complete excision of the gland

**What microbes are commonly implicated in Bartholin gland abcesses?**

*Escherichia coli*, *Neisseria gonorrhoeae*, *Chlamydia trachomatis*, and several anaerobes

**How are Bartholin gland abscesses managed and treated?**

An aspirate and culture of the abscess should be done. Treatment includes antibiotics such as ceftriaxone and clindamycin, and surgical drainage of the pus (with possible supplementation of a Word catheter)

**For the following descriptions, list the most appropriate type of cyst or cyst-related condition**

1. Occurring mostly beneath the labia majora, this cyst occurs when the **sebaceous gland duct becomes obstructed**. They are multiple, smooth, and palpable masses that are generally asymptomatic. Acute infection can be treated with incision and drainage

**1. Sebaceous cyst**

2. These cysts are lined by **squamous epithelial cells and contain oily material**. They occur in the setting of vulva surgery or arise from obstruction of pilosebaceous ducts. They are usually small, solitary, and asymptomatic

**2. Epidermal cyst**

3. Apocrine sweat gland cysts are mainly found in the labium majus and become functional after puberty. They are usually small, multiple, and extremely pruritic. This disease occurs when **keratin obstructs the duct**

**3. Fox-Fordyce disease**

4. This condition occurs with chronic infection of the apocrine glands and is manifested by multiple painful, pruritic, and subcutaneous abscesses. It may be treated with antibiotics or incision

**4. Hidradenomas**

5. This cystic vulvar tumor is a rare **congenital anomaly** and located near the urethral meatus. It can be treated with partial excision

**5. Skene duct cyst**

6. Occlusion of a **persistent processus vaginalis** may cause this hydrocele or cystic tumor

**6. Cyst of the canal of Nuck**

7. These lateral vaginal wall cysts result from dilation of the **mesonephric duct remnants**

**7. Gartner duct cyst**

8. This is a benign outgrowth of normal skin. More of a solid tumor than a cyst, it must be removed when it causes discomfort

**8. Acrochordon (skin tag)**

## PYODERMAS AND OTHER NONSEXUALLY TRANSMITTED INFECTIONS OF THE VULVA AND VAGINA

**What are the specific types of pyodermas?**

Cellulitis, impetigo, folliculitis, furuncles, and carbuncles

**What is the most common bacterial etiology for all of these pyodermas?**

*Staphylococcus aureus*

**How does impetigo manifest?**

Vesicles and pustules form in an area that was recently traumatized. They often rupture and form a characteristic golden crusting

**How is it treated?**

Erythromycin or dicloxacillin (oral)

**What is folliculitis? How does it manifest?**

An infection of the hair follicles. It can occur with exposure to whirlpools/hot tubs, antibiotic therapy, and shaving of pubic hair. The lesions are multiple, ″ 5 mm, cluster in groups, erythematous, and pruritic

**What is the recommended treatment for folliculitis?**

Warm saline compresses and topical antibiotics

**What other pyodermas can occur after an episode of folliculitis? Describe them.**

Furuncules: a painful nodular lesion that involves the hair follicle and drains pus

Carbuncles: clusters of furuncles or subcutaneous abscesses that drain pus through multiple hair follicle openings

**What is the preferred treatment for furuncules and carbuncles?**

Warm compresses to promote spontaneous drainage in furunculosis. Patients with systemic symptoms of furuncules and/or carbuncles warrant empiric oral antibiotic therapy followed by guided therapy based on cultures and sensitivity

**What is erysipelas?**

Rapidly spreading erythematous lesions of the skin caused by **invasion of the superficial lymphatics by β-hemolytic streptococci**. It usually occurs after trauma or a surgical procedure to the vulva. Pustules, vesicles, and bullae may appear

**How is erysipelas treated?**

Oral penicillin or tetracycline

**What is hidradenitis suppurativa? How is it treated?**

A more severe condition of hidradenomas that occurs when the cysts develop into abscesses and rupture. **Draining sinus tracts develop deep within the skin, and scars, fibrosis, hyperpigmentation, and pitting** can be seen over the vulva. It is treated by drainage and antibiotic therapy

**What is the agent that commonly causes nocturnal perineal itching in children? How is it diagnosed and what is the treatment?**

*Enterobius vermicularis* (pinworm). Apply adhesive tape to the perineum and look for ova under the microscope for diagnosis. Mebendazole is the treatment of choice

## OTHER VULVAR DISORDERS

**Trauma to the vulva can occur in both children and women. Straddle-type injuries are the most common cause of vulvar hematomas in children whereas trauma incurred during vaginal delivery is the main etiology in women of reproductive age.**

**What vessels are most commonly involved in vulvar hematomas?**

Branches from the pudendal artery

**What are the common symptoms?**

Severe perineal pain within the first 24 hours is usually the first symptom of a rapidly expanding vulvar hematoma. Rapid appearance of a tense, palpable, fluctuant, and sensitive tumor of varying size covered by discolored skin readily gives a diagnosis of vulvar hematoma

**How are vulvar hematomas managed?**

The two primary modalities are

1. Conservative management with analgesia and ice packs
2. Surgical drainage is warranted for large hematomas (>3 cm)

CHAPTER 5

# Gynecologic Oncology

## Cervical Cancer

### INTRODUCTION

**Describe the three histologic regions of the cervix**

1. **Ectocervix:** the inferior portion of the cervix that is continuous with the vagina; covered with **squamous epithelium**
2. **Squamocolumnar junction (SCJ):** separates two regions of the cervix (often with overlap)
3. **Endocervix:** the superior portion of the cervix that begins at the external os and continues to the endocervical canal; covered with mucin-secreting **columnar epithelium** and continues into the cuboidal epithelium of the endometrium

**Describe the location of the SCJ**

It varies between the ectocervix, the cervical canal, and the vaginal fornices. Throughout a woman's life, the SCJ **migrates internally** toward the endocervix via the metaplasia

**What is the transformation zone?**

The 1–3 cm area of **squamous metaplasia** that separates the endocervix from the ectocervix created from the internal migration of the SCJ. It is the area **most susceptible to the development of cervical neoplasia** because of the metaplastic changes.

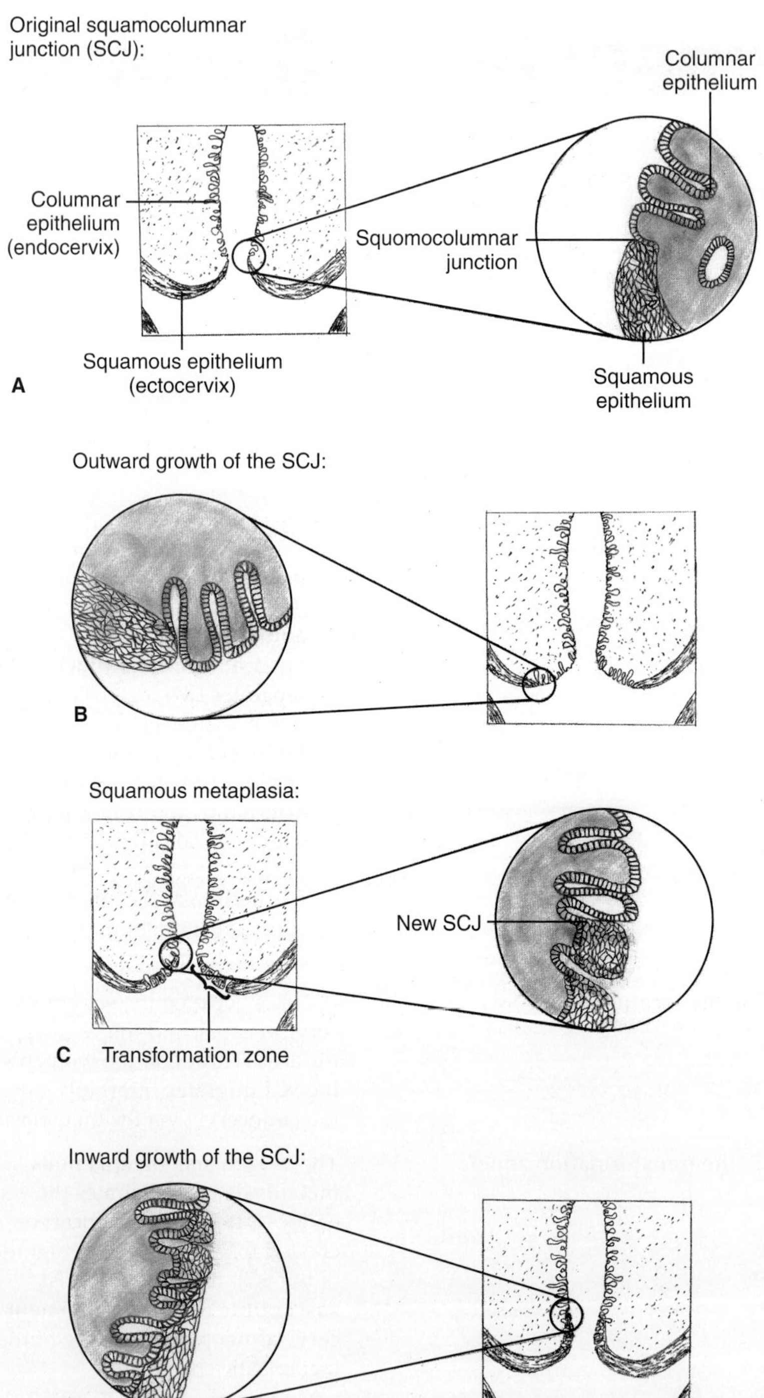


**Figure 5-1** The cervical transformation zone.

**What is the incidence of cervical cancer?**

It is the second leading cause of malignancy in women worldwide but comprises only 1% of all cancer deaths of women in the United States

**Who does cervical cancer affect?**

Sexually active women, usually in a bimodal age distribution with peaks in the late 30s and in the early 60s

**What are the risk factors for cervical cancer?**

**HPV infection**

**Sexual history:** Early onset of sexual activity; multiple sexual partners; history of sexually transmitted infections (STIs); sex with high-risk partners

**Smoking**

**High parity**

**Immunosuppression**

Low socioeconomic status

Pelvic radiation

Prior history of vulvar or vaginal squamous dysplasia

**What is the epidemiologic relationship between HPV infection and cervical cancer?**

**Human papillomavirus** (HPV) is found in nearly all cases of squamous cell cervical cancer and is thought to **contribute to the pathogenesis of dysplasia.** While most HPV infections self-resolve, some progress to genital warts or cervical dysplasia. HPV infection is therefore deemed **necessary but not sufficient** for the development of cervical cancer

**How does HPV infection lead to cervical cancer?**

HPV initially infects the basal layer cervical cells, forming **koilocytes** within the cells. HPV can then **integrate into the cells genome,** altering the expression of the cell's regulatory genes. This leads to intraepithelial neoplasia and/or cancer

**What serotypes of HPV most commonly cause cervical cancer?**

**HPV 16, 18, 31, 33, and 45**

**In what other types of neoplasia is HPV thought to be a causative agent?**

1. **Vaginal intraepithelial neoplasia** (VAIN) and **vaginal malignancies**
2. **Vulvar intraepithelial neoplasia** (VIN) and **vulvar malignancies**
3. **Penile neoplasia**

**What are the types of cervical cancer, how common are each worldwide, and where in relation to the SCJ do they occur?**

1. **Squamous cell carcinomas:** 80–90% of all cervical cancers, occur below the SCJ
2. **Adenocarcinomas:** 15% of all cervical cancers, occur above the SCJ
3. **Adenosquamous carcinomas:** 3–5% of all cervical cancers
4. Neuroendocrine, small cell carcinomas, clear cell carcinomas, melanomas, lymphomas, and sarcomas can all originate in the cervix but are rare

**What are the signs/symptoms of cervical cancer?**

Early stages of cervical dysplasia and cancer are asymptomatic. There is **no classic presentation for cervical cancer** but the most common symptom is **abnormal vaginal bleeding** (either postcoital, postmenopausal, or intermentrual)

Symptoms of late stage disease include: **vaginal discharge** pain (usually pelvic or lower back pain), weight loss, hematuria (vaginal passage of blood in urine) or hematochezia (passage of blood in stool)

Signs on cervical examination can range from a normal gross appearance with aberrant cytology to a cervix entirely replaced with tumor

**What is the differential diagnosis of these symptoms?**

Cervicitis, vaginitis, STI

**How is the definitive diagnosis of cervical cancer made?**

**Cervical biopsy** if the lesion is grossly visible. If the lesion is only diagnosable microscopically, a **colposcopy-directed biopsy** or diagnostic **conization** (for microinvasive disease) are modalities for diagnosis

**Upon diagnosis, what other tests need to be done?**

1. A comprehensive physical examination to evaluate metastases, including cervical and vaginal inspection, a rectovaginal examination, and palpation of the liver and lymph nodes (inguinal and supraclavicular)
2. Lab and imaging tests to evaluate for metastases

**What do each of the following contribute to the evaluation of cervical cancer?**

**Chest x-ray:** Identifies lung metastasis

**Intravenous pyelogram:** Identifies bladder involvement, but has been largely replaced by CT, MRI, or cystoscopy

**MRI, CT, or lymphangiography:** Identifies nodal involvement, tumor size, and abdominal/retroperitoneal spread; CT and MRI cannot be used for staging purposes

**Renal function tests:** Identifies urinary tract metastasis

**Liver function tests:** Identifies liver metastasis

**Barium enema:** Identifies colonic metastasis

**How and to where does cervical cancer spread?**

1. **Direct extension** to contiguous structures
2. **Lymphatic dissemination** to any of the pelvic lymph node groups
3. **Hematogenous dissemination** most commonly to the **lungs, liver,** and **bone** although it can spread to the large intestine, adrenals, spleen, or brain as well
4. **Intraperitoneal implantation**

**What are the stages of cervical cancer?**

The **FIGO system** is based on the histological assessment, the physical examination, and the laboratory results. See Table 5-1.

**What are the overall survival rates for cervical cancer?**

The survival rates **depend most significantly on the stage of disease** at diagnosis. The 5-year survival rates for each stage are:

Stage I: over 90%

Stage II: 75%

Stage III: 40%

Stage IV: under 15%

**What is the differential diagnosis of a cervical mass?**

Nabothian cysts

Glandular hyperplasia

Mesonephric remnants

Reactive glandular changes

Endometriosis

**Table 5-1** The Stages of Cervical Cancer

|  |  |  |  |
|---|---|---|---|
| I | | | **Carcinoma confined to the cervix** |
| | IA | | Invasive carcinoma diagnosable only by microscopy |
| | | IA1 | Minimal microscopic invasion <3 mm deep and <7 mm horizontally |
| | | IA2 | Microscopic lesions <5 mm deep and <7 mm horizontally |
| | IB | | Clinically visible lesions that are confined to the cervix |
| II | | | **Carcinoma extends beyond the cervix, but not to the pelvic wall or lower third of the vagina** |
| | IIA | | No parametrial involvement |
| | IIB | | Parametrial involvement |
| III | | | **Carcinoma extends to the pelvic wall and/or lower third of the vagina. Also includes all cases with hydronephrosis** |
| | IIIA | | No extension to pelvic wall, but involvement of lower third of vagina |
| | IIIB | | Extension to pelvic wall or hydronephrosis |
| IV | | | **Carcinoma extends beyond the true pelvis or clinically involves the mucosa of the bladder or rectum** |
| | IVA | | Spread to adjacent pelvic organs |
| | IVB | | Spread to distant organs |

## CERVICAL CANCER SCREENING AND PREVENTION

**What is a Pap smear and how is it done?**

A cytological examination of the cervix. A small brush scrapes cells from the endocervix and ectocervix. These cells are either spread on a microscopic slide and fixed or placed in a liquid medium for evaluation

**What is the difference between a Pap smear and the thin-layer liquid-based cytology (ThinPrep, SurePath)?**

In a **traditional Pap smear,** a spatula or brush is used to collect cells on the ectocervix and then from the endocervix. The specimen is rolled or smeared onto a slide and rapidly fixed. A single slide can be used to examine both ectocervical and endocervical cells

**Liquid-based cytology** involves taking cells from the ectocervix and endocervix and placing the specimens in vials containing preservative solutions. The vials are placed in a ThinPrep processor machine and ultimately, the cells are transferred to a slide. This technique results in a monolayer of cells on the slide, which can be read more quickly than conventional cytology slides

**How often should a Pap smear be done?**

The general consensus to date is an **annual examination beginning at coitus or by the age of 21.** If a female is low-risk and has three negative Pap smears, she can then get repeat evaluations every 3 years

**What are some of the limitations of Pap smear screening?**

Not all patients have access (the most important limiting factor); it is less successful in diagnosing adenocarcinoma; it has a low sensitivity and therefore a high false-negative rate

**Describe the histologic definition of cervical intraepithelial neoplasia (CIN) and of each of the stages**

CIN refers to precancerous pathology that can slowly progress to cervical cancer.

**CIN I:** formerly known as mild dysplasia, is a **cellular dysplasia confined to the basal one-third of the epithelium**

**CIN II:** refers to **lesions confined to the basal two-thirds of the epithelium** that used to be referred to as moderate dysplasia

**CIN III:** formerly known as severe dysplasia and carcinoma in situ (CIS), is a **cellular dysplasia that affects more than two-thirds of the epithelium**

**Describe the cytological definitions of the Bethesda system?**

Low-grade squamous intraepithelial lesion (**LSIL** or LGSIL): includes CIN I and condylomatous atypia

High-grade squamous intraepithelial lesion (**HSIL** or HGSIL): includes CIS, CIN II, and CIN III

Atypical squamous cells of undetermined significance (**ASCUS**)

Atypical squamous cells that cannot exclude HSIL (**ASCH**). See Table 5-2.

**How rapidly does cervical dysplasia progress to cervical cancer?**

Cervical cancer in general progresses slowly and mild dysplasia (CIN I or LSIL) often spontaneously regresses

It is estimated that is takes 3–10 years for women with CIN III to progress to cervical cancer

**Table 5-2** The Bethesda System

| Bethesda System | Dysplasia/CIN System |
|---|---|
| Atypical squamous cells of undetermined significance | Squamous atypia |
| Low-grade squamous intraepithelial lesion | HPV atypia |
| High-grade squamous intraepithelial lesion | CIN I |
| | CIN II |
| | CIN III |

**What is colposcopy?**

A binocular stereomicroscope that **magnifies the cervix** that is used to visualize changes consistent with dysplasia, allowing for directed biopsy

**What must be seen in order to consider colposcopy satisfactory?**

**The entirety of the SCJ and the entire lesion in question**

**What findings on colposcopy are suggestive of cervical cancer?**

Abnormal blood vessels; abnormal appearing surface of the cervix; color change

**What is endocervical curettage?**

**A sampling procedure of the endocervix** used to retrieve cells further inside the cervical canal that can be visualized with colposcopy

**What should be done if the ECC is positive?**

Because there is no tissue orientation, **a positive ECC warrants conization**

**What is cervical conization?**

A **cone-shaped biopsy of the entire SCJ** that allows diagnosis via histologic criteria

**How is cervical conization done?**

**Cold knife conization** (via scalpel); **Loop electrosurgical excision procedure** (LEEP) (via heated wire)

**What are the four common indications for conization in order of their frequency?**

1. CIN III
2. Unsatisfactory colposcopy
3. Positive endocervical curettage
4. A discrepancy between Pap smear and biopsy results

**What are the risks of cervical conization?**

Infection, blood loss, risks from anesthesia, cervical stenosis, and cervical incompetence

**What is the appropriate workup of each of the following abnormal Paps?**

**LSIL:** **Colposcopy with local ablation** or **repeat Pap smears** to rule out a high-grade lesion. If ≤CIN I, the patient can be just followed-up over time. Conization can also be used, both diagnostically and therapeutically, but it is not necessary

**HSIL:** Warrants a **colposcopy followed by direct ablation or excision**

**ASCUS:** **HPV DNA testing.** If high-risk HPV+, colposcopy should be done. If high-risk HPV−, then a repeat Pap smear can be done in 12 months. Alternatively, a repeat Pap smear can be done every 3–4 months until there are three consecutive negative smears

Menopausal women may have an atrophic component leading to this cytology, and they can be given **intravaginal estrogen** and followed up every 3–4 months

Women with an infection should be reexamined once their infection is treated

Immunosuppressed women with ASCUS need colposcopy

**Glandular cell abnormalities:** All glandular cell abnormalities warrant **colposcopy and endocervical sampling**

**How often should patients be followed up after treatment of noninvasive abnormalities?**

Because of the greater risk of recurrence, patients need to be followed **every 3–6 months for 2 years after ablation or excision**

**What types of vaccination is now available to prevent cervical cancer?**

**Gardasil,** a quadravalent vaccine protecting against HPV 6, 11, 16, and 18

**Who should get this vaccination?**

Females ages 9–26. Whether males should also be vaccinated is controversial and it is not FDA approved for males

**Do vaccinated individuals still need to get Pap smears?**

**Yes!** The vaccine only protects against four of the many HPV serotypes that cause cervical cancer

## SQUAMOUS CELL CARCINOMA OF THE CERVIX

**Who gets squamous cell carcinoma (SCC) of the cervix?**

There is a bimodal age distribution with peaks between 35 and 40 and between 60 and 65

**What are the five prognostic indicators for SCC?**

1. **Stage of disease** (most important)
2. Lymph node involvement
3. Tumor size
4. Depth of stromal invasion
5. Invasion of lymphovascular space

**What are the treatment options for invasive SCC of the cervix and what are the indications of each?**

1. **Cervical conization:** used for women with stage Ia1 with no involvement of the lymphovascular space who wish to preserve fertility
2. **Radical trachelectomy:** involves surgical removal of the cervix and parametria and placement of a cerclage, and can be combined with a laparoscopic or open diagnostic/therapeutic lymphadenectomy with para-aortic lymph node sampling; used for women with stage Ia1 with involvement of the lymphovascular space, stage Ia2 or Ib1 disease who wish to preserve fertility
3. **Radical hysterectomy:** used for premenopausal women with early stage (up to stage IIa) cervical cancer who wish to preserve ovarian function
4. **Chemoradiotherapy alone:** used for women with stage Ia, Ib, or IIa cancer who are poor surgical candidates or who decline a surgical approach
   Chemoradiotherapy versus surgery for Ib2 is controversial
5. **Chemoradiotherapy and hysterectomy:** women with advanced disease. Can be done via:
   a. Chemoradiotherapy followed by hysterectomy
   b. Neoadjuvant chemotherapy followed by hysterectomy and, if indicated, radiation

c. Hysterectomy followed by chemoradiotherapy

*This is rarely an ideal choice as the morbidity is increased when this combination is used.

Patients with locally advanced disease should be treated with primary chemoradiotherapy. Women with PID, another pelvic mass, or anatomic alterations should be treated with primary hysterectomy.

**What is the recommended treatment for each of the following stages of cervical cancer?**

**Ia1:** Conization or simple hysterectomy
**Ia2–early IIb:** Radical hysterectomy with a pelvic lymphadenectomy or chemoradiotherapy
**Late IIb–IV:** Chemoradiotherapy or combination chemotherapy

**What are the indications for adjuvant radiotherapy without chemotherapy?**

Patients with any two of the following risk factors should be considered candidates for adjuvant radiotherapy without chemotherapy: large tumor size; deep stromal invasion; lymphovascular space invasion

**What are the indications for adjuvant chemoradiotherapy?**

If a patient has any of the following:

Positive resection margins

Positive lymph nodes

Parametrial involvement

**What types of chemotherapy are used for cervical cancer treatment and how do they work?**

**Cisplatin** with or without **5-FU.** Cisplatin is a cycle-nonspecific alkylating agent that cross-links DNA. 5-FU is a cycle-specific DNA synthesis inhibitor

**What are the main side effects of the following?**

Cisplatin:

Leukopenia, ototoxicity, nephrotoxicity, and peripheral neuropathy

5-FU:

Fatigue, diarrhea, nausea, vomiting, and myelosuppression

**The two main methods of radiation delivery for cervical cancer are external photon beam radiation therapy (RT) and intracavitary brachytherapy. When is each indicated?**

Intracavitary brachytherapy alone is adequate treatment for stage Ia1 disease, external beam RT is generally added to brachytherapy to improve pelvic control with more advanced disease, such as stage Ib and IIa disease

**What are the side effects of radiation?**

Acute side effects: nausea, diarrhea, and skin damage

Long-term complications: **cystitis, proctitis,** vaginal foreshortening, stenosis, and dryness (which leads to **sexual dysfunction**), development of fistulae, small bowel obstruction

**What are the complications of surgery?**

Postoperative complications: hemorrhage, fever, sepsis, pulmonary embolus, and infection

Long-term complications: bladder dysfunction, strictures of the ureter, lymphocyst formation, and fistula formation

**What type of surveillance is indicated in posttreatment for SCC?**

Patients need to be evaluated **every 3 months for the first 2 years** after treatment. After these 2 years, they must be seen every 4 months in the third year, every 6 months for 5 years, and annually thereafter. These evaluations must include careful attention to the supraclavicular and inguinal lymph nodes, a rectovaginal examination, and an abdominal examination. A Pap smear must be done at each visit

**What is the treatment for recurrence?**

Depends on patient and presentation, however in general, patients who were initially surgically treated may receive radiotherapy. Patients initially treated with radiotherapy may be surgically treated if their recurrence is localized or they may receive chemotherapy

**What are the 5-year survival rates for the following stages of SCC?**

**Stage I:** 85–90%

**Stage II:** 60–80%

**Stage III:** 30%

**Stage IV:** 10%

## ADENOCARCINOMA OF THE CERVIX

**What are the types of adenocarcinoma?**

Mucinous; endometrioid; clear cell; serous

**What is the incidence of cervical adenocarcinoma?**

Accounts for 15% of cervical cancers, however this rate has been rising

**What are the risk factors for the development of cervical adenocarcinoma?**

The same risk factors as for SCC

**How is cervical adenocarcinoma classified?**

Using the **Bethesda 2001 system** which divides it into four subgroups:

1. **Atypical glandular cells** (AGC)—either endocervical, endometrial, or unspecified
2. **AGC favoring neoplasia**—either endocervical, endometrial, or unspecified
3. **Endocervical adenocarcinoma in situ** (AIS)
4. **Adenocarcinoma**

**What are some of the theories for the rise in the diagnosis of AIS?**

1. Improved detection
2. An increase in the prevalence of the pathogenic serotype of HPV (HPV 18)
3. An increase in oral contraceptive use (more associated with adenocarcinoma than SCC)

**What is the epidemiologic relationship between AIS and SCC of the cervix?**

About 50% of women found to have adenocarcinoma have concomitant SCC or CIN

**How is AIS diagnosed?**

It is usually asymptomatic and is found through the following:

1. **Cervical cytology** with **colposcopy-directed biopsy** (not sensitive)
   a. cold knife conization—best method
   b. electro-excision—may obscure margins
2. **Endocervical curettage** (improves the detection rate if used with the above methods)

**What is the microscopic appearance of cervical adenocarcinoma?**

Endocervical glands crowded together in a cribiform pattern, lined by atypical columnar epithelial cells. **Multifocal** disease is often found

**What is the gross appearance of cervical adenocarcinomas?**

Half are exophytic, some are ulcerative, and some have the lesion within the endocervical canal (and so it is not visible)

**What are the treatment options for microinvasive disease/carcinoma in situ?**

There is not a consensus; however the following options are acceptable:

1. **Simple hysterectomy** (generally recommended if fertility need not be preserved)
2. Radical hysterectomy
3. Conization (however, margins have poor predictive value for residual disease)
4. Radical trachelectomy

**How should a patient be followed after the diagnosis of AIS if she does not have a hysterectomy?**

With cervical cytology and endocervical sampling, every 6 months indefinitely

**What are the treatment options for adenocarcinoma?**

Similar to that of SCC. However, adenocarcinomas tend to be more bulky and therefore more often warrant radiotherapy, even with earlier stage disease

**What are the prognostic indicators for adenocarcinoma?**

Prognosis primarily depends on **stage**. However, in general, adenocarinoma is more aggressive than SCC and so survival rates are slightly lower

**What are the 5-year survival rates for the following stages of adenocarcinoma?**

**Stage I:** 70–75%

**Stage II:** 30–40%

**Stage III:** 20–30%

**Stage IV:** <15%

# Vulvar and Vaginal Cancer

## VULVAR CANCER OVERVIEW

**What are the designations of preinvasive vulvar malignancy?**

**Vulvar intraepithelial neoplasia**, classified into three levels:

**VIN-I**: mild dysplasia

**VIN-II**: moderate dysplasia

**VIN-III**: severe dysplasia or carcinoma in situ

**How do each of the preinvasive lesions typically present?**

VIN-I and VIN-II present most commonly with **itching, chronic irritation,** and development of a **palpable lesion**. The lesion typically appears as localized, isolated, raised, whitish areas found most commonly along the posterior vulva and perineal body. Perineal pain and dysuria can also be presenting symptoms. VIN-III typically presents with **intractable itching and irritation** along with the gross lesion(s) described above. Occasionally, the vuvlar involvement is extensive

**How is VIN treated?**

**Complete excision**. Early cases with limited involvement can be treated with local excision, cryocautery, electrodesiccation, or laser ablation. VIN-III is treated with wide local excision with/without laser ablation

**What is the incidence of vulvar cancer?**

Vulvar cancer is the fourth most common gynecologic cancer that affects almost 4000 women in the United States annually

**Whom does vulvar cancer affect?**

Typically, postmenopausal women, usually around 65 years of age

**What are the risk factors for vulvar cancer?**

Infection with certain types of HPV history of cervical cancer

Immunocompromise; northern European ancestry

Cigarette smoking; diabetes

Vulvar dystrophy; obesity

Vulvar intraepithelial neoplasia; hypertension

**How is the diagnosis of vulvar cancer made?**

Careful history-taking and inspection are essential. Inspection must include all of the vulvar skin, peri-anal skin, cervix, and vagina. A **biopsy** of each lesion leads to a definitive diagnosis as gross appearance is often inconsistent with the underlying cellular morphology. If there is no obvious lesion, **colposcopy** may be used. Also, the skin can be washed with a dilute **acetic acid solution** to accentuate any lesions or aberrant vascular patterns

**What other test should be ordered after biopsy?**

A synchronous secondary malignancy is found in over 20% of patients with vulvar cancer and so screenings for a secondary malignancy as well as for metastasis should be done

Screenings may include: **CXR; IVP; LFTs; renal function tests; CT scan.**

If the lesion is located near the anus then a **barium enema** is warranted and if the lesion is located near the urethra then **cystoscopy** is warranted

**What is the differential diagnosis of a suspected vulvar cancer?**

Epidermal inclusion cysts; seborrheic keratoses

Lentigo condyloma acuminata

Bartholin gland disorders; lichen sclerosus

Acrochordons; hidradenomas

**What are the types of vulvar cancer?**

Over 90% of vulvar cancers are primary cancers.

Types of primary vulvar cancers include: **squamous cell carcinomas** (90%); **melanomas** (5%); Bartholin's gland carcinomas; basal cell carcinomas; sarcomas; lymphomas; endodermal sinus tumors

Metastasizing cancers to the vulva include **cervical, endometrial, renal, and urethral cancers**

## SQUAMOUS CELL VULVAR CANCER

**What are the signs/symptoms of squamous cell vulvar cancer?**

**Itching, burning, irritation**, and/or the development of a **palpable lesion** (plaque, ulcer, or mass) usually on the labia majora. Bleeding, ulceration, abnormal discharge, dysuria, or an enlarged groin lymph node are usually associated with more advanced disease

**What are the two subtypes of squamous cell carcinoma of the vulva?**

1. **Keratinizing type**—occurs in older women; associated with other vulvar dystrophies such as lichen sclerosis but not with HPV; usually unifocal
2. **Warty or basaloid type**—found in younger women; associated with HPV, VIN, and cigarette smoking; usually multifocal

**How does squamous cell vulvar cancer spread?**

1. **Direct extension:** to the vagina, urethra, or anus
2. **Lymphatic dissemination:** occurs via the superficial inguinal nodes into the deep inguinal and femoral nodes and finally into the pelvic lymphatics
3. **Hematogenous dissemination:** rare; occurs mostly in patients who also have lymphatic dissemination; spreads to lung, liver, and bone

**How common is lymphatic spread and what factors predict whether it occurs?**

Lymphatic spread **occurs in 30%** of vulvar cancers and its likelihood increases with the size of the lesion and the depth of invasion

**What are the stages of vulvar cancer?**

The FIGO system is used to stage vulvar cancer and is based on both the microscopic evaluation of the removed tumor as well as of the regional lymph nodes. See Table 5-3.

**How is squamous cell vulvar cancer treated?**

In general, treatment needs to be **individualized** using the most conservative treatment that will lead to cure of the disease. The possible modalities are listed below:

1. **Groin node dissection** with either **wide local excision** or **radical vulvectomy** is the mainstay of treatment
2. **Adjuvant radiation therapy** can be added postoperative in patients with either positive inguinal nodes or close/positive surgical margins or preoperatively in patients with advanced disease

## Table 5-3 The Stages of Vulvar Cancer

| | | |
|---|---|---|
| **Stage 0** | | |
| | Tis | Carcinoma in situ; intraepithelial carcinoma |
| **Stage I** | | |
| | T1 N0 M0 | Tumor confined to the vulva and/or perineum; <2 cm in diameter; no palpable nodes |
| **Stage II** | | |
| | T2 N0 M0 | Tumor confined to the vulva and/or perineum; >2 cm in diameter; no palpable nodes |
| **Stage III** | | |
| | T3 N0 M0<br>T3 N1 M0<br>T1 N1 M0<br>T2 N1 M0 | Tumor of any size with: (1) adjacent spread to the lower urethra and/or the vagina, or the anus; and/or (2) unilateral regional lymph node metastasis |
| **Stage IVA** | | |
| | T1 N2 M0<br>T2 N2 M0<br>T3 N2 M0<br>T4 N-any M0 | Tumor invades any of the following: upper urethra, bladder mucosa, rectal mucosa, pelvic and/or bilateral regional lymph node metastasis |
| **Stage IVB** | | |
| | T-any N-any M1 | Any distant metastasis including pelvic lymph nodes |

3. **Chemoradiotherapy** can be used for advanced stage disease where surgery is associated with high morbidity and mortality
4. Adjunctive chemotherapy alone is only of limited value

**When is node dissection warranted and how is it done?**

All patients with more than 1 mm of stromal invasion require an inguinal femoral lymphadenectomy. Unilateral lesions only need node dissection on the ipsilateral side if these nodes are negative. Midline or bilateral lesions warrant bilateral node dissection. Sentinel node biopsy is currently under investigation as a method to evaluate degree of treatment

**What is the difference between the following:**

**Wide local excision:**

Surgical excision of the lesion down to the layer of underlying fascia that must include at least 1 cm negative surgical margins

**Radical vulvectomy:**
Excision of both the labia majora and the mons pubis down to the layer of underlying fascia

**What are the complications of radical vulvectomy and groin dissection?**
1. **Wound infection, necrosis,** and **breakdown** (occurs in 40–50% of cases)
2. **Chronic leg edema** (occurs in 30% of cases)
3. **Depression,** poor body image, sexual dysfunction
4. Less commonly: UTIs, deep vein thrombosis (DVT), PE, MI, seromas, hemorrhage, femoral nerve injury, chronic cellulitis, femoral hernias, and fistula development

**What are the most important predictors of recurrence and survival?**
**Lymph node involvement** (most important predictor); **lesion size**

**What is the treatment for recurrent disease?**
**Further surgical resection** or **radiotherapy.** Metastatic recurrences are treated with chemotherapy (usually cisplatin, cyclophosphamide, methotrexate, bleomycin, or mitomycin C)

**What type of surveillance is indicated posttreatment for vulvar cancer?**
Biannual gynecologic evaluations. They must include a thorough inspection as well as palpation of the vulva and inguinal lymph nodes

**What are the survival rates for squamous cell vulvar cancer?**
The average 5-year survival rate for all stages is around 70%. If there is no lymphatic spread, survival rates reach up to 90%, but if spread has extended to the deep pelvic nodes, 5-year survival rate drops below 20%

**What is a verrucous carcinoma and how does it present?**
A type of squamous cell cancer that grossly has a cauliflower-like appearance

**Who develops verrucous carcinoma?**
Usually postmenopausal women; it is associated with HPV infection

**How is verrucous carcinoma treated?**
Radical local excision

**What is the prognosis for verrucous carcinoma?**
Good—it grows slowly, does not metastasize often. However it can be locally destructive

## Vulvar Melanoma

| | |
|---|---|
| **How does vulvar melanoma present?** | Typically in postmenopausal Caucasian women as a **raised pigmented lesion,** usually on the labia minora or clitoris. It is often asymptomatic, however it can present with **itchiness, irritation,** or **bleeding** |
| **What is the etiology of a vulvar melanoma?** | Melanomas can arise either de novo or from a prior nevus. They are rare (2–10% of vulvar cancers) |
| **How is vulvar melanoma staged?** | Using the **Breslow** criteria. Because of the direct association of survival with depth, this system measures the thickness of the lesion from the surface to the deepest point of invasion. The Clark and Chung staging system are also used |
| **How is vulvar melanoma treated?** | **Local excision** with wide margins<br>**Groin lymph node dissection** is needed for lesions with more than 1 mm invasion<br>**Sentinal lymph node sampling** may also be warranted in women with central primary lesions<br>Chemotherapy and radiotherapy do not have good results |
| **What are survival rates for vulvar melanoma?** | Survival is near 100% if the melanoma has not invaded more than 1 mm, but rates decline with increasing dermal depth |

## Bartholin Gland Carcinoma

| | |
|---|---|
| **What is Bartholin gland carcinoma?** | An uncommon type of **adenocarcinoma** that arises mainly from either the squamous epithelium of the Bartholin's ducts/glands |
| **How does a Bartholin gland carcinoma present?** | It typically presents either as an **asymptomatic vulvar mass** or as **perineal pain**, usually in women in their 50s. Because of this, any Bartholin gland enlargement in postmenopausal women must be biopsied |

**What are the criteria required to diagnose a vulvar tumor as a Bartholin gland carcinoma?**

1. Tumor in the posterior vulva
2. Tumor is deep in the labia majora
3. The overlying skin is infracted
4. There is some recognizable normal gland present

**How is Bartholin gland carcinoma treated?**

Because metastasis is common, treatment usually involves a **radical vulvectomy, bilateral lymphadenectomy,** and postoperative **radiation therapy**

**What is the survival rate for a Bartholin gland carcinoma?**

The 5-year survival is only 50–60% as recurrences are common

## Basal Cell Carcinoma

**What is basal cell carcinoma of the vulva and how does it present?**

A rare vulvar cancer that typically presents in postmenopausal Caucasian women as a **vulvar lesion** that has **rolled edges** with **central ulceration** (a "**rodent ulcer**") usually on the labia majora. While usually asymptomatic, symptoms can include pruritus, bleeding, soreness, or irritation

**How is basal cell carcinoma treated?**

**Wide local excision** without lymph node dissection. They are associated with the presence of other antecedent or concomitant malignancies, so treatment also involves a search for concomitant disease

**What are the survival rates for basal cell carcinoma?**

Survival rates are overall good; while they are locally aggressive, lymphatic metastasis is rare

**How is basal cell carcinoma diagnosed?**

Via biopsy

## Vulvar Sarcoma

**What are the most common types of vulvar sarcoma?**

**Leiomyosarcoma** and **rhabdomyosarcoma**

**How does leiomyosarcoma usually present?**

As an **enlarging, painful lesion** of the labia majora

**How is a leiomyosarcoma treated?**

Wide local excision (lymph node involvement is rare)

**In whom is vulvar rhabdomyosarcoma most common?**
Children

**How is vulvar rhabdomyosarcoma treated?**
Primary chemotherapy followed by surgery

## Paget Disease of the Vulva

**What is Paget disease of the vulva and how does it present?**
**An extensive intraepithelial adenocarcinoma**. It is most commonly found in white women aged 60–80 and it grossly appears as **multifocal, well-demarcated areas of a bright red background with white, hyperkeratotic areas**

**How does Paget disease usually present?**
With **pruritis** and **vulvar soreness**

**What is the histological appearance of Paget lesions?**
Similar to Paget disease of the breast—large pale apocrine cells directly below the epithelium

**What is the diagnostic workup for Paget disease?**
About 20–30% of Paget disease patients will have a noncontiguous carcinoma (especially of the breast, colon, cervix, bladder, or gallbladder) and so evaluation should include an extensive evaluation

**What is the treatment for Paget disease?**
Either wide local excision or a simple vulvectomy. Long-term follow-up and lifelong surveillance for tumors at other sites are warranted

**What is the prognosis of Paget disease?**
Local recurrence is common. Increased depth of invasion and involvement of the lymph nodes lead to a poorer prognosis

# VAGINAL CANCER OVERVIEW

**Describe preinvasive vaginal malignancy**
Called **vaginal intraepithelial neoplasia** (**VAIN**). It is squamous atypia without invasion and is classified by depth of involvement

**What are the designations of preinvasive vaginal malignancy?**
**VAIN I:** involves lower one-third of the epithelium

**VAIN II:** involves lower two-thirds of the epithelium

**VAIN III:** involves more than two-thirds of the epithelium; includes carcinoma in situ

**How does VAIN typically present?**

Usually **asymptomatic**, but can present as **postcoital spotting** or **vaginal discharge**

**What are the options for VAIN treatment and what are the benefits of each?**

1. **Excision:** the mainstay of therapy; allows histologic diagnosis
2. **Ablation:** well tolerated but may require repeat administration
3. **Topical chemotherapy:** good for multifocal disease or difficult to access lesions
4. **Radiation therapy:** a last resort therapy if all else has failed or is contraindicated
5. **Observation:** for mild cases

**What factors should be considered when deciding on therapeutic modalities for VAIN?**

Previous treatment failures; presence of multifocal disease; risks of surgery; desire to preserve sexual function; whether invasive disease has been definitively excluded

**What is the incidence of vaginal cancer and VAIN?**

One case per 100,000 women in the United States; 3% of all female genital malignancies. However, the diagnosis of VAIN has been steadily increasing (likely secondary to increased awareness)

**What is the most common type of vaginal cancer?**

Metastatic cancer from other primary sites, especially cervix

**What are the types of primary vaginal cancer?**

**Squamous cell carcinomas** (most common); melanoma; sarcoma; adenocarcinoma

**How is the diagnosis of vaginal cancer made?**

**Digital palpation** and **colposcopy** (with acetic acid and Lugol's iodine to enhance visualization). **Biopsy** of suspicious areas is the definitive diagnostic tool

**In whom should you aggressively search for VAIN/vaginal cancer?**

Postmenopausal women with an abnormal Pap smear; any woman with an abnormal Pap smear without any cervical lesions

## Squamous Cell Vaginal Carcinoma

**What are the risk factors for squamous cell vaginal cancer?**

HPV infection; HIV infection; increased number of sexual partners; early age at coitarche; smoking; prior lower genital neoplasia

**What are the explanations for the association between squamous cell vaginal cancer and other genital neoplasia?**

1. **Extension of disease** → CIN of VIN may spread contiguously to the vagina
2. **Common etiologic factors** → vulvar, cervical, and vaginal cancer share many common etiologies (such as HPV exposure)
3. **Prior radiation** → treatment of prior neoplasia increases susceptibility to later cancers

**What are the symptoms of squamous cell vaginal cancer?**

Up to one-fifth of all women are **asymptomatic** but are found to have a vaginal mass or atypical Pap smear. Symptoms can include **abnormal vaginal bleeding, vaginal discharge**, vaginal mass, urinary/GI complaints, pelvic pain

**Where are squamous cell vaginal lesions typically located?**

In the **upper one-third of the vagina**, especially the **posterior wall**

**How is vaginal cancer staged?**

Using the FIGO system which is clinically done using information obtained from the physical examination, cystoscopy, proctoscopy, and x- rays. See Table 5-4.

**What are the common primary sites for metastatic vaginal cancer?**

Endometrium, breast,
Cervix, rectum,
Vulva, kidney, ovary

### **Table 5-4** The Stages of Vaginal Cancer

|  |  |
|---|---|
| I | **Carcinoma confined to the vaginal mucosa** |
| II | **Submucosal infiltration into parametrium, but not extending out to pelvic wall** |
| IIA | Subvaginal infiltration; no parametrial involvement |
| IIB | Parametrial infiltration; not extending to pelvic wall |
| III | **Carcinoma extends to the pelvic wall** |
| IV | **Carcinoma extends beyond the true pelvis** |
| IVA | Infiltration of the mucosa of bladder or rectum or extends outside true pelvis |
| IVB | Distant metastatic disease |

**How do these cancers spread to the vagina?**

Either through direct extension or via lymphatic or hematogenous spread

**To where and by what routes does primary vaginal cancer spread?**

1. **Direct extension** to bladder, rectum, urethra, parametria, and bony pelvis
2. **Lymphatic spread** to pelvic and paraaortic lymph nodes
3. **Hematogenous dissemination** to lungs, liver, and bone (usually occurs late)

**What are the treatment options for vaginal cancer and when is each used?**

1. **Radiation:** the main treatment modality; used with or without surgery for large stage I or all stage II–IV lesions
2. **Surgery:** used for small, localized stage I cancer in the upper vagina
3. **Chemotherapy:** sometimes used in combination with radiation with advanced disease, however not shown to be more effective

**What are the side effects of treatment?**

Fistulas (rectovaginal or vesicovaginal); vaginal or rectal strictures; radiation cystitis or proctitis; vaginal stenosis; radiation-induced menopause

**What considerations need to be taken into account when deciding on a treatment modality?**

Stage of tumor; proximity of tumor to structures that preclude radiotherapy; anatomical constraints of surgery; future sexual function

**What predicts survival rates?**

Stage of cancer at presentation

**What are the average 5-year survival rates for each stage?**

1. Stage 0: 95%
2. Stage 1: 67%
3. Stage 2: 39%
4. Stage 3: 33%
5. Stage 4: 19%

**What is a verrucous carcinoma?**

An uncommon variant of squamous cell carcinoma that presents as a **large, verrucous mass**. It has a low **malignant potential**, although it is locally aggressive

## Other Vaginal Cancers

**What is vaginal melanoma and how does it typically present?**

A rare but aggressive malignancy of the vaginal mucosa. Occurs in middle-aged Caucasian women and presents as a **dark-colored mass or ulceration,** usually in the distal one-third of the vaginal wall

**What is the 5-year survival rate of vaginal melanoma?**

A dismal 10%

**When does adenocarcinoma of the vagina typically present?**

Usually in women under 20

**In utero exposure to what leads to vaginal adenocarcinoma?**

**DES** (diethylstilbestrol)—it leads to the **clear cell variant** of adenocarcinoma

**What is the risk of developing clear cell adenocarcinoma if exposed?**

1 in 1000; higher risk is associated with those exposed before 12 weeks of gestation

**How does clear cell carcinoma of the vagina present?**

As a polypoid vaginal mass in a young woman; DES was discontinued in 1971 and so most cases have already been discovered

**What are the major types of vaginal sarcomas?**

Rhabdomyosarcomas; leiomyosarcomas; endometrial stromal sarcomas; malignant mixed Müllerian tumors

**What is the most common form of vaginal sarcoma?**

**Embryonal rhabdomyosarcoma** or **sarcoma botryoides**

**What is sarcoma botryoides and how does it present?**

A **very aggressive malignant** tumor that presents in early childhood as a vaginal mass that resembles a **bunch of grapes**

**How is sarcoma botryoides treated?**

Preoperative chemotherapy followed by surgery or radiation

# Uterine Cancer

## ENDOMETRIAL CANCER

**What is endometrial cancer?**

An **estrogen-dependent neoplasm** of the endometrium that begins with proliferation of normal endometrial tissue. Over time, hyperplasia of the glandular elements becomes anaplastic and then neoplastic, with invasion of the underlying stroma, myometrium, and vascular spaces

**There are two types of endometrial cancer based on light microscopic appearance, clinical behavior, and epidemiology, Type 1 and Type II. What are these types?**

**Type 1:** These have an endometrioid histology and comprise 70–80% of newly diagnosed cases of endometrial cancer in the United States. They are associated with unopposed estrogen exposure and are often preceded by premalignant disease

**Type II:** These have nonendometrioid histology (usually papillary serous or clear cell) with an aggressive clinical course. Hormonal risk factors have not been identified, and there is no readily observed premalignant phase

**How common is endometrial cancer and in whom does it occur?**

It is the **most common** gynecologic cancer; 75% of these cancers occur in **postmenopausal women**

**What are the major symptoms of endometrial cancer?**

Abnormal uterine bleeding (primarily postmenopausal bleeding)

**What are the roles of estrogen and progesterone in endometrial cancer?**

**Estrogen stimulates endometrial growth** while **progesterone has anti-proliferative** effects. Long-term unopposed estrogen stimulation can eventually lead to atypical endometrial hyperplasia and endometrial cancer

**What are the main etiologies for chronically elevated estrogen levels?**

Exogenous unopposed estrogen (i.e., estrogen replacement therapy); chronic anovulation (i.e., polycystic ovarian syndrome [PCOS]); estrogen producing tumors (i.e., granulosa cell tumors); obesity

**What are the risk factors for endometrial cancer?**

Obesity; diet; diabetes; hypertension; early menarche/late menopause; nulliparity; PCOS (infertility); tamoxifen treatment for breast cancer; family predisposition (hereditary nonpolyposis colorectal cancer [HNPCC]/Lynch syndrome II)

**What are protective factors against endometrial cancer?**

Combined oral contraceptives; exercise; multiparity; smoking (through increased hepatic metabolism of estrogen)

**What is the relationship between endometrial hyperplasia and endometrial cancer?**

Endometrial hyperplasia is a benign condition associated with hyperestrogenic states. Atypical hyperplasia is a precancerous condition

**What characteristics are used to classify endometrial hyperplasia?**

1. Glandular/stromal architecture (simplex or complex)
2. Nuclear atypia (present or absent)

**Which histologic feature of endometrial hyperplasia confers the greatest risk for cancer?**

**Nuclear atypia**

**What are the four types of endometrial hyperplasia and what is the risk of cancer for each?**

1. Simple hyperplasia without atypia 1% (penny)
2. Complex hyperplasia without atypia 3% (nickel)
3. Simple hyperplasia with atypia 8% (dime)
4. Complex hyperplasia with atypia 40% (~quarter)

**What are the general guidelines for the treatment of endometrial hyperplasia?**

If nuclear atypia is absent, treat with progesterone. If nuclear atypia is present, hysterectomy is recommended

**Describe your classic patient diagnosed with endometrial cancer**

A **postmenopausal woman** who is **obese, nulliparous/infertile, diabetic,** and **hypertensive**

**How should atypical endometrial cells on a Pap smear be worked up?**

They are not diagnostic for endometrial cancer, but they do warrant an endometrial biopsy for further evaluation

**What is the differential diagnosis for abnormal uterine bleeding in the premenopausal woman?**

Complications of early pregnancy; other gynecologic neoplasms; leiomymata; endometrial hyperplasia/polyps; cervical polyps; Intrauterine device; hemophilias

**What are your differential diagnoses for abnormal uterine bleeding in the postmenopausal woman?**

Atrophic vaginitis; exogenous estrogens; other gynecologic neoplasms; endometrial hyperplasia/polyps

**What is the gold standard for diagnosing endometrial cancer?**

Hysteroscopy with dilation and curettage (**D&C**)

**Is CA-125 a useful laboratory test to help with diagnosis?**

In advanced disease, CA-125 may be elevated; however, it is not useful in the diagnosis or management

**What are the different subtypes of endometrial cancer?**

1. **Endometrioid adenocarcinoma** (80%)

2. Papillary serous carcinoma (5–10%)
3. Clear cell carcinoma (1–5%)

**How does endometrial cancer spread?**

Most commonly through **direct extension**, but it can also spread transtubally, lymphatically, or hematogenously

**What lymph nodes are involved in endometrial cancer metastases?**

Pelvic and paraaortic lymph nodes

**How is tumor grading for endometrial cancer determined?**

By tumor histology (architecture and nuclear atypia)

**What are the three different tumor grades for endometrial cancer?**

1. Grade 1: Well differentiated (~95% glandular tissue, 5% solid pattern)
2. Grade 2: Moderately differentiated (~50–95% glandular tissue, 5–50% solid pattern)
3. Grade 3: Poorly differentiated (<50% glandular tissue, >50% solid pattern)

**How is endometrial cancer staged?**

Surgically (by the spread of the cancer) based on **abdominal exploration, pelvic washings, total abdominal hysterectomy with bilateral salpingo-oophorectomy (TAH/BSO), and pelvic and periaortic lymph node biopsies**

**What is the staging system for endometrial cancer?**

See Table 5-5.

**How is endometrial cancer treated?**

TAH/BSO with lymph node dissection

**What is the role of adjuvant therapy in endometrial cancer?**

It is dependent on whether the patient is at low, intermediate, or high risk for disease recurrence. Below are general guidelines for adjuvant postoperative treatment:

1. Low risk (Stage Ia, Ib): no adjuvant treatment warranted (Stage Ia, grade 3) Vaginal brachytherapy
2. Intermediate-risk (Stage Ic, Stage II): vaginal brachytherapy
3. High risk (Stage III, IV): pelvic/abdominal radiation therapy ± chemotherapy

**Table 5-5** Stages of Endometrial Cancer

| Stage | Description | Endometrial tumors | 5-Year survival |
|---|---|---|---|
| Stage I: Involvement limited to the uterus | Ia: tumor limited to the endometrium<br>Ib: invasion < half of myometrium<br>Ic: invasion > half of myometrium | 75% | 80–95% |
| Stage II: Extension to and involvement of the cervix | IIa: extension to endocervical glands only<br>IIb: cervical stromal invasion | 11% | 65–75% |
| Stage III: Local spread | IIIa: invasion of serosa and/or adnexa, and/or positive peritoneal cytology<br>IIIb: vaginal metastases<br>IIIc: metastasis to pelvic and/or para-aortic lymph nodes | 11% | 30–60% |
| Stage IV: Distant spread | IVa: invasion of the bladder and bowel<br>IVb: distant metastasis including intra-abdominal and/or inguinal lymph nodes | 3% | 5–20% |

**Name the chemotherapeutic agents used in endometrial cancer and their major toxicities**

1. Doxorubicin (cardiotoxicity)
2. Cisplatin (ototoxicity, neuropathy, nephrotoxicity, nausea)
3. Paclitaxel (bone marrow suppression, allergic reaction)

**What is the recommended treatment for women who have early-stage disease and wish to preserve their fertility?**

Trial of progestins after careful counseling

**What factors worsen the prognosis for endometrial cancer?**

Advanced stage; higher pathologic grade; histologic subtype; increase in myometrial invasion; lymph/vascular space invasion

**What is the appropriate follow-up after treatment of endometrial cancer?**

Monitor patients every 3–4 months for the next 2–3 years, then twice yearly with a comprehensive pelvic examination

**What is the overall prognosis for endometrial cancer?**

Without major adverse risk factors, treatment with a TAH/BSO may result in a 5-year survival greater than 95%

**What is the screening recommendation for the general population?**
Screening is not warranted for women who are asymptomatic

**What is the screening recommendation for women with/at risk for HNPCC?**
Annual endometrial biopsies by age 35

## UTERINE SARCOMA

**What is a uterine sarcoma?**
A very aggressive tumor that arises from the myometrium

**How common is it and who does it affect?**
It is a very rare cancer (3–4% of all uterine malignancies) and commonly affects women over age 40

**What are risk factors for uterine sarcoma?**
History of pelvic radiation; Long-term use of tamoxifen

**What are the main types of sarcomas?**
Mixed müllerian tumors (carcinosarcoma); leiomyosarcoma; endometrial stromal sarcoma (ESS); undifferentiated sarcoma

**How do uterine sarcomas present clinically?**
**Abnormal uterine bleeding; rapidly enlarging uterus;** malodorous vaginal discharge; pelvic pressure and pain; part of the tumor may protrude from the cervical os

**What is the major differential diagnosis of uterine sarcoma?**
Uterine leiomyomas

**What preoperative examinations may help with the diagnosis of a uterine sarcoma?**
Endometrial biopsy; dilation and fractional curettage

**How is the definitive diagnosis of uterine sarcoma made?**
Exploratory laparotomy with a pathologic diagnosis

**What is the role of imaging studies in uterine sarcomas?**
Imaging studies cannot distinguish between a sarcoma or other uterine tumors. A CT scan of the thorax is recommended because uterine sarcoma commonly metastasizes to the lung

**What is the staging system for uterine sarcomas?**
Staging is done surgically and is a modification of the system used for endometrial cancer

**What is the treatment for uterine sarcomas?**
TAH/BSO, pelvic/paraaortic lymph node dissection, and pelvic washings

**What is the role of adjuvant therapy?**

Stage I and II pelvic radiation therapy

**What is the overall prognosis for sarcomas?**

Generally they have worse prognosis than endometrial cancers of a similar stage

# Ovarian Cancer

## INTRODUCTION

**How common is ovarian cancer?**

It is the second most common gynecologic malignancy, but the **leading cause of mortality** among women who develop a gynecologic malignancy, and the **fifth most common cause of cancer-related female deaths in the United States**. The lifetime risk of developing ovarian cancer is 1.4% (1 in 70)

**Why is ovarian cancer the leading cause of mortality among women with gynecologic cancers?**

Symptoms of early-stage ovarian cancer are ill-defined and many women will not seek medical attention. Often, the cancer is detected at its advanced stages when it has spread beyond the ovaries

**How are ovarian tumors categorized?**

**Epithelial origin; germ cell tumors; sex cord-stromal tumors; cancer metastatic to the ovary** (usually from primary tumors of the breast, GI tract, or genital tract)

**Which ovarian tumor is the most common?**

Epithelial (~90% of all ovarian tumors)

## EPITHELIAL OVARIAN CANCER

**What age group does EOC affect?**

Predominantly **postmenopausal** women. Median age is 62 years old

**What is thought to be the underlying hypothesis in the development of EOC?**

It is not well understood, but one hypothesis is that repetitive ovulation where disruption and repair of the ovarian epithelium may allow opportunity for genetic mutation and malignant transformation

**What are the risk factors for development of EOC?**

**Family history of breast cancer or EOC; history of breast cancer; advanced age**; obesity/high fat diet; infertility; nulliparity; talc; endometriosis

**What factors are protective against development of EOC?**

**OCPs; tubal ligation;** breastfeeding (history of); pregnancy; multiparity

**What percent of EOC develops sporadically? What percent are because of genetic predisposition?**

90% are sporadic; 10% are genetic predisposition

**What is one feature that distinguishes hereditary ovarian cancer from a somatic cause?**

The onset of ovarian cancer occurs **10 years earlier** in hereditary syndromes

**With what hereditary syndromes has ovarian cancer been associated? Describe them.**

1. **Breast and ovarian cancer (BOC):** associated with BRCA-1 mutation (autosomal dominant), more susceptibility to BOC, higher frequencies in Ashkenazi Jews
2. **Lynch II Syndrome (hereditary nonpolyposis colon cancer—HNPCC):** colorectal cancer is hallmark, also commonly found are endometrial, urogenital, and other GI primaries
3. **Site-specific ovarian cancer:** strong genetic link, autosomal dominant, usually two or more first-degree relatives have the disease

**What are current screening recommendations for women at high risk?**

1. Prophylactic genetic screening
2. CA-125 and transvaginal ultrasound every 6–12 months beginning between ages 25 and 35 years

**What other preventative surgical procedure is recommended for women with a presumed hereditary ovarian cancer syndrome?**

Prophylactic oophorectomy who have completed childbearing or by age 35

**With what other gynecologic disease is ovarian cancer associated?**

Endometriosis (25%)

**What are the subtypes of EOC and how common is each type?**

Serous 75–80%

Mucinous 10%

Endometrioid 10%

Clear cell <1%

Transitional cell <1%

Undifferentiated <10%

**What are some key features that describe each tumor type?**

Serous: often bilateral if malignant, resembles the endosalpinx, extraovarian spread common, histological finding of **psammoma bodies**

Mucinous: unilateral, **large size,** resembles the endocervix

Endometrioid: resembles the endometrium

Clear cell: "mesonephroid," **"clear cells"** similar to renal carcinoma, **hypercalcemia**

Transitional cell: "Brenner tumors," **transitional epithelium,** unilateral, benign, or malignant

Undifferentiated: No distinguishable histologic features

**At what cancer stage is EOC usually diagnosed?**

75% of ovarian cancers are detected at **stage III or IV**. Five-year survival rate is 5–35%

**What is the typical presentation of a patient with ovarian cancer?**

A **postmenopausal woman** who presents with any or a combination of these:

1. **Abdominal distension** from ascites or pelvic mass
2. **Pelvic pressure**
3. **Nausea, early satiety,** weight loss, bowel obstruction
4. Dyspnea because of a pleural effusion (metastasis to the lungs)

**How does ovarian cancer spread?**

Ovarian cancer cells are found in peritoneal fluid (ascites) which carries them to distant abdominal sites

**Should the ovaries on a postmenopausal woman be palpable on examination?**

Women who are more than 1 year postmenopause should have atrophic, nonpalpable ovaries. An ovarian enlargement in a postmenopausal woman is cancer until proven otherwise

**What findings on the physical examination would lead you to believe this is an ovarian malignancy?**

A **solid, fixed, irregular pelvic mass** associated with an upper abdominal mass (omental caking) and/or ascites

**What is the following?**

**Omental caking:** ovarian cancer metastasis to the omentum causing a fixed upper abdominal mass with ascites, very common in advanced disease

**What is the initial step to evaluate an ovarian lesion?**

Ultrasound

**What other radiographic tests should be ordered in a patient suspected of having EOC?**

**Abdominal-pelvic CT:** to determine the extent of metastases

**Chest x-ray:** to determine the presence of a pleural effusion

**What tumor marker is often elevated in advanced stage ovarian cancer? What is its value?**

CA-125 is elevated in 80% of cases with advanced ovarian cancer. It is not as useful in premenopausal women or for early stage disease. It is most useful to **evaluate the progression/regression of disease following treatment**

**What is the "gold standard" to diagnose EOC?**

Exploratory laparotomy/laparoscopy and histopathologic diagnosis

**How is ovarian cancer staged?**

Surgically

**Describe the stages of ovarian cancer and their prognoses**

See Table 5-6.

## Table 5-6 The Stages of Ovarian Cancer

| Stage | Description | 5-Year survival |
|---|---|---|
| Stage I: Tumor limited to the ovaries | 1a: one ovary involved and capsule intact<br>1b: both ovaries involved and capsule intact<br>1c: 1a or 1b and tumor on the ovary; ruptured capsule; malignant ascites and positive peritoneal washings for malignant cells | >90% |
| Stage II: Spread of the tumor to the pelvis | IIa: uterus/oviducts are involved<br>IIb: other pelvic structures are involved<br>IIc: IIa or IIb and tumor on the ovary; ruptured capsule; malignant ascites and positive peritoneal washings for malignant cells | 60–75% |
| Stage III: Spread to the abdominal cavity | IIIa: microscopic seeding of the abdominal peritoneal surfaces; negative nodes<br>IIIb: <2 cm implants on the abdominal peritoneal surface<br>IIIc: >2 cm implants on the abdominal peritoneal surface and/or positive retroperitoneal or inguinal lymph nodes | 25–40% |
| Stage IV: Distant metastasis | Liver, splenic, or pulmonary parenchymal metastasis<br>Malignant pleural effusion<br>Metastases to the supraclavicular lymph nodes or skin | 5% |

**Which lymph nodes are typically involved in advanced ovarian cancer?**

Pelvic and para-aortic lymph nodes

**What is the optimal treatment for advanced ovarian cancer disease?**

Surgical debulking and chemotherapy. Debulking includes TAH/BSO, omentectomy. In epithelial tumors, cytoreductive surgery does not include uterus removal

**What is the most effective chemotherapeutic regimen?**

A combination of **paclitaxel plus cisplatin**

**What are the most common side effects of chemotherapy?**

Nausea, vomiting, alopecia, diarrhea, nephrotoxicity, myelosuppression

**What are poor prognostic factors?**

Stage III or IV disease; advanced age; short disease-free interval; residual tumor after primary surgery

## NONEPITHELIAL OVARIAN CANCER

### Ovarian Germ Cell Tumors

**What percent of all ovarian neoplasms are germ cell tumors (GCTs)?**

20–25%

**From what embryologic origin do ovarian GCTs (OGCTs) arise?**

They arise from the totipotential germ cells that normally differentiate into the three germ layers

**What are the OGCT subtypes?**

Dysgerminoma; endodermal sinus tumor (yolk sac tumor); immature teratoma; mature teratoma; embryonal carcinoma; choriocarcinoma; mixed GCTs

**At what age do these malignancies occur?**

It is a disease of children and young women (usually between 10 and 30 years)

**What are the typical clinical symptoms and signs?**

Acute abdominal pain (from rupture or torsion); rapid abdominal enlargement (because of either the mass or ascites); fever; vaginal bleeding

**How does the time of diagnosis differ from that of EOC?**

**Patients usually present at Stage Ia**

**For each of the following scenarios, identify the correct GCT:**

A **20-year-old** woman presents with acute onset of lower abdominal pain and pelvic mass. Serum tests reveal an **elevated level of alpha-fetoprotein**

**(AFP).** Intraoperative examination reveals **bilateral ovarian masses and intraperitoneal dissemination.** Tumor biopsy reveals **Schiller-Duval bodies**

*Endodermal sinus tumor (yolk sac tumor)*

These tumors are **rare,** found in **young females**. They may **secrete estrogen,** causing **precocious puberty** and **abnormal vaginal bleeding. β-hCG is commonly elevated** and serves as a tumor marker

*Embryonal carcinoma and choriocarcinoma*

A **young female** presents with abdominal enlargement. Radiographic films reveal a **unilateral mass with calcification.** Tumor markers are not present. Histology of the removed specimen reveals the presence of a poorly differentiated tumor consisting of **hair, teeth, cartilage, bone, and muscle**

*Immature (malignant) teratoma*

This dysgerminoma is the **female counterpart of the male seminoma** and commonly occurs in **adolescents** and young females. It is the most common of the malignant OGCTs and typically presents as a rapidly growing unilateral mass. Lactic dehydrogenase **(LDH) may be elevated**

*Dysgerminoma*

A young female presents with **tachycardia, palpitations, anxiety, and tremors.** The pituitary and thyroid appear normal on examination and radiographic films. The patient is later found to have a **mature teratoma consisting of thyroid tissue**

*Mixed GCTs*

These neoplasms contain **two or more germ cell elements.** A dysgerminoma and endodermal sinus tumor occur together most frequently. **LDH, AFP, and β-hCG may be elevated**

*Struma ovarii*

| | |
|---|---|
| **Which GCTs are benign?** | Gonadoblastomas and mature cystic teratomas |
| **What laboratory test should be ordered prior to definitive diagnosis and treatment?** | Serum ovarian tumor marker panel for **β-hCG, AFP, LDH** |
| **What is the treatment plan for malignant OGCTs?** | Unilateral adnexectomy (fertility preserving) and complete surgical staging; adjuvant chemotherapy |
| **How are OGCTs staged?** | Similar to EOC staging |
| **How effective is chemotherapy in malignant GCTs?** | GCTs are very chemosensitive. 90% of patients with early-stage OGCTs and 80% of patients with advanced disease are long-term survivors |
| **For which tumors is chemotherapy recommended?** | For all resected Stage I GCTs except Stage Ia dysgerminoma and Stage Ia, grade 1 unruptured immature teratoma |
| **What chemotherapeutic agents are used?** | **Bleomycin, etoposide, cisplatin** is the preferred regimen |
| **List the chemotherapeutic agent that causes the toxicities listed below:** | |
| **Nephrotoxicity** | Cisplatin |
| **Pulmonary fibrosis** | Bleomycin |
| **Blood dyscrasias** | Etoposide |
| **How do you monitor the response to chemotherapy?** | Based on the physical examination and decrease in the serum tumor marker levels (if initially elevated) |
| **What is the prognosis of GCTs?** | Much better than EOC. Depending on the GCT, 5-year survival ranges from 60% to 95% |

## Ovarian Sex Cord-Stromal Tumors

| | |
|---|---|
| **What percent of all ovarian tumors are sex cord-stromal tumors?** | 5–8% of all primary ovarian neoplasms |
| **From what embryologic origin do ovarian sex cord-stromal tumors arise?** | They develop from the cells that surround the oocytes, including those that **produce ovarian hormones** |
| **What are the ovarian sex cord-stromal tumor subtypes?** | Granulosa cell tumors; ovarian thecoma; ovarian fibroma; Sertoli-Leydig cell tumors |

**What are the typical clinical symptoms and signs?**

Estrogen-producing tumors may cause **precocious puberty** in young girls, and **endometrial hyperplasia** and **abnormal vaginal bleeding** in postmenopausal women. Androgen-producing tumors cause **virilization, acne**, and **gynecomastia**

Most women present with a **unilateral adnexal mass** between the second and third decade. **Virilization, hirsutism, acne,** and **menstrual abnormalities** commonly occur. **Testosterone** levels may be elevated

*Sertoli-Leydig cell tumors*

**In the following scenarios, identify the correct sex cord-stromal tumor**

A postmenopausal woman presents with a **unilateral benign solid mass** that is not hormone secreting

*Ovarian fibroma*

These tumors are **estrogen producing** and cause **precocious puberty** in young females and **abnormal vaginal bleeding** in postmenopausal women. **Inhibin** may be elevated

*Granulosa/thecoma*

**What is Meigs' syndrome?**

It is the association of an **ovarian fibroma** with **ascites** and/or **pleural effusion**

**With what other syndrome are ovarian fibromas associated?**

**Gorlin syndome** (nevoid basal cell carcinoma syndrome): an autosomal dominant disease characterized by its association with **basal cell cancers, brain tumors, odontogenic keratocysts,** and **mesenteric cysts**

**What are Call-Exner bodies and for what tumor are they nearly pathogonomic?**

They are small, fluid-filled cavities in between granulosa cells of ovarian follicles that contain eosinophilic fluid. They are associated with **granulosa cell tumors**

**What other cancer is associated with granulosa cell tumors/ovarian thecomas?**

With estrogen-producing tumors, **endometrial adenocarcinoma** must be considered. **These women must have an endometrial biopsy**

**How are ovarian sex cord-stromal tumors staged?**

Similarly to EOC

| | |
|---|---|
| **What is the surgical treatment?** | TAH/BSO or unilateral oophorectomy for women who wish to preserve their fertility and who have low-stage/grade neoplasms. A dilation & curettage or an endometrial biopsy must be performed for estrogen-secreting tumors |
| **Is adjuvant therapy recommended?** | Chemotherapy is not recommended for low-stage/grade neoplasms. Data is inconclusive for more advanced stages |
| **What is the prognosis for these tumors?** | In general, very good. For early-stage cancers, 5-year survival rates range between 70–90% |
| **What follow-up procedures are recommended for the hormone-producing cancers?** | Serial pelvic examinations and serum tumor marker levels |

## Tumors Metastatic to the Ovary

| | |
|---|---|
| **What percent of ovarian tumors are metastatic?** | 5% |
| **What are the primary tumors that metastasize to the ovary?** | **Breast; gastrointestinal tract**; acute leukemia and lymphoma (rare) |
| **How do metastatic tumors to the ovary clinically present?** | Gastrointestinal cancers present like primary ovarian: pelvic mass, ascites, early satiety, and change in bowel habits. Recurrent metastatic breast cancer may present as an asymptomatic pelvic mass |
| **What are gastric tumors metastatic to the ovaries called?** | Krukenberg tumors |
| **What primary ovarian tumor do Krukenberg tumors resemble in histology?** | Mucin-secreting adenocarcinoma of the ovary |
| **What histologic feature is pathognomonic for Krukenberg tumors?** | Signet ring cells |
| **What can be used to differentiate between a primary mucinous ovarian tumor and metastastic colon cancer?** | Immunohistochemistry (cytokeratin expression) |
| **Describe the cytokeratin expression pattern of each of the following:** | Primary mucinous ovarian: CK7 positive; CK20 negative |

| | |
|---|---|
| | Metastases from a primary mucinous adenocarcinoma of the colon: CK7 negative; CK20 positive |
| **What is the overall prognosis in patients who have cancers metastatic to the ovary?** | Survival following surgery and chemotherapy is very poor, ranging from 4 to 12 months |

# Fallopian Tube Cancer

| | |
|---|---|
| **How common is fallopian tube cancer?** | Primary carcinoma is **very rare,** accounting for 0.3% of primary gynecologic malignancies. Secondary carcinoma from metastases of ovarian, endometrium, gastrointestinal (GI), or breast cancers are more common |
| **What are risk factors for fallopian tube cancers?** | A mutation in the BRCA1 or BRCA2 gene. Women with these mutations who are planning prophylactic oophorectomies should also have their oviducts removed |
| **What is the most common type of fallopian tube cancer?** | Papillary serous adenocarcinoma |
| **What other types of fallopian tube cancers are there?** | Adenosquamous carcinoma and sarcoma |
| **How does the cancer spread?** | It spreads through the tubal ostia into the peritoneal cavity and also through lymphatics to the para-aortic and pelvic lymph nodes |
| **Where does fallopian tube cancer commonly metastasize?** | Ovaries, uterus, and pelvic and para-aortic nodes |
| **What is the classic clinical presentation?** | A woman between the ages of 40 and 60 who presents with **Latzko triad: serosanguineous vaginal discharge, pelvic pain, and pelvic mass.** However, this triad is seen in less than 15% of patients |
| **What is hydrops tubae profluens?** | The spontaneous or pressure-induced release of clear or blood-tinged vaginal discharge followed by shrinkage of an adnexal mass and relief of cramping pain. It is pathognomonic for fallopian tube cancer |

**What preoperative evidence suggests fallopian tube cancer?**

Positive vaginal cytology for abnormal cells with a negative workup for endometrial or cervical cancer suggests fallopian tube carcinoma

**What is the role of CA-125 in fallopian tube cancer?**

Preoperative CA-125 levels may determine prognosis. CA-125 levels are also sensitive markers for response to chemotherapy and recurrence

**How is staging for fallopian cell cancers determined?**

Surgically; it is staged similarly to epithelial ovarian cancer

**What is the treatment?**

Total abdominal hysterectomy with bilateral salpingo-oophorectomy (TAH/BSO) and tumor debulking. Retroperitoneal lymph node sampling, infracolic omentectomy, and peritoneal washings should also be performed for staging purposes. Chemotherapy consisting of carboplatin and paxlitaxel is recommended after surgery

**What is the prognosis?**

Similar to ovarian cancer. The overall 5-year survival rate is 56%

CHAPTER 6

# Urogynecology

## Urinary Infections

### ACUTE CYSTITIS

**What is the prevalence and incidence of acute cystitis?**

50–60% of women report having had cystitis at some point in their life. Young, sexually active women have on an average 0.5 episodes per year; postmenopausal women have on an average of 0.1 episodes per year

**Describe the symptoms of acute cystitis**

Abrupt onset of: **dysuria, urinary frequency and urgency, suprapubic or low back pain,** possible hematuria (in hemorrhagic cystitis)

**What is the differential diagnosis for these symptoms?**

**Urethritis; vaginitis; pyelonephritis**

**For each differential diagnosis, list the main symptoms/signs that would differentiate it from acute cystitis**

Urethritis: urethral discharge, more gradual onset, history of new sexual partner

Vaginitis: vaginal discharge/odor, pruritis, dyspareunia, external dysuria, absence of frequency or urgency

Pyelonephritis: elevated temperature, costovertebral angle (CVA) tenderness, nausea/vomiting

**How is the diagnosis of acute cystitis definitively made?**

1. Most cases can be diagnosed on **history and physical examination alone**. The examiner should specifically look for signs of vaginitis, cervicitis, urethral discharge, or herpetic ulcerations
2. **Gonococcus (GC) and *Chlamydia* cultures** should be done if urethritis is suspected

3. **Urinalysis** should also be done, looking for pyuria or hematuria. Urine culture is typically not always needed, unless the infection is complicated or it is a recurrent infection

**Describe the pathophysiology of acute cystitis**

Coliform bacteria from the rectum colonize the vaginal introitus, enter the urethra, and ascend toward the bladder. This migration can be facilitated by sexual intercourse

**What are the most common pathogens that cause acute cystitis?**

***Escherichia coli*** (80% of cases); ***Staphylococcus saprophyticus*** (5–15% of cases); *Proteus mirabilis, Klebsiella,* enterococci, *Pseudomonas, Serratia, Providencia,* staphylococci, and fungi (rare, more common in complicated cases)

**What are the risk factors for the development of acute cystitis?**

Increased sexual intercourse; newly sexually active; postmenopausal; diabetes, sickle cell anemia, immunosuppressed conditions; abnormalities of the genitourinary tract; use of spermicide, especially with a diaphragm; history of a recent UTI; recent hospitalization

**What factors suggest the presence of a complicated urinary infection?**

Patient characteristics: elderly patient; pregnancy

Medical history: hospital-acquired infection; indwelling catheter/recurrent instrumentation; functional or anatomic abnormality of the urinary tract; recent antibiotic use; diabetes; immunosuppression

**What is the prognostic significance of a complicated urinary infection?**

Complicated infections are associated with increased rates of failing therapy

**What are the treatment options for uncomplicated acute cystitis?**

1. **Trimethoprim-sulfamethoxazole** for 3 days is first line therapy in geographic regions with resistance rates <20%
2. **Nitrofurantoin** for 3-5 days
3. **Fluoroquinolone** for 3 days

No follow up is needed unless symptoms recur

**What are the treatment options for complicated acute cystitis?**

Treat initially with **broad spectrum antibiotics** (such as fluoroquinolones) and then tailor therapy based on the culture results. These patients should be treated for **7 to 14 days** and they need to be followed up to ensure resolution of symptoms

**How often does cystitis recur?**

In 20% of premenopausal women; the vast majority of these are because of exogenous reinfection. Postmenopausal women also have frequent reinfections

**What is considered recurrent cystitis?**

More than three UTIs per year or more than two UTIs within a 6-month period

**What are the risk factors of recurrent cystitis?**

Sexual intercourse; use of spermicide, especially with a diaphragm; recent antimicrobial use; genetic predisposition; in postmenopausal women: urinary incontinence, cystocele, elevated post-void residual volume

**How is recurrent cystitis treated?**

Cultures need to be taken to rule out resistance to prior treatment

For patients with multiple reinfections, treatment consists of one of three options:

1. **Behavioral changes** (change contraceptive methods, early postcoital voiding)
2. **Continuous low-dose antibiotic prophylaxis**
3. **Postcoital low-dose antibiotic prophylaxis**
4. **Self-start therapy** when symptoms begin

In postmenopausal women with frequent infections, **topical estrogen** is often used, with or without concomitant use of prophylactic antibiotics

**Is cranberry juice an effective home remedy for preventing UTIs?**

There is some evidence which suggests that cranberry juice inhibits pathogens from adhering to uroepithelial cells, which can reduce the incidence of UTI. Cranberry has not been found to be effective in the treatment of UTI

**What percentage of reproductive-age women have asymptomatic bacteriuria?**

3–6%

**What are the risk factors for the development of asymptomatic bacteriuria?**

Diabetes; advanced age; presence of an indwelling bladder catheter

**Should asymptomatic bacteriuria be treated?**

**No**, unless the woman is high risk

**Who are the high-risk women that need treatment for their asymptomatic bacteriuria?**

Pregnant women; women with indwelling catheters; renal transplant recipients; women with spinal cord injury; prior to invasive procedures

## UTI IN PREGNANCY

UTI is the most common medical complication of pregnancy.

**Why is pregnancy considered a high-risk condition with asymptomatic bacteriuria?**

Both hormonal and mechanical changes predispose the pregnant woman with asymptomatic bacteriuria to develop acute pyelonephritis, which is associated with preterm birth and perinatal death. Pyelonephritis in pregnancy will lead to septicemia in 10–20% and acute respiratory distress syndrome (ARDS) in 2% of cases

**How prevalent is asymptomatic bacteriuria in pregnancy?**

It is estimated to occur in 4–7% of pregnant patients. If left untreated, up to 40% of cases will progress to pyelonephritis

**How is this condition detected?**

Screening for asymptomatic bacteriuria using urine culture is recommended at the first prenatal visit

**How is asymptomatic bacteriuria treated?**

Nitrofurantoin for 70 days is first line. If ineffective, amoxicillin, trimethoprim-sulfamethoxazole or a cephalosporin can be used for 3 days. Quinalones are generally not used during pregnancy.

A urine culture should be done 1-2 weeks after completion of therapy. Monthly urine cultures should be done and suppressive antibiotics should be considered.

**How is symptomatic cystitis treated in pregnancy?**

Treatment and follow up are similar to asymptomatic bacteriuria. Acute pyelonephritis should be treated with intravenous (IV) antibiotics and hospitalization. Suppressive antibiotics should be given following treatment to any pregnant patient treated for acute pyelonephritis

## URETHRITIS

**Describe the signs and symptoms of urethritis**

Dysuria, but with a more **gradual** onset and **milder** symptoms than with acute cystitis. **Hematuria is rare** and points to cystitis more than urethritis. Urethritis is often associated with abnormal vaginal discharge or bleeding (because of related cervicitis). A **mucopurulent discharge from the urethral os** is usually found on examination

**What are the risk factors for urethritis?**

History of an STD; new sexual partner in past weeks; partner with urethral symptoms

**How is the diagnosis definitively made?**

Pyuria on urinalysis and mucopurulent cervicitis or herpetic lesions are usually found. A positive GC, *Chlamydia,* or herpes test result can confirm the diagnosis

**What are the most common pathogens that cause urethritis?**

Most common: ***Chlamydia trachomatis*** (5–20%)
***Neisseria gonorrhea*** (<10%)
**Genital herpes**

Others: *Candida, Trichomonas*

**What is irritant urethritis?**

Dysuria that occurs as a reaction to an irritant such as a condom, tampon, or any other product inserted into the vagina

## ACUTE PYELONEPHRITIS

**Describe the symptoms of acute pyelonephritis**

Typical presentation: flank pain, fever (>38°C), CVA tenderness, nausea/vomiting, ± cystitis symptoms

**What is the differential diagnosis for acute pyelonephritis?**

Gastrointestinal: **cholecystitis, appendicitis, pancreatitis, diverticulitis**

Gynecologic, pelvic inflammatory disease **(PID), ectopic pregnancy**

Pulmonary: **lower lobe pneumonia**

Genitourinary: **urinary calculi**

**How is the diagnosis definitively made?**

Most patients can be diagnosed based on history and physical examination alone

Urinalysis: **pyuria** is almost always found; **white cell casts**, if found, indicate renal origin; **gram-negative bacteria** on Gram stain

Urine cultures and possible blood cultures should be taken at time of diagnosis for antimicrobial susceptibility

**What is the most common pathogen that causes acute pyelonephritis?**

***E. coli*** (70–95%); ***S. saprophyticus*** (5–20%)

**Describe the pathophysiology of acute pyelonephritis**

Uropathogens from the fecal flora colonize the vaginal introitus and infect the urethra. They then ascend via the urethra to the bladder and then into the kidneys. It is also possible that the kidneys could be seeded from bacteria in the lymphatics

**What are the risk factors associated with developing uncomplicated acute pyelonephritis?**

Increased sexual intercourse; history of UTI within past year; diabetes; stress incontinence within the past 30 days; a new sexual partner within the past year; spermicide use; family history of UTIs

**How is acute pyelonephritis treated?**

Outpatient treatment: **trimethoprim-sulfamethoxazole** or a **quinolone** for 10–14 days; if enterococcus is suspected, add amoxicillin until cultures return

Inpatient treatment: indicated if patient is noncompliant, cannot tolerate PO, is severely ill, or is pregnant; initial treatment is **ceftriaxone, ampicillin** and **gentamycin**, or **aztreonam**

**What should be done if flank pain does not resolve after 2–3 days?**

An ultrasound or CT to rule out perinephric or intrarenal abcess or ureteral obstruction

**When should a patient be followed up after treatment for acute pyelonephritis?**

Two weeks after completion of therapy or as soon as symptoms recur

# Pelvic Organ Prolapse

**How significant is pelvic organ prolapse (POP) in women in the United States?**

Approximately 200,000 procedures for POP are performed annually. The lifetime risk for undergoing surgery for urinary incontinence or prolapse is 11%. The risk of requiring a repeat procedure may be as high as 29%

**What is meant by POP?**

Refers to the relaxation of the normal connective tissue supports of any of the pelvic organs (uterus, vaginal apex, bladder, rectum) and its associated vaginal segment from its normal anatomic location

**What are the most common POP abnormalities? Describe each defect**

**Cystocele:**

An anterior vaginal wall defect/prolapse that includes the bladder. See Fig. 6-1.

**Enterocele:**

An apical vaginal wall defect/prolapse in which bowel is contained within the prolapsed segment. See Fig. 6-2.

**Rectocele:**

A posterior vaginal wall defect/prolapse that includes the rectum. See Fig. 6-3.

**Uterine prolapse:**

An apical vaginal wall defect where the cervix/uterus descend with strain from its normal anatomic site. Sometimes associated with cervical elongation

**Vault prolapse:**

A defect of the apex of the vagina, most commonly found posthysterectomy

**Defects in which pelvic floor muscles/supporting structures allow POP?**

The uterosacral and cardinal ligaments, the levator ani muscles, and the endopelvic connective tissue. See Figs. 6-4 and 6-5.

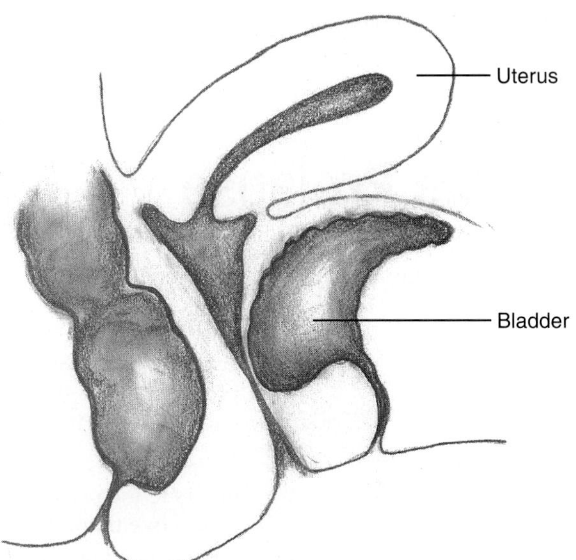


**Figure 6-1** Anterior vaginal prolapse—cystocele.

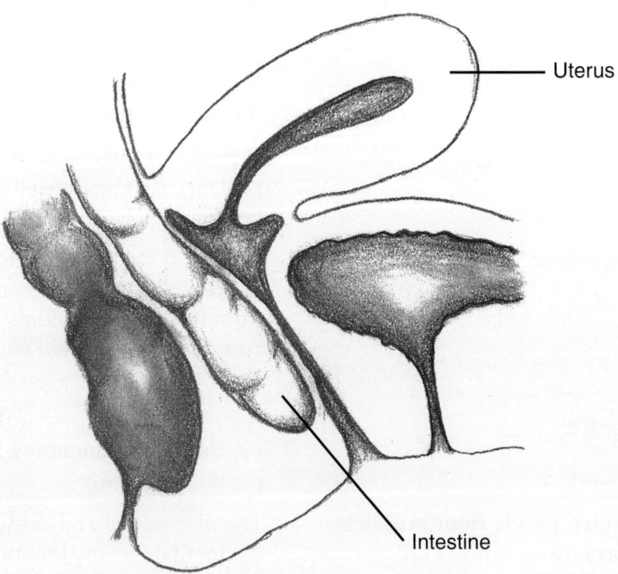


**Figure 6-2** Apical prolapse—enterocele.

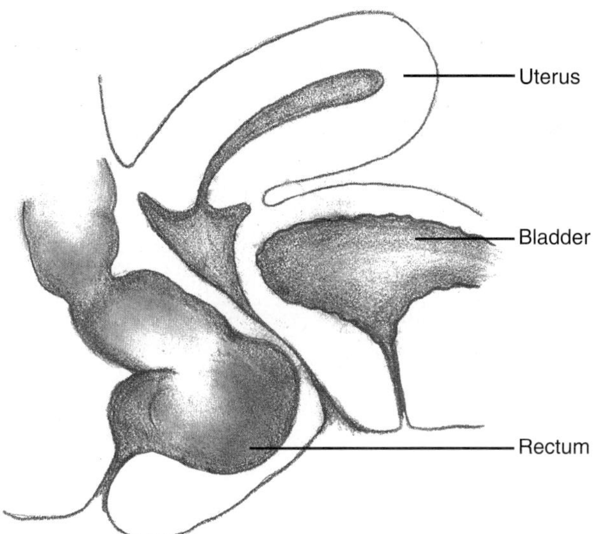


**Figure 6-3** Posterior vaginal wall prolapse—rectocele.

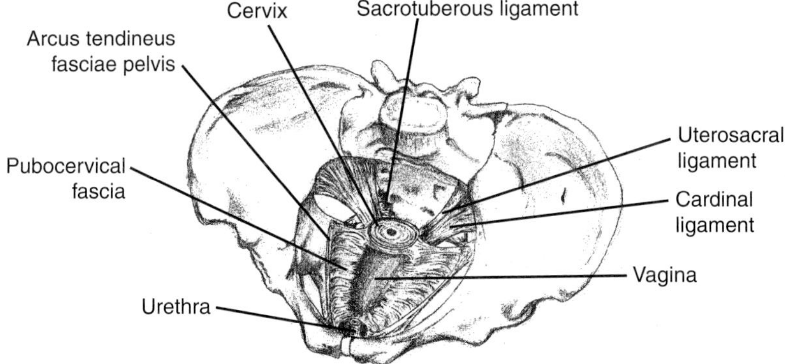


**Figure 6-4** Ligaments of the female pelvis.

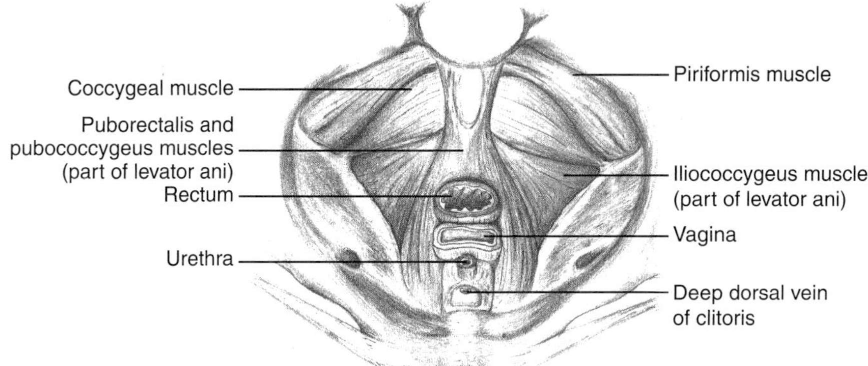


**Figure 6-5** Pelvic diaphragm—superior view.

**What are the risk factors for POP?**

Advancing age; multiparity (vaginal delivery route); obesity; history of pelvic surgery (particularly hysterectomy); increased intra-abdominal pressure (i.e., chronic straining during constipation, chronic coughing (COPD), heavy lifting); postpartum muscle weakness (i.e., levator ani); loss of innervation; connective tissue disorders; tumor/masses; genetic predisposition

**What is the most common symptom of POP?**

Many women are asymptomatic and are found to have prolapse on exam. **The most specific complaint for POP is when the woman can see or feel a bulge of tissue that protrudes to or past the vaginal opening.** Patients sometimes describe this as a pressure or heaviness. This may be relieved by lying down, may be less noticeable in the morning and worsen later in the day because of extended exertion or standing

**Other symptoms include:** stress incontinence, urinary frequency or hesitancy, feeling of incomplete emptying of the bladder, defecatory symptoms, coital laxity

**How is POP diagnosed?**

It is based upon the findings of physical examination. The patient should be examined in both upright and recumbent (dorsal lithotomy) positions and each area of vaginal anatomy should be described separately

**What are the grading systems used to evaluate and diagnose POP?**

While there are several different classifications, currently the two most commonly used are:

(1) The Pelvic Organ Prolapse Quantification (POPQ) system
(2) The Baden–Walker system

**What does the POPQ system involve?**

The POPQ system was created to use objective measurements in centimeters using the hymenal ring as a reference point. It involves quantitative measurements of various points representing anterior, apical, posterior, and basal vaginal prolapse. These points are then used to determine the stage of the prolapse

**Pro:** it is helpful in standardizing the reporting of prolapse outcomes by relying on objective measurements

**Con:** it can be confusing to those not familiar with the system

**Explain the Baden–Walker System**

It is a less detailed grading system for evaluation of POP displacement compared to the POPQ system, but it is still widely used in clinical practice. See Table 6-1

**Pro:** it is straightforward and familiar to most practitioners

**Con:** it uses a subjective description of the prolapse that is not quantifiable

**What is the management for women with asymptomatic POP?**

Reassurance and observation at regular intervals. Pelvic floor muscle exercises (i.e., Kegel exercises) can in theory be of some benefit by improving the tone of the muscular floor upon which the pelvic organs rest

**Table 6-1** Baden–Walker System for the Evaluation of POP on Physical Examination

| Grade | Displacement of Prolapse |
|---|---|
| 0 | No prolapse |
| 1 | Halfway to the hymen |
| 2 | At the hymen |
| 3 | Halfway out of the hymen |
| 4 | Total prolapse |

**What is the management for women with symptomatic POP?**

(1) Nonsurgical treatment such as pessaries and symptom-directed therapies (i.e., weight loss, pelvic floor muscles rehabilitation, behavior modifications)
(2) Surgical intervention

**What is a pessary?**

It is a prosthesis usually made out of rubber or silicone-based material with a spring frame that is placed in the vaginal vault to support the prolapsing vaginal walls or uterus. There are several types available which come in varying shapes and sizes. See Fig. 6-6.

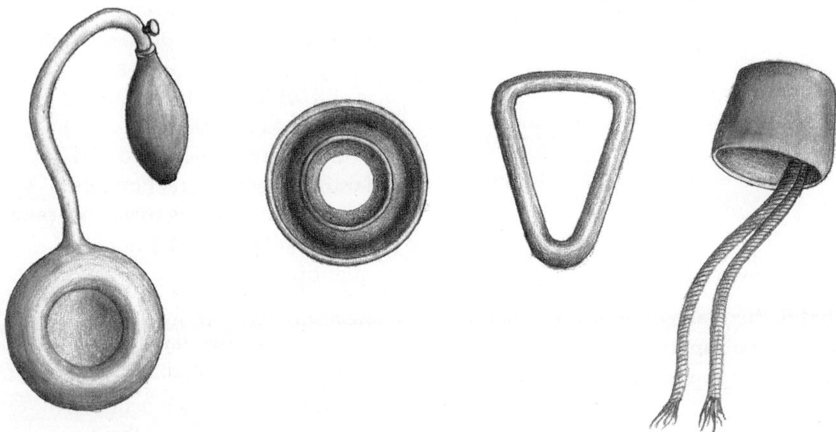

**Figure 6-6** Types of pessaries.

**When is a pessary contraindicated?**

There are few contraindications to using a pessary: allergy to the product material untreated vaginitis or pelvic inflammatory disease and in a patient who is unable/unlikely to follow up

**When is surgery indicated?**

When a patient is symptomatic from her prolapse and has been counseled regarding her treatment options

**What is the traditional procedure for an anterior vaginal prolapse (cystocele)? What does it involve?**

**Anterior vaginal colporrhaphy**. It involves dissecting the vaginal epithelium from the underlying fibromuscular connective tissue and bladder, and plicating the vaginal muscularis across the midline

**What is the traditional procedure for a posterior vaginal prolapse (rectocele)? What does it involve?**

**Posterior vaginal colporrhaphy.** It involves dissecting the vaginal epithelium from the underlying fibromuscular connective tissue and rectum, and plicating the vaginal muscularis across the midline.

If a site-specific defect is noted, this is repaired

**What are the different surgical options for treatment of an apical prolapse (enterocele)?**

**Colpocleisis:** usually reserved for severe uterovaginal prolapse. It is an obliterative procedure that closes off the genital hiatus, and therefore should only be considered in patients who do not desire future sexual intercourse. It is minimally invasive, so it is a good consideration for patients in whom major surgery is contraindicated

**Sacrospinous ligament fixation:** attachment of the vaginal apex to the sacrospinous ligament, usually unilaterally

**Iliococcygeus suspension:** attachment of the vaginal apex to the iliococcygeus muscle, either uni- or bilaterally

**Uterosacral ligament suspension:** attachment of the vaginal apex to the uterosacral ligament bilaterally

**Abdominal sacral colpopexy:** an abdominal procedure attaching the vaginal apex to the sacral promontory

**When is a hysterectomy warranted?**

For treatment of uterine prolapse or if concomitant uterine pathology is present at the time of prolapse surgery

# Urinary Incontinence

## INTRODUCTION

**Name the factors involved in normal urethral closure**

Extrinsic factors: the levator ani muscles, endopelvic fascia, ligamentous attachments
Intrinsic factors: striated and smooth muscle of the urethral wall, vascular congestion of the submucosal venous plexus, urethral epithelial folds, urethral elasticity, α-adrenergic receptors in the urethra (urethral tone)

**Describe the factors involved in normal bladder function**

Bladder filling: increased outlet resistance via muscle fiber recruitment; the detrusor is inactive

Full bladder: a micturition reflex is sent to the brain by tension-stretch receptors, cortical control mechanisms then permit or do not permit this reflex

Bladder emptying: voluntary relaxation of the pelvic floor and urethra, sustained contraction of the detrusor muscle

**Describe the action of the detrusor muscle?**

It is the **involuntary smooth muscle** wall of the bladder that **reflexively contracts** after voluntary relaxation of the pelvic floor and urethral musculature

**Describe the innervation to the lower urinary tract**

1. **Sympathetic** system—controls **bladder storage**
   a. α-receptors: located mainly in the urethra and bladder neck, stimulation increases urethral tone (promotes closure)
   b. β-receptors: located mainly in the bladder body, stimulation decreases bladder tone
2. **Parasympathetic** system—controls **bladder emptying**
   a. stimulation of muscarinic receptors increases bladder contraction

3. Somatic system—innervation of the pelvic floor and the external urethral sphincter

**What is the prevalence and incidence of urinary incontinence?**

Over 13 million Americans carry the diagnosis, with approximately 1 million new cases diagnosed each year

**What are some of the causes of urinary incontinence?**

Anatomic abnormalities; infection; drugs; atrophy; neurologic issues

**What is the differential diagnosis of urinary incontinence?**

Infection: cystitis

Anatomic: fistula (vesicovaginal or ureterovaginal), ectopic ureter

Neuro/Psych: dementia, normal pressure hydrocephalus

Medications: diuretics, caffeine, sedatives

Endocrine: diabetes mellitus, diabetes insipidus

**What is meant by the following symptoms?**

**Urgency:** sudden pressing desire to urinate

**Nocturia:** waking at night more than one time to urinate

**Overactive bladder:** a syndrome of urgency, frequency, and nocturia ± urge incontinence

**Continuous urinary incontinence:** constant dribbling of small amounts of urine

**Daytime frequency:** subjective voiding too often by day

**Name and describe the symptoms of the following major types of incontinence**

**Stress incontinence:** involuntary leakage with increased intra-abdominal pressure (e.g., with exertion, sneezing, or coughing)

**Urge incontinence:** involuntary leakage immediately preceeded by a feeling of urgency; often precipitated by running water, hand washing, or cold temperatures

**Mixed incontinence:** involuntary leakage associated with urgency and increased intra-abdominal pressure

**Overflow incontinence:** leakage associated with significant urinary retention which exceeds the storage capacity of the bladder (usually associated with neurogenic conditions)

**What type of incontinence do the following symptoms suggest?**

**Leakage when coughing/sneezing/laughing/exercising:** stress incontinence

**Leakage associated with a strong desire to void:** urge incontinence

**Many voids per day:** urge or overflow incontinence or possible infection

**Continual dripping with shifting positions:** overflow incontinence or sphincter impairment

**Nocturia or incontinence associated with intercourse:** urge incontinence

**Painful urination:** obstruction, infection, or urge incontinence

**What are the known risk factors for urinary incontinence?**

Childbearing; advanced age; obesity; family history; chronic cough; ascites; pelvic masses

**What age-related changes contribute to the development of urinary incontinence?**

1. The prevalence of detrusor overactivity increases with age
2. Total bladder capacity diminishes
3. Urinary flow rate decreases
4. Postvoiding residual increases
5. The urethral mucosal epithelium becomes atrophic secondary to low estrogen levels

**Is incontinence a part of normal aging?**

No, however the prevalence and severity of incontinence increases with age. Thus, patients should be queried regarding the presence of these symptoms. Infection should be ruled out when there is any sudden change or onset of incontinence symptoms

## PATIENT EVALUATION

**What are the pertinent factors to ask about when taking a history?**

Review of symptoms: how often leakage occurs, what provokes urine loss, how much urine is leaked, what makes the problem better/worse, any prior treatment that has been tried

General medical history: systemic illnesses (such as diabetes, vascular insufficiency, chronic pulmonary disease, or any neurologic condition)

Past surgical history

Current medications

**What types of medications can sometimes cause urinary incontinence?**

Benzodiazepines; α-agonists (OTC cold medications); α-antagonists (antihypertensives); calcium channel blockers; ACE inhibitors (by increasing cough); alcohol

**What should be done on physical examination and what tests should be done?**

**General examination:** look for signs of other medical problems as well as for alertness/functional status

**Pelvic examination:** look for signs of atrophy, infection, fistulae, diverticulum, pelvic organ prolapse

**Urinalysis:** routine urinalysis and culture, urine cytology (in women over 50 with urinary tract irritation or hematuria)

**Labs:** metabolic panel (renal function, glucose, calcium), vitamin $B_{12}$ (in the elderly), glucose

Measurement of **postvoid residual urine** (especially in high-risk patients)

Give out a frequency/volume **bladder diary** for the patient to record her symptoms

**What are normal values for the following?**

**Daily urine output:** 1500–2500 mL

**Average void volume:** 250 mL

**Functional bladder capacity:** 400–600 mL

**Voids per day:** 7–8 times

**Is routine urodynamic testing indicated in the evaluation of urinary incontinence?**

No. While it is the gold standard, it is not always necessary to make the diagnosis. It should be considered if empiric therapy has failed or prior to any surgical intervention

**Describe the following urodynamic tests:**

**Multichannel urodynamic testing:** produces a biophysical profile of the patient's bladder and urethra. Used for patients with mixed incontinence, prior bladder surgeries, or suspected intrinsic sphincter deficiency

**Cystometry:** measures the pressure-volume relationship of the bladder. **Filling cystometry** measures bladder pressure during filling; fluid is infused while pressure is continually monitored. The point of urgency, point of leakage, and total capacity are recorded. **Voiding cystometry** (also known as pressure-flow study) measures the urine flow rate and correlates it with the detrusor pressure

**Urethral pressure profile:** measures urethral closure and sphincteric integrity

**During a bladder filling test, what type of incontinence does a woman have if:**

**She feels urinary urgency and involuntary voiding upon filling?**

Urge incontinence

**She leaks small amounts upon coughing?**

Stress incontinence

## STRESS INCONTINENCE

**What are the typical symptoms of stress incontinence?**

Leakage of a small amount of urine with any activity that increases intra-abdominal pressure (coughing, sneezing, laughing, etc)

**What is the prevalence of stress incontinence?**

20–30% of women complain of stress incontinence. It is the **most common type** of urinary incontinence in younger women and the second most common cause of incontinence in older women

**Describe the pathophysiology of stress incontinence**

With weakening of the pelvic muscles and endofascia, **urethral support is impaired**. With rising intra-abdominal pressure (because of sneezing, coughing, or exercise), the intravesicular pressure rises higher than the pressure of the urethral closure mechanism, leading to urine leakage

**What are the risk factors for the development of stress incontinence?**

**Advanced age; Denervation and/or connective tissue injuries** from childbirth or surgery; **previous surgery for prolapse and/or incontinence; low estrogen levels; chronically increased intra-abdominal pressure; collagen vascular disorders**

**What is intrinsic urethral sphincter deficiency?**

A less common cause of stress incontinence wherein there is **complete failure of urethral closure**; usually because of **scarring** from a past operation or occasionally from severe atrophy in postmenopausal women

**Does demonstration of urine leakage during coughing always indicate stress incontinence?**

No. It could also be detrusor overactivity, detrusor hyperactivity with impaired contractility (DHIC), or overflow incontinence

**What is the Q-tip test?**

Insertion of a cotton swab into the urethra at the bladder neck. It is positive (indicates stress incontinence) if the angle of the cotton swab changes by more than 30° with strain

**How does the timing between the increased pressure and incontinence affect the diagnosis?**

**Immediate leakage** with pressure suggests **stress incontinence. A delay** between the maneuver and the leakage suggests **detrusor overactivity**

**What is the treatment for stress incontinence?**

Nonsurgical: muscle strengthening, pessaries, medications (usually ineffective)

Surgical: **pubovesical sling** or **collagen injections**

## URGE INCONTINENCE

**What are the typical symptoms of urge incontinence?**

Leakage of urine preceded by a feeling of urgency

**How common is urge incontinence?**

It is the second most common form of incontinence and the most common form of incontinence in older women

**Describe the pathophysiology of urge incontinence**

Involuntary **detrusor overactivity** or bladder contractions

**What are some of the causes of detrusor overactivity?**

**Advanced age; disruption of inhibitory pathways** (stroke, cervical stenosis, diabetes, Alzheimer disease, Parkinson disease); **bladder irritation** (infection, stones, cancer); **idiopathic**

**What is interstitial cystitis?**

A spectrum of symptoms, characterized by **urgency** and **frequent voiding of small amounts** of urine and often associated with dysuria or pain. Most commonly diagnosed in younger women

**What is DHIC?**

Detrusor hyperactivity with impaired contractility. It is characterized by both urgency and an elevated post-void residual

**What is the treatment for urge incontinence?**

Behavioral: bladder retraining

Medication: anticholinergics and/or β-adrenergics; botox injections into the detrusor

Surgical: neuromodulation implants; surgical denervation (usually ineffective); correction pelvic organ prolapse if significant

## MIXED INCONTINENCE

**What are the symptoms of mixed incontinence?**

Leakage associated with urgency and with increased intra-abdominal pressure

**Describe the pathophysiology of mixed incontinence**

Combination of both **detrusor overactivity and stress incontinence, sometimes compounded by impaired urethral sphincter function**

**What is the treatment for mixed incontinence?**

Individualized care based on the primary complaint and the individual's characteristics

## OVERFLOW INCONTINENCE

**What are the symptoms of overflow incontinence?**

Continual **dribbling** associated with incomplete bladder emptying

**Describe the pathophysiology of overflow incontinence**

There is **underactivity of the detrusor muscle** resulting in failure of full bladder emptying. This leaves a **large postvoid residual** which leads to leakage with increased intra-abdominal pressure. It can also be caused by bladder outlet **obstruction**, usually in women with significant pelvic organ prolapse

**What are some of the causes of underactivity of the detrusor muscle?**

Neurogenic bladder (e.g., from diabetes, vitamin $B_{12}$ deficiency, Parkinson's disease); prior bladder surgery; chronic, long-standing overdistention

## TREATMENT

**What are the three categories of treatment options for urinary incontinence?**

Lifestyle/behavioral changes; medications; surgery (should be tried in that order)

**What types of lifestyle changes are associated with an improvement in urinary incontinence?**

1. Limiting fluid intake (no more than 2 L/day)
2. Avoidance of caffeine and alcohol
3. Smoking cessation
4. Treatment of cough (for stress incontinence)
5. Treatment of constipation
6. Weight loss and increased physical activity

**What types of behavioral changes are associated with an improvement in urinary incontinence?**

**Bladder training; pelvic muscle exercises**

**Describe bladder training**

**Timed voiding** while awake, with gradually increasing intervals between voids; **relaxation and distractive techniques** to suppress urgency in between voids

**What is the theory behind bladder training?**

The central nervous system and pelvic musculature can be **trained to inhibit detrusor contractions by becoming gradually accustomed to accommodating larger bladder volumes**

**What is supplemental biofeedback?**

Vaginal or anorectal biofeedback mechanisms used to help patients identify and use their pelvic musculature in response to a sense of urgency. It can be used as a primary therapy or as a supplement to either medication or bladder training therapy

**For which type of incontinence is bladder training most useful?**

Urge incontinence

**What are pelvic muscle exercises?**

Also known as **Kegel** exercises, they involve isometric repetitions of exercises in order to strengthen the levator ani muscles, which support the pelvic organs and significantly contribute to urethral closure mechanisms

**For which types of incontinence are pelvic muscle exercises effective?**

Urge, stress, or mixed incontinence

**In which types of incontinence is pharmacotherapy warranted?**

Urge and mixed incontinence. They are often ineffective in treating stress incontinence

**What types of medications are used to treat urinary incontinence?**

Antimuscarinics: oxybutynin; tolterodine; trospium; solifenacin; darifenacine

α-adrenergic agonists: duloxetine; tricyclic antidepressants (TCAs) (imipramine); topical estrogens; botulinum toxin

**What is a continence pessary?**

A device that can be used to treat incontinence because of pelvic floor prolapse

**What types of surgical options are effective for urge incontinence?**

Sacral nerve modulation; augmentation cystoplasty

**What types of surgical options are effective for stress incontinence?**

1. Minimally invasive midurethral anti-incontinence procedures

| | |
|---|---|
| | 2. Retropubic bladder neck suspension (Burch or Marshall–Marchetti–Krantz [MMK] colposuspension)<br>3. Sling procedures<br>4. Periurethral bulking injections |
| **Should an indwelling urinary catheter be used to alleviate symptoms of incontinence?** | As these are associated with high morbidity, they should only be considered in select cases as a last resort |
| **Describe the midurethral anti-incontinence procedures** | These are minimally invasive, vaginal surgical procedures using synthetic mesh material placed at the level of the midurethra in a tension-free manner |
| **What complications are associated with the midurethral anti-incontinence procedures?** | Postoperative voiding dysfunction<br>Urinary retention<br>Erosion of mesh material |
| **Describe the retropubic bladder neck suspension procedures** | An abdominal procedure that uses the periurethral vaginal tissue to support the urethrovesical junction via sutures to Cooper's ligament (Burch) or to the pubic symphysis (MMK) |
| **What complications are associated with the retropubic bladder neck suspension procedure?** | Enterocele formation; postoperative voiding dysfunction; urinary retention |
| **Describe suburethral sling procedures** | Elevation of the urethrovesical junction and introduction of mechanical compression of the urethra using autologous or synthetic graft material |
| **What are the complications of a sling procedure?** | Postoperative voiding dysfunction; urinary retention; erosion of graft material |
| **Describe periurethral bulking agents procedures** | Elevation of the urethrovesical junction and introduction of mechanical compression of the urethra using autologous or synthetic graft material |

CHAPTER 7

# Reproductive Endocrinology and Infertility

## Adolescent Development

### INTRODUCTION

**What types of changes occur during puberty?**

1. Development of secondary sexual characteristics
2. Growth
3. Changes in body composition
4. Achievement of fertility

**What is meant by the following terms?**

1. **Thelarche:** breast development
2. **Pubarche:** development of pubic hair
3. **Menarche:** beginning of menses

**What is the typical sequence of events in puberty for girls?**

**Thelarche** (breast development) → **pubarche** (pubic hair growth) → peak growth spurt → **menarche**

**What is the average time duration of puberty and when does it start?**

4.5 years is the average duration of puberty. On an average, thelarche begins at 10 years and menarche at 12 years of age

**What are the Tanner stages?**

A **staging system** for the sequence of **pubertal development**. Divides the development of secondary sex characteristics into five stages

**Describe the Tanner stages for breast development in females**

1. Stage 1: Prepubertal
2. Stage 2: Elevation of breast and papilla; enlargement of areola; breast bud stage
3. Stage 3: Further enlargement of breast and areola; increased glandular tissue
4. Stage 4: Areola and papilla project above the breast
5. Stage 5: Recession of areola, projection of papilla only, mature stage

**Describe the Tanner stages for pubic hair development**

1. Stage 1: Velus hairs only, prepubertal
2. Stage 2: Sparse growth of slightly pigmented hair
3. Stage 3: Hair growth spreads and becomes darker, coarser, and more curly
4. Stage 4: Adult hair type, but no spread to medial thigh
5. Stage 5: Medial spread with inverse triangle distribution

**What happens to the external genitalia during puberty?**

**Estrogen stimulation** leads to thickening of the mons pubis, growth of the labia majora, rounding of the labia minora, thickening of the hymen, elongation of the vagina

**What happens to the uterus during puberty?**

The myometrium thickens, altering the uterine shape. The endometrium thickens gradually and then more rapidly before menarche

**Describe the pattern of growth that occurs in puberty**

Growth affects both the trunk and the limbs, with the limbs (especially the distal portions thereof) growing before the rest of the body. Girls have their growth spurt before boys and the peak growth occurs approximately 6 months prior to menarche

**What happens to the long bones during puberty?**

Long bones lengthen and their epiphyses close

**What are some of the unwelcome physiological changes that occur as a result of puberty?**

Acne; psychological changes—boys develop a more positive and girls experience a diminished self-image; scoliosis; myopia

## CONGENITAL ANOMALIES

| | |
|---|---|
| **What is suggested by clitoral enlargement?** | Exposure to high levels of **androgens**. Proper evaluation to exclude any intersex conditions is warranted |
| **What is imperforate hymen?** | **A persistent urogenital membrane** |
| **What are the symptoms of an imperforate hymen?** | It is rare to make this diagnosis before puberty. Symptoms include **primary amenorrhea, pelvic pain,** and difficulty with urination/defecation |
| **What are some of the potential complications associated with an untreated imperforate hymen?** | Endometriosis and vaginal adenosis |
| **What is a vaginal septum?** | An absence of fusion of the müllerian ducts and/or urogenital sinuses leading to an obstructive lesion in the vagina. This leads to obstructive symptoms similar to those of an imperforate hymen |
| **What is vaginal agenesis?** | Usually associated with Mayer-Rokitansky-Kuster-Hauser syndrome. It involves normal-appearing external genitalia with agenesis of the vagina superior to the hymen. It is usually associated with uterine and cervical agenesis. Also associated with testicular feminization, yet these patients have testes instead of ovaries and need to have them removed |
| **What are the symptoms of vaginal agenesis?** | **Primary amenorrhea** and **pelvic pain** |
| **How is vaginal agenesis treated?** | Creation of a vagina by use of either **serial vaginal dilation** or surgical reconstruction with a **vaginoplasty procedure** |
| **What are the various congenital anomalies of the uterus and how common are each? Describe each** | Arcuate uterus (15%): small septum with minimal cavity indentation<br>Incomplete septum (13%): partial fusion resulting in a septum that does not completely divide the horns |

Complete uterine septum (9%): partial fusion that completely divides the uterine horns

Bicornate uterus (37%): partial fusion leading to a midline septum (can be partial or complete)

Uterine didelphys (11%): failure of fusion resulting in two separate uterine bodies

Unicornuate uterus (4%): agenesis of one Müllerian duct, with an absence of the corresponding fallopian tube and round ligament

**What are the symptoms of these uterine anomalies?**

Usually asymptomatic; can occasionally cause **retention of menstrual flow** or **infertility**

**What does the palpation of an inguinal mass in an adolescent patient suggest?**

Possible aberrant gonad (often with testicular elements)

**How should an aberrant gonad be managed?**

A **karyotype** should be done and a **biopsy** of the gonad should be done. If it is an ovary, it should be returned to the peritoneal cavity. If it is a testis, it should be removed

## ACCELERATED SEXUAL MATURATION

**What is premature thelarche and how is it managed?**

Isolated development of breasts before 8 years of age. No intervention is required if other signs of precocious puberty do not develop

**What is premature pubarche and how is it managed?**

Isolated appearance of public or axillary hair before 6–7 years of age. It generally represents premature secretion of androgens from the adrenal gland. Evaluation of the adrenal and gonadal function should be done to exclude precocious puberty

**What is premature menarche and how is it managed?**

Isolated cyclic vaginal bleeding without any other signs of sexual development. It is usually related to increased end-organ sensitivity to estrogen and it does not require any intervention

| | |
|---|---|
| **What is sexual precocity?** | Onset of sexual maturation before 2.5 times the standard deviation of the normal age for that population |
| **How is precocious puberty classified?** | GnRH dependent and GnRH independent |
| **What is GnRH-dependent precocious puberty?** | Also called central precocious puberty (CPP); premature activation of the hypothalamic-pituitary axis with premature gonadotropin secretion |
| **What is GnRH-independent precocious puberty?** | Sex steroids are present independent of the release of pituitary gonadotropins. This is a pseudoprecocious puberty |
| **What are some of the causes of GnRH-independent precocious puberty?** | Congenital adrenal hyperplasia; tumors of the adrenal gland; tumors of the gonads; hCG-secreting tumors; mcCune-Albright syndrome; Exogenous steroids |
| **What is the workup for precocious puberty?** | 1. History: age of onset, progression, family history<br>2. Physical examination (PE): growth velocity changes, acne, breast development, genital changes<br>3. Laboratory: luteinizing hormone (**LH**), follicle-stimulating hormone (**FSH**), **estradiol**, **GnRH-stimulation test**<br>4. Imaging: skeletal survey and **bone scan** to determine bone age, pelvic ultrasound, abdominal CT (of adrenals), brain MRI |
| **What are the results of the laboratory tests in GnRH-dependent precocious puberty?** | Normal pubertal range |
| **What is the treatment for GnRH-dependent precocious puberty?** | GnRH analogues, which induce down-regulation of the receptor function, creating an inhibition of the hypothalamic-pituitary-ovarian axis |
| **What is McCune-Albright syndrome?** | A genetic disorder with a classic triad of **precocious puberty**, polyostotic **fibrous dysplasia**, and **café-au-lait skin lesions** |

## DELAYED SEXUAL MATURATION

**What is delayed sexual maturation?**

Absence of pubertal changes after 2.5 times the standard deviation of the mean age for a population (e.g., absence of thelarche by age 13 and menarche by age 15)

**What is the proper evaluation for a patient with delayed sexual maturation?**

1. History: previous growth patterns and pubertal development, other medical disorders
2. PE: height and weight, Tanner staging, pelvic examination (for congenital anomalies and obstruction)
3. Labs/imaging: vaginal smear (for cytohormonal evaluation), karyotype, pelvic ultrasound, FSH

**What does breast development signify?**

Prior gonadal function

**What does the absence of pubic hair signify?**

Androgen insensitivity

**What is the differential diagnosis of a patient with delayed menarche and adequate secondary sexual characteristics?**

Pregnancy; anatomic genital abnormalities; inappropriate positive feedback; complete androgen insensitivity syndrome

**How are patients with delayed menarche and inadequate secondary sexual characteristics classified?**

By their FSH level

**What is the differential diagnosis of a patient with delayed menarche and inadequate secondary sexual characteristics?**

Low FSH: constitutional delay; weight loss (extreme dieting, drug abuse, extreme exercise); kallman syndrome; pituitary destruction
High FSH: Turner syndrome; Ovarian destruction (chemotherapy, radiation, infection, autoimmune); Resistant ovary syndrome

**What is Kallman syndrome?**

A rare genetic syndrome causing **hypogonadotropic hypogonadism** and **anosmia**

**What is the differential diagnosis of a patient with delayed menarche and virilization?**

1. Enzyme deficiency (such as 21α-hydroxylase deficiency)
2. Neoplasia
3. Male pseudohermaphroditism

# Disorders of the Menstrual Cycle, Uterus, and Endometrium

## PMS

**What is premenstrual syndrome?**

Premenstrual syndrome (PMS) is a cyclical pattern of **emotional, physical, and/or behavioral** changes that occur in the **luteal phase** of the menstrual cycle and remit during menses. Symptoms cause **significant disability**, and it is *not* an exacerbation of an underlying psychiatric disorder. It is best characterized as an abnormal response to normally fluctuating hormones. A more severe variant is described in the *Diagnostic and Statistical Manual of Mental Disorders*, Fourth Edition (DSM-IV) as **premenstrual dysphoric disorder**.

**What is the incidence of PMS and in whom does it occur?**

The reported incidence of PMS ranges from 5% to 90% of women. Approximately 70% have some symptoms of PMS and 5% have the more severe PMDD. It occurs mostly in women in their mid-20s to 40s

**What are the symptoms of PMS?**

PMS is characterized by various constellations of symptoms including at least one of the following which is temporally related to the menstrual cycle:

1. **Affective lability**
2. **Anxiety or tension**
3. **Depressed mood, hopelessness,** or **self-deprecating thoughts**
4. **Persistent anger** or **irritability**

Other symptoms include decreased interest/avoidance of usual activities, decreased productivity, lethargy, changes in appetite/cravings, reproducible patterns of physical complaints (such as headaches, weight gain, breast tenderness), difficulty concentrating, sleep disturbances (hypersomnia or insomnia), and a sense of being overwhelmed

**How is PMS diagnosed?**

The patient is asked to keep a daily **menstrual diary** to document her symptoms and their severity. The patient must demonstrate at least 5 of the above symptoms. She also must demonstrate a **symptom-free follicular phase** and problems with notable changes in the **luteal phase**. A comprehensive history and physical examination must be done to rule out any other illness

**What are the treatment options for PMS?**

**Education** of the patient and her family, **dietary changes** (emphasizing fresh foods), **exercise**, medications to **prevent ovulation** (such as oral contraceptive pills), **progesterone suppositories**, **NSAIDs**, **diuretics**, **anxiolytic/antidepressant medications**, and **vitamin** $B_6$. **GnRH agonists** and surgical intervention are a last resort for severe refractory PMS

## Dysmenorrhea

**What is dysmenorrhea and what are the two types?**

Dysmenorrhea is **pain with menses** either due to **pelvic pathology** (**secondary dysmenorrhea**) or **without pelvic pathology** (**primary dysmenorrhea**)

**What is the incidence of dysmenorrhea and in whom does it occur?**

Dysmenorrhea occurs in approximately **15% to 75% of women. Primary dysmenorrhea** is most common in **younger** women, whereas the incidence of **secondary dysmenorrhea** increases with age

**What is the etiology of primary dysmenorrhea?**

Primary dysmenorrhea is caused by an excess of **prostaglandin** $F_{2\alpha}$ produced in the endometrium. It stimulates smooth muscle, leading to uterine contractions and uterine ischemia

**What are the clinical signs and symptoms of primary dysmenorrhea?**

Pain typically begins **at menstruation** and subsides after

1–3 days. It is characterized as **cramping, labor-like pain**, typically in the **lower abdomen** and **suprapubic** area, radiating to the back. The pain can be associated with **nausea, vomiting**, and **diarrhea**. **Fatigue** and **headache** are often also associated. In general, the physical examination is normal

**What is the treatment of primary dysmenorrhea?**

**NSAID** therapy is first line. Other options include **heat, exercise**, and **oral contraceptives**. In severe, refractory cases, **presacral neurectomy** is a last resort. However, secondary dysmenorrhea should be suspected if symptoms are refractory to NSAIDs or OCPs

**How do NSAIDs and OCPs work to treat dysmenorrhea?**

**NSAIDs** work by **inhibiting prostaglandin production**. **OCPs** work by **decreasing prostaglandin production** through suppression of ovulation

**What are the gynecologic causes of secondary dysmenorrhea?**

**Extrauterine causes:** Endometriosis

Neoplasm
Inflammation (e.g., PID)
Adhesions
**Intramural causes:** Adenomyosis
Leiomyomata

**Intrauterine causes:** Leiomyomata
Polyps
IUDs
Infection
Cervical stenosis/lesions

**For a patient with dysmenorrhea, what primary diagnosis do each of the following findings suggest:**

**Uterine asymmetry**

Myomas or other tumors

**Symmetrical enlargement of uterus**

Adenomyosis

**Painful nodules in posterior cul-de-sac**

Endometriosis

**Restricted motion of the uterus**

Endometriosis or pelvic scarring/adhesions from prior infection

**What is the treatment for secondary dysmenorrhea?**

Treatment of the underlying condition is the primary modality.

However, when this is not possible, **NSAIDs** and low-dose **oral contraceptives** offer symptomatic therapy

**What other underlying diseases are exacerbated by menstruation?**

Women with **migraines**, tension, or vascular can have increased frequency of headaches at the time of menstruation. Asthma patients occasionally report worsening of symptoms with menses. These effects are thought to be due to increased prostaglandin production

## DYSFUNCTIONAL UTERINE BLEEDING

**Describe what is meant by the following patterns of abnormal bleeding:**

**Hypomenorrhea**

A **decreased amount** of bleeding at **regular intervals**

**Intermenstrual bleeding**

Bleeding of variable amounts occurring **between regular menstrual periods**

**Menorrhagia**

**Prolonged or excessive** uterine bleeding occurring at **regular** intervals. Synonymous with **hypermenorrhea**

**Metrorrhagia**

Uterine bleeding occurring at **irregular intervals**

**Polymenorrhea**

Uterine bleeding occurring at **intervals of less than 21 days**

**Oligomenorrhea**

**Menstrual bleeding** at intervals of **longer than 35 days**

**What is dysfunctional uterine bleeding?**

Dysfunctional uterine bleeding (DUB) is a diagnosis of exclusion that consists of **irregular menstruation unrelated to anatomic lesions***

**What is the physiologic cause of DUB?**

Women with DUB may be in a **hyperestrogenic** state. Because of

*Patients may also bleed from lack of estrogen (atrophy), or too much or too little progesterone

**anovulation**, these women have **noncyclic estrogen** levels that **stimulate endometrial growth**. Once the **endometrium outgrows its blood supply**, it sloughs off, leading to irregular, often heavy bleeding

**How can you clinically differentiate between ovulatory cycles and anovulatory cycles?**

**Ovulatory cycles** are **regular** in their length, duration of menses, and amount of bleeding. Anovulatory cycle bleeding is much more **irregular**

**What must be ruled out before the diagnosis of DUB can be made?**

**Organic causes of abnormal bleeding** such as **leiomyomas**, **inflammation** (cervicitis, endometritis), **carcinomas**, **cervical/endometrial polyps**, **vaginal lesions**, **blood dyscrasia**, and **iatrogenic causes** (IUDs, fertility drugs)

**Note: Abnormal uterine bleeding in a postmenopausal woman is cancer until proven otherwise**

**What conditions are often associated with DUB?**

**Obesity**

**Polycystic ovarian disease**

**Adrenal hyperplasia**

**Perimenopause**

**In whom does DUB occur?**

**Half** of all patients with DUB are **peri- or postmenopausal**. Another **20%** are **adolescents**

**What type of bleeding pattern is seen in women with high estrogen levels and with low estrogen levels?**

**High** levels of **estrogen** cause the endometrium to build up beyond its blood supply. This leads to **prolonged amenorrhea followed by profuse bleeding**

**Low** levels of **estrogen** cause **intermittent spotting of a prolonged duration, but can cause heavy bleeding from denuded, dysynchronous endometrium**

**What is the initial workup for abnormal bleeding?**

All women with abnormal uterine bleeding need a thorough **menstrual**

**history**, **bimanual examination**, and **Pap smear**. A TSH may also be ordered as thyroid disease can affect bleeding patterns.

**In each scenario, what additional tests should be done and why?**

**An ovulatory woman**

**Transvaginal ultrasound**, **sonohysterogram**, or **D&C with hysteroscopy** (gold standard) should be done to rule out anatomic causes of abnormal bleeding

**An anovulatory woman**

**β-hCG:** pregnancy

**CBC:** infection

**Coagulation profile:** blood dyscrasia

**Endocrine tests** (FSH, LH, TSH, prolactin): premature ovarian failure, polycystic ovarian syndrome (PCOS), prolactinoma, hypothyroidism

**All postmenopausal women**

**Endometrial biopsy:** endometrial carcinoma

**What are the risks of unrecognized DUB?**

**Hemorrhage**, **endometrial hyperplasia**, and/or **cancer**

**What is the goal of treatment for DUB?**

**To convert the proliferative endometrium into secretory endometrium**

**How is anovulatory DUB treated?**

Anovulatory DUB is treated with **OCPs** or **cyclic progesterone therapy** (such as medroxyprogesterone daily for 10 days of each month)

DUB associated with heavy bleeding is treated with **high-dose estrogen or progestins. Endometrial ablation** can also be used for treatment if patient is refractory to oral and IV estrogen therapy. A **D&C** can be done if patient is hemodynamically unstable

**How is ovulatory DUB treated?**

Ovulatory DUB is treated primarily with OCPs

## AMENORRHEA

**What is amenorrhea and what are the two subtypes?**

Amenorrhea is the **absence of menstruation**. It can be subdivided into two subtypes. If a woman has **never menstruated**, she has **primary amenorrhea,** whereas if she has previously menstruated but has **failed to menstruate within 6 months** or **for 3 cycle intervals** she has **secondary amenorrhea**

**What are the four main etiologies of amenorrhea?**

**Pregnancy:** Since it is the most common cause of amenorrhea, this is an essential diagnosis to exclude via a pregnancy test

**Hypothalamic-pituitary dysfunction:** When the pulsatile secretion of GnRH is altered, the pituitary gland ceases secreting FSH and LH. This results in the absence of regular ovulation and menstruation. Most hypothalamic-pituitary dysfunction is of functional origin

**Ovarian dysfunction:** The ovarian follicles are resistant to stimulation by FSH and LH

**Anatomic dysfunction:** Genital outflow tract obstruction can be congenital or from the development of scar tissue. The most common cause of obstruction is scarring of the uterine cavity (Asherman syndrome)

**What are the common causes of hypothalamic-pituitary dysfunction?**

Functional: Weight loss

Excessive exercise
Obesity
Drug induced: Marijuana
Sedatives

Malignancy: Prolactinoma
Craniopharyngioma
Hypothalamic hamartoma
Psychogenic: Anxiety
Anorexia
Other: Head injury

Chronic disease
Empty sella syndrome
Sheehan syndrome

**How is amenorrhea due to hypothalamic-pituitary dysfunction diagnosed?**

A history of any of the above conditions suggests this etiology. However, **low serum levels** of **FSH** and **LH** are diagnostic. **Prolactin** is usually normal, except in a prolactinoma

**What are the common causes of ovarian dysfunction that lead to primary amenorrhea?**

Gonadal dysgenesis: Turner syndrome
Mosaicism
17-hydroxylase deficiency

Gonadal agenesis

**What are the common causes of ovarian dysfunction that lead to secondary amenorrhea?**

Pregnancy

Menopause

Autoimmune ovarian failure (Blizzard syndrome)

Premature ovarian failure

Alkylating chemotherapy

**How is amenorrhea due to ovarian dysfunction diagnosed?**

As the ovaries fail, serum FSH level rises

**How can estrogen deficiency due to hypothalamic-pituitary failure be differentiated from that due to ovarian failure?**

Estrogen deficiency secondary to **hypothalamic-pituitary failure** usually does **not** cause **hot flashes**. **Ovarian failure** may **cause hot flashes**

**What genital outflow obstructions lead to primary amenorrhea?**

Müllerian anomalies (e.g., imperforate hymen)
Müllerian agenesis

**What genital outflow obstructions lead to secondary amenorrhea?**

Asherman syndrome

**What laboratory tests are indicated in the evaluation of a patient with secondary amenorrhea?**

**β-hCG**

**TSH**

**Prolactin**

**FSH**

**Progesterone challenge test**

**What diagnoses are suggested by the following lab results:**

**↑ β-hCG?**

Pregnancy

**↑ TSH?**

Hypothyroidism

| | |
|---|---|
| **↑ Prolactin?** | Hyperprolactinemia from a pituitary tumor, idiopathic, or due to medications (e.g., dopamine antagonists) |
| **↑ FSH ?** | Postmenopausal state or ovarian failure |
| **↓ FSH ?** | Hypothalamic disorder or pituitary dysfunction |
| | **Key: In general, if the gonadotropins are high, the problem is at the level of the ovary. If the gonadotropins are low, the problem is in the hypothalamus or pituitary** |
| **What further test must be done if the patient is found to be hypogonadotropic?** | Imaging of the sella turcica, either via **CT scan** or **MRI**. Abnormal imaging suggests a pituitary tumor, whereas normal imaging is assumed to signify a hypothalamic problem |
| **What further test must be done if the patient is found to be hypergonadotropic?** | A **karyotype** to diagnose mosaicism with a Y chromosome |
| **What is the progesterone challenge test and what is the procedure?** | A test done if all the preceding lab test are found to be normal. It assesses if an amenorrheic patient has **adequate estrogen** levels and an **intact outflow tract**. The patient is given oral **progesterone**. **Withdrawal bleeding** is observed after a few days |
| **What does withdrawal bleeding in the progesterone challenge test indicate?** | Withdrawal bleeding indicates that the patient is **chronically anovulatory** or **oligo-ovulatory**. Ovulation had not occurred and so no endogenous progesterone was made. The exogenous progesterone allowed menses to occur after withdrawal. Causes of anovulation include hypothalamic dysfunction, polycystic ovarian syndrome, Cushing syndrome, or an ovarian tumor |
| **What does the absence of withdrawal bleeding in the progesterone challenge test indicate?** | The absence of withdrawal bleeding indicates that the patient is either **hypoestrogenic** or has an **anatomic obstruction** |
| **What is the next step if withdrawal bleeding does not occur?** | An **estrogen-progesterone test, imaging** |

**What is an estrogen-progesterone test and what do the results indicate?**

The estradiol and progesterone test entails giving a small dose of **estradiol daily for 28 days** and adding **progesterone for the last 7 days**. This differentiates a hypoestrogenic state from an anatomic obstruction. **Withdrawal bleeding** indicates **inadequate estrogen**. If withdrawal bleeding does **not** occur within a few days, **anatomic obstruction** is the diagnosis

**What is the treatment for amenorrhea due to the following?**

**Hypothalamic anovulation?**

Induction of ovulation with **gonadotropins if pregnancy desired, otherwise OCPs**

**A prolactinoma?**

**Dopamine agonists. Rarely, surgical excision**

**Premature ovarian failure?**

Exogenous **estrogen** replacement

**Genital tract obstruction?**

**Surgery** to restore genital tract integrity

# Infertility

## EVALUATION OF INFERTILITY

**How is infertility defined?**

It is defined as the **inability to conceive after 12 months** of frequent intercourse without use of contraception

**What is the definition of fecundability?**

It is the probability of achieving pregnancy in one menstrual cycle

**What is the prevalence of infertility?**

About 13%, with a range from 7% to 28% depending on the age of the woman

**What is the difference between primary and secondary infertility?**

Primary infertility pertains to those who have never conceived, whereas secondary infertility is applied to those who have conceived in the past

**What percent of infertility is because of male factors, female factors, both and unknown etiology?**

1. Male factor (23%)
2. Female factors (40–50%)
3. Both (27%)
4. Unknown etiology (15–20%)

**What are the most common factors that comprise female factor infertility?**

- Ovulatory disorders (25%)
- Endometriosis (15%)
- Pelvic adhesions (12%)
- Tubal blockage (11%)
- Other tubal abnormalities (11%)
- Hyperprolactinemia (7%)

**What is the first test to perform for infertility if the history and physical from the infertile couple offer no clues?**

Semen analysis

**What are the relevant characteristics of normal semen?**

Volume: 2–5 mL

Concentration: ≥20 million per mL

Motility: 50% should be motile, 25% should have rapid progressive motility

Morphology: lower limit of normal is 10–15%

**What hormone tests should be ordered if the sperm concentration is less than 5 million per ml?**

Follicle-stimulating hormone (FSH), luteinizing hormone (LH), and testosterone

**What is the next step in evaluation of infertility if the semen analysis is normal?**

Ovulatory function

**What percent of female factor fertility can be attributed to ovulatory dysfunction?**

25%

**What are risk factors for premature ovarian failure?**

Exposure to cytotoxic drugs, pelvic radiation therapy, autoimmune diseases, previous ovarian surgery, family history of early menopause

**What are the methods to evaluate ovulatory function?**

Menstrual history, basal-body-temperature (BBT) chart, serum progesterone levels in the mid-luteal phase, sonogram, and/or endometrial biopsy

**How is anovulation classified and what is the mechanism of that type of anovulation?**

1. **Hypogonadotropic hypogonadal anovulation (hypothalamic amenorrhea)**—low secretion of GnRH or pituitary unresponsiveness to GnRH, resulting in low serum FSH and estradiol levels. Can be seen in stress- or exercise-related amenorrhea, anorexia nervosa, Kallman syndrome, or CNS tumors

2. **Normogonadotropic normoestrogenic anovulation**—most prevalent subtype. Normal GnRH secretion, estradiol and FSH levels with either normal or elevated LH concentrations. Includes women with polycystic ovary syndrome (PCOS)
3. **Hypergonadotropic hypoestrogenic anovulation**—ovarian failure is the primary cause
4. **Hyperprolactinemic anovulation**—hyperprolactinemia inhibits gonadotropin and, therefore, estrogen secretion

**What other endocrine abnormalities may result in infertility?**

Hypothyroidism, androgen excess, diabetes/obesity, starvation

**How do each of these methods help evaluate a woman's ovulatory function?**

A **menstrual cycle history** that reveals amenorrhea indicates anovulation and a cause of infertility, whereas a normal monthly menstrual cycle is a strong indicator of normal ovulation

A **basal-body-temperature chart** that indicates normal ovulation is reflected by a biphasic curve during ovulation, with a rise in temperature by 0.5–1.0°F during the luteal phase (because of an increased level of progesterone). The highest temperature in one menstrual cycle occurs during ovulation

**Urinary LH kits.** Over-the-counter monitors that detect the LH surge in the urine. This method allows for appropriate timing of intercourse

Measurement of a **serum progesterone level in the mid-luteal phase** (18–24 days after the onset of menses) is the definitive confirmation for ovulation. Normal levels are between >5 ng/mL

**Sonogram and/or endometrial biopsy** may be used to evaluate whether the endometrium is optimal for normal implantation of the egg

**If a female's ovulatory function is intact, what other factors may cause female factor infertility and what is their relative frequency?**

1. Tubal damage (14%)
2. Endometriosis (9%)
3. Coital problems (5%)
4. Cervical factor (3%)

**What is the major cause of tubal infertility and by what method may tubal abnormalities and/or other uterine cavity abnormalities be evaluated?**

Pelvic inflammatory disease. Hysterosalpingogram should be obtained for evaluation

**What are other causes of tubal infertility?**

Prior abdominal or pelvic surgery, ectopic pregnancy, severe endometriosis

**When should laparoscopy be used?**

It should be considered for couples with otherwise unexplained infertility or in women with known or suspected endometriosis and/or pelvic adhesions

**How should a woman who presents with infertility and early stage endometriosis be treated for fertility?**

Surgical resection of endometriosis lesions and other pelvic adhesions, followed by a trial of clomiphene or gonadotropin plus IUI (intrauterine insemination)

**What is meant by assessing a female's ovarian reserve and what are the most commonly used tests to evaluate this?**

This assessment is to determine quantity and possibly quality of remaining oocyte pool. The most commonly used tests are the day 3 FSH test and the clomiphene citrate challenge test (CCCT)

## TREATMENT OF INFERTILITY

**What is the general approach to treatment of infertility?**

A stepwise approach, from least to most invasive (and expensive). It may start with use of clomiphene citrate to induction with gonadotropins, and then to in vitro fertilization (IVF). For patients with anovulation, the goal is monofollicular development with ovulation. For patients over 35 and those with unexplained infertility, the goal may be 2–4 follicles, with ovarian stimulation

**What modifications in lifestyle habits may improve fertility?**

Smoking and alcohol cessation, decrease in caffeine consumption, increased frequency of coitus. Maintaining a healthy weight and diet not only helps with conception but predicts a healthier pregnancy

**What is clomiphene citrate and in which patients is it used?**

It is a selective estrogen receptor modulator (SERM) that ultimately increases gonadotropin release. It is the agent of choice for women less than 36 years of age and in normogonadotrophic normo-estrogenic anovulation. It has been effective in inducing ovulation for 60–85% of anovulatory women

**When is induction with human menopausal gonadotropins (hMG) indicated?**

Subcutaneous injection of hMG, specifically FSH, is used in women who have failed with clomiphene and in women with hypothalamic amonorrhea with hypopituitarism

**How is follicle development and ovulation induced in women in hypogonadotropic hypogonadal anovulation with normal pituitary function?**

Pulsatile administration of GnRH stimulates endogenous production of FSH and LH

**What agent should be used in women who have anovulation because of hyperprolactinemia?**

Dopamine agonists such as bromocriptine or cabergoline

**Do these induction agents have an associated risk for ovarian cancer and breast cancer?**

Although historical evidence may indicate an association between clomiphene use and ovarian cancer, more recent well-controlled studies do not support the concept of increased risk. However, it is recommended that induction with clomiphene be limited to 12 cycles. There has been no reported risk between fertility drugs and breast cancer

**What is intrauterine insemination (IUI)?**

It consists of collecting a specimen of ejaculated sperm, followed by washing and concentration of the sperm. The concentrated sperm is then injected directly into the upper uterine cavity using a small catheter through the cervix. The pregnancy rate is 4–6% per cycle when used alone. It is frequently used in combination with ovulation induction to achieve pregnancy rates of 5–15%

## ASSISTED REPRODUCTIVE TECHNOLOGIES

**What are the different modalities of assisted reproductive technologies (ARTs)?**

1. In vitro fertilization-embryo transfer (IVF-ET)
2. Intracytoplasmic sperm injection (ICSI)
3. Gamete intra-fallopian tube transfer (GIFT)
4. Zygote intra-fallopian tube transfer (ZIFT)
5. Oocyte donation

**What is the mechanism of each of the following technologies and their success rate of pregnancy?**

**IVF-ET:** The female's ovary is hyperstimulated by daily FSH injections. Multiple mature eggs are collected by a transvaginal procedure and combined with sperm in the laboratory to allow fertilization to occur. After fertilization selected embryos are placed in the female's uterus to allow development. Pregnancy is achieved 28% of the time and 82% result in one or more births

**ICSI:** This procedure combines the technique of IVF and involves taking a single sperm from the male partner and injecting it directly into the cytoplasm of the egg in the laboratory. It is commonly used as treatment for male infertility factor. Overall fertilization rate is 60%

# Osteoporosis

**What is osteoporosis?**

A disorder of the skeleton that involves **low bone mass** and **micro-architectural disruption**, both of which lead to skeletal fragility and increased fracture risk

**What is the prevalence of osteoporosis?**

Over 30% of women over 50 years have radiographic evidence of osteoporosis; over 44 million men and women are currently diagnosed with osteoporosis in the United States

| | |
|---|---|
| **Who does osteoporosis affect?** | Predominately **thin, postmenopausal** women and more often **Caucasian** and **Asian** women |
| **Why does osteoporosis affect women more than men?** | Women have a **lower peak bone mass** and have **accelerated bone loss** after menopause |
| **When does bone mass peak?** | At age 30–35 |
| **What is the pathogenesis of osteoporosis?** | Bone loss, which is a result of a mismatch between bone resorption and bone formation. Most is a result of either age-related or menopause-related bone loss |
| **How does osteoporosis typically present?** | Often with **hip fracture**, a **vertebral compression fracture** (leading to kyphosis), or a **wrist fracture** after minimal trauma |
| **What is the differential diagnosis of osteoporosis?** | Osteomalacia<br>Hyperparathyroidism<br>Multiple myeloma<br>Pathological fracture secondary to metastatic cancer |
| **What is "high turnover" osteoporosis and what are the causes?** | Osteoporosis primarily secondary to **increased bone resorption**<br>Caused by **estrogen deficiency,** hyperparathyroidism, hyperthyroidism, hypogonadism, cyclosporine, heparin |
| **What is "low turnover" osteoporosis and what are the causes?** | Osteoporosis primarily secondary to **decreased bone formation**<br>Caused by **advanced age,** liver disease, heparin |
| **What drug causes both decreased formation and increased resorption of bone, leading to osteoporosis?** | Glucocorticoids |
| **What drugs are known to cause osteoporosis?** | Glucocorticoids; heparin; medroxyprogesterone acetate; vitamin A; certain retinoids |
| **Describe age-related bone loss** | Loss of both the cortical and trabecular bone that begins around age 30–40 in both men and women; partially because of **decreased calcium absorption** |

| | |
|---|---|
| **Describe menopause-related bone loss** | Loss of all but especially trabecular bone that occurs for 10 years beginning after the onset of menopause because of the **decline in estrogen levels** |
| **Can estrogen be used to prevent menopause-related bone loss?** | Yes, however it is not first-line therapy because of its cardiovascular and breast cancer risks |
| **What is the relationship between lactation and bone loss?** | Lactation is associated with a 1–4% bone loss; however, it is regained after lactation is completed. There is no association between osteoporosis and lactation earlier in life |
| **What is the relationship between calcium and osteoporosis?** | Calcium has been shown to reduce bone loss when a, 1000–1500 mg supplement is taken by postmenopausal women daily |
| **How is osteoporosis diagnosed?** | Either by the **presence of a fragility fracture** or by testing for **bone mineral density** (BMD) with a dual-energy x-ray absorptiometry (**DEXA**) scan of the spine and/or hip. Osteoporosis is defined as a BMD of less than 2.5 standard deviations below the mean |
| **Are there any abnormal lab tests in osteoporosis?** | No |
| **What is osteopenia?** | Decreased BMD; diagnosed on a DEXA scan as a BMD between 1 and 2.5 standard deviations below the mean |
| **Who should be screened for osteoporosis using a DEXA scan?** | Women under 65 years who have one or more risk factors for osteoporosis (in addition to menopause); All women over 65 years of age |
| **In women with osteoporosis, what are risk factors for fracture?** | Medical history: **previous fracture or fracture in first-degree relative**, inflammatory bowel disease (IBD), celiac disease, cystic fibrosis, history of hyperthyroidism, use of anxiolytic, anticonvulsant, or neuroleptic drugs, type II diabetes mellitus (DM), dementia<br>Social history: **cigarette smoking,** consumption of lots of caffeine, |

sedentary lifestyle, inadequate calcium intake

Physical examination: **low body weight,** tall stature

**What are the categories of treatment for osteoporosis?**

Reduce risk of falls; nonpharmacologic therapies; drug therapies

**What types of nonpharmacologic therapies are useful for the treatment of osteoporosis?**

1. Diet: adequate calcium/vitamin D intake
2. Exercise: any weight-bearing exercise (including walking) at least 30 minutes three times per week
3. Cessation of smoking
4. Avoidance of drugs that increase bone loss

**Who should be considered for pharmacologic therapy?**

Postmenopausal women with diagnosed osteoporosis or with high risk for its development

**What types of drugs are available?**

**Bisphosphonates; selective estrogen receptor modulators** (SERMs); **estrogen; calcitonin; vitamin D**

**How do bisphosphonates work?**

They **increase bone mass** and **reduce the incidence of fracture by inhibiting resorption of bone**. They are **first-line therapy** for osteoporosis treatment

**What are the side effects of bisphosphonates?**

Pill-induced **esophagitis, osteonecrosis of the jaw** (rare)

**How do SERMs work?**

They **increase BMD** and **reduce the risk of vertebral fractures**

**What other benefits do SERMs confer?**

Lower risk of breast cancer; decrease total cholesterol and LDL

**What are the side effects of SERMs?**

Increased risk of venous thromboembolism

**What are the indications for estrogen/progesterone therapy?**

Persistent menopausal symptoms

Inability to tolerate other antiresorptive medications

**How does parathyroid hormone (PTH) work and how is it administered?**

If given intermittently, PTH stimulates bone formation more than it causes resorption

**When is calcitonin used?**

Not a first-line treatment; used in women with pain secondary to a fracture because it offers analgesia in addition to its antiosteoporotic effects

**What are the potential side effects of calcitriol that limit its use?**

Hypercalcemia, hypercalciuria, and renal insufficiency

**What are isoflavones?**

A type of phytoestrogen; a micronutrient substance that has many similar properties to estrogen. Their effectiveness has not been proven

**How are thiazide diuretics used in the prevention of osteoporosis?**

Used in postmenopausal women with hypertension because they decrease bone loss slightly

**What is tibolone and how is it used in osteoporosis?**

A **synthetic steroid** that metabolizes to have the effects of estrogens, androgens, and progestins. It **improves BMD;** however, it may increase the risk of stroke

# Perimenopause and Menopause

**How is menopause defined?**

**12 months of amenorrhea after the final menstrual period** because of a loss of ovarian activity

**What is the average age of menopause in the United States?**

51 years

**What are some factors that cause an earlier age of onset for menopause?**

Smoking

Genetic factors

Nulliparity

Hysterectomy

Living at higher altitudes

**What is premature menopause?**

Also known as premature ovarian failure; the **spontaneous cessation of menses before the age of 40**

**What are the other phases of menopause?**

**Perimenopause**: the phase preceding menopause; reflected by menstrual cycle irregularities

**Postmenopause**: phase of life that follows menopause

| | |
|---|---|
| **When does perimenopause begin?** | Between 5 and 10 years before menopause |
| **How does the menstrual cycle length change in the perimenopause?** | Early phase: the menstrual cycle remains regular but is shortened by 7 days or more<br>Late phase: more menstrual cycle variability; may skip two or more cycles |
| **How do the following hormones change during the perimenopausal state?** | |
| **FSH/LH** | **Increases** |
| **Estrogen** | **Remains normal** (until follicular growth stops) |
| **Progesterone** | **Decreases** |
| **Why does FSH change during perimenopause?** | The decline in the number of follicles and the irregular maturation of follicles leads to a **decreased concentration of inhibin** (which normally inhibits FSH secretion). This causes the rise in FSH levels |
| **What are the symptoms of perimenopause?** | Hot flashes (episodic sensation of warmth on chest/face that becomes generalized; associated with sweating)<br>Sleep disturbances |
| **How do the following hormones change at menopause?** | |
| **Androstenedione** | Decreases |
| **FSH/LH** | Markedly increases |
| **Testosterone** | Increases |
| **Estrogen** | Decreases (to <20 pg/mL) |
| **Why do estrogen levels change during menopause?** | Because of the loss of ovarian follicles |
| **Compare the changes in the levels of FSH and LH during menopause** | Both increase; however **FSH >> LH** |
| **Why does FSH increase more than LH?** | Renal clearance of FSH is less than that of LH |
| **What disorder presents with the same hormonal abnormalities as menopause (increased serum FSH > LH)?** | **Primary ovarian failure**, which can be seen in Turner syndrome |

| | |
|---|---|
| **What are the chief complaints from women going through menopause?** | Hot flashes<br>Hair/skin changes<br>Atrophic urogenital system (symptoms of urinary tract infection, dyspareunia)<br>Vaginitis (atrophic)<br>Variable moods<br>Osteoporosis<br>Coronary artery disease<br>***Can be remembered by the mnemonic "menopause causes HHAVVOC"** |
| **Describe the pathophysiology and the treatment for each of the symptoms of menopause** | See Table 7-1 |
| **What complaint is often associated with hot flashes?** | Insomnia (because symptoms often occur at night) |
| **What are the clinical manifestations of an atrophic urogenital system?** | Symptoms similar to those seen in UTIs (including urinary frequency, urgency, dysuria, pyuria, and urge incontinence) |
| **Where does menopause-associated osteoporosis typically begin?** | In the spine |
| **What is the rate of bone loss associated with osteoporosis?** | Before menopause, bone loss occurs at a rate of 0.5% per year; after menopause it increases to over 1% per year |
| **What type of bone is most sensitive to the changes in estrogen levels associated with menopause?** | Trabecular bone |
| **What diagnosis is most likely when a postmenopausal woman presents with severe itching around the vagina? How is it diagnosed and how is it treated?** | **Lichen sclerosis**. A **biopsy** is required for diagnosis. Treatment is **high-potency corticosteroids** |
| **What are the two most commonly used hormone replacement therapies?** | Unopposed estrogen therapy<br>Continuous combined therapy with conjugated estrogen and medroxyprogesterone acetate |
| **Is there cardiovascular benefit to using unopposed estrogen therapy (ET) and continuous combined oral estrogen-progestin therapy (CCE-MPA)?** | According to data from the Women's Health Initiative (WHI) study, there is no benefit from estrogen therapy and a slight increased risk with combined therapy |

**Table 7-1** The Pathophysiology and Treatment for Symptoms of Menopause

| Symptom/Condition | Pathophysiology | Treatment |
| --- | --- | --- |
| Hot flashes | Estrogen withdrawal → thermoregulatory dysfunction | Short-term estrogen replacement therapy |
| Hair and skin changes | Decreased collagen → wrinkles<br>Decreased estrogen, no change in testosterone → male growth patterns | Estrogen replacement therapy |
| Atrophic urogenital system | Decreased estrogen → atrophy of urethral epithelium → loss of urethral tone, shrinkage of the uterus, cervix, vagina, ovaries, and bladder | Estrogen replacement therapy |
| Vaginitis (atrophic) | Decreased estrogen → epithelial atrophy → soreness, burning, dyspareunia, sexual dysfunction | Lubricants (mild) vaginal estrogen (severe) |
| Variable moods | Hormonal/life changes → nervousness, anxiety, depression | Estrogen replacement therapy |
| Osteoporosis and joint pain | ↑Bone resorption phase and ↑ osteoclasts; ↓ bone formation phase and ↓ osteoblasts | Raloxifene or bisphosphonates |
| Coronary heart disease | ↑ LDL, ↓HDL → increased atherosclerosis | Hormone replacement therapy does not have any benefit |
| Cognitive decline | Change in areas important for memory → memory loss, possible link to Alzheimer's disease | Estrogen or combined hormonal therapy has no benefit |

**What is the risk of breast cancer when using unopposed estrogen therapy or combined estrogen-progestin HRT?**

In the WHI **unopposed estrogen trial, there is no increase in risk of breast cancer** in 10,000 women who had a hysterectomy. In the **combined estrogen-progestin group, there was a significant increase in the risk of breast cancer.** The presence of breast cancer was seen in year 3 in women who had previously used menopausal hormones and in year 4 who had no history of previous use

**What are the relative risks of endometrial cancer when using unopposed estrogen therapy versus combined estrogen-progestin hormone therapy?**

Treatment with estrogen alone greatly increases the risk of endometrial hyperplasia and cancer. Adding a progestin diminishes this excess risk of endometrial hyperplasia and carcinoma

**When is estrogen replacement therapy (ERT)/hormone replacement therapy (HRT) contraindicated?**

Women who have abnormal vaginal bleeding

History of breast cancer

History of coronary heart disease (CHD)

History of estrogen-dependent neoplasia

History of DVTs or thromboembolic event

History of liver dysfunction/disease

**What are complications of estrogen replacement therapy?**

Endometrial cancer

Breast cancer

Thromboembolic disease

Stroke

Uterine bleeding

Gallbladder disease

# Hirsutism, Virilization, and Polycystic Ovarian Syndrome

## HIRSUTISM AND VIRILIZATION

**What is hirsutism?**

Excessive growth of **androgen-dependent** hair (e.g., on the upper lip, chest, chin)

**What is virilization?**

Excessive androgen-induced changes in addition to hirsutism. These include clitoromegaly, voice deepening, increasing muscle mass, and other masculinizing signs

**What is hypertrichosis?**

It is a rare disease that refers to **diffusely increased androgen-independent** fine body hair, usually caused by drugs or systemic illnesses. It does not represent hirsutism

**How does the clinical presentation of hirsutism differ from that of virilization?**

***Hirsutism*** manifests with **increased "midline" hair** on the upper lip, chin, ear, cheeks, lower abdomen, chest, back, and upper arms. Amenorrhea is seen in severe cases. ***Virilization*** is excess hair and additional characteristics such as **deepening of the voice, acne, breast atrophy, clitoromegaly, balding, and increased strength**

**Which androgens cause and are elevated in hirsutism?**

Testosterone and dehydroepiandrosterone sulfate (DHEAS)

**What two organs may be involved in hirsutism and what steroid does each mainly secrete?**

**Ovary:** testosterone

**Adrenal gland:** DHEAS

**What is the role of 17OH progesterone in the development of hirsutism?**

17OH progesterone is a precursor to the biosynthesis of cortisol and can be converted peripherally into androgens if found in excess

**What is the most common disorder that causes hirsutism?**

Polycystic ovarian syndrome (PCOS)

**What other underlying diseases may cause hirsutism?**

**Congenital adrenal hyperplasia** (CAH; 21-hydroxylase deficiency)

**Androgen-secreting ovarian tumors** (Sertoli-Leydig or granulosa-theca tumors)

Adrenal tumors

Cushing syndrome

Exogenous androgens (danazol)

Hyperprolactinemia

Other rare disorders (hyperthecosis)

**What is idiopathic hirsutism?**

It is a diagnosis given to women with hirsutism without adrenal or ovarian dysfunction, normal serum androgen concentrations, normal menstrual cycles, and no other identifiable cause of their hirsutism. There is often a positive family history

**How may the presenting signs and symptoms of a patient help specify the disorder causing hirsutism?**

**Ovarian tumor:** pelvic mass, sudden onset of amenorrhea, virilization

**PCOS:** obesity, acne, long history of irregular menses, slow onset of hirsutism beginning at puberty, acanthosis nigricans

**Theca-lutein cysts:** hirsutism develops during pregnancy

**CAH:** gradual onset of anovulation, positive family history

**Adrenal tumor:** rapid onset, virilization, abdominal-flank mass

**Cushing syndrome:** moon facies, buffalo hump, centripetal obesity, striae, extremity wasting

**Hyperprolactinemia:** galactorrhea or visual changes with menstrual irregularities

**What laboratory studies assist in the diagnosis of the etiology of hirsutism?**

**Testosterone >200 ng/mL** → androgen-secreting ovarian tumor

**DHEAS >700 ug/dL** → androgen-secreting adrenal tumor

**17α-hydroxyprogesterone > 200 ng/dL** → 21-hydroxylase deficiency

**LH:FSH ≥ 3** → PCOS

Prolactin > 200 μg/dL → prolactinoma

24-hour urinary free cortisol > 100 ng/24 h → Cushing syndrome

**What imaging studies are warranted?**

**Pelvic ultrasound** may reveal polycystic ovaries or ovarian tumors/cysts

**CT/MRI of the abdomen** to look for an adrenal mass when DHEAS levels are elevated

**How is hirsutism generally treated?**

Treat the underlying disorder. The most common medications are **oral contraceptives (OCPs)**, GnRH analogs, and antiandrogens (first-line spironolactone, second-line flutamide, finasteride)

**What are the specific treatments for each of the following causes of hirsutism?**

**Ovarian tumor:** surgical removal

**PCOS:** combination OCPs

**CAH:** continuous corticosteroid replacement

**Adrenal tumor:** surgical removal

**Idiopathic hirsutism:** spironolactone

**How do combination OCPs work as antiandrogens?**

They suppress LH stimulation of the theca cells and they increase sex hormone-binding globulin (SHBG) (thus decreasing free testosterone)

**How does spironolactone act as an antiandrogen?**

It is an androgen receptor blocker and it suppresses 5α-reductase in hair follicles

## Polycystic Ovarian Syndrome (Stein-Leventhal Syndrome)

**Describe polycystic ovarian syndrome (PCOS)**

It is the most common chronic endocrine condition characterized by **persistent anovulation** which leads to **secondary amenorrhea** and other menstrual irregularities, and **androgen excess** which may cause hirsutism and virilization

**What is the pathophysiology behind PCOS?**

It is a **dysfunction of the hypothalamic-pituitary axis. Increased pulsatile secretions of GnRH→ excess production of LH→** excess production and secretion of androgens→ virilization

**How does PCOS lead to anovulation?**

Some of the excess androgens are converted to estrogen. High estrogen levels increase LH (by blocking the inhibitory feedback mechanism of progesterone on the pituitary). High LH levels stimulate the immature follicles to produce more androgens, which then become converted to estrogen. The cycle then repeats

**FSH is inhibited** by high estrogen levels. This allows the early growth of multiple follicles, but **failure of the development of the mature follicle and its ovulation**

**What are the two most common presenting complaints of patients with PCOS?**

Hirsutism and infertility

**What other clinical manifestations are associated with PCOS?**

Chronic anovulation

Obesity

Insulin resistance

Irregular bleeding (from a chronically estrogen-stimulated endometrium)

**What dermatologic condition may be associated with PCOS?**

Acanthosis nigricans

**How is the diagnosis of PCOS made?**

It is suspected in the presence of menstrual irregularity (anovulation), evidence of androgen excess, and exclusion of other causes of menstrual irregularities and hyperandrogenism

**What test should be ruled out first in a woman who presents with secondary amenorrhea?**

Pregnancy test (β-hCG)

**What biochemical test confirms the diagnosis of PCOS?**

**An LH/FSH ratio > 3:1**

**How do polycystic ovaries appear on pelvic ultrasound?**

They appear with eight or more, small (2–8 mm), subcapsular fluid-filled follicle cysts that look like a **"black pearl necklace"**

**How is infertility in PCOS patients treated?**

**Weight loss** is recommended first. Ovulation induction with **clomiphene citrate** can be used. **Metformin** and/or gonadotropins can be added if clomiphene alone fails

**How is hirsutism treated in PCOS patients?**

**Combination OCPs** are first line (for women who do not desire pregnancy)

Antiandrogen therapy (spironolactone, flutamide, finasteride)

**What are complications associated with PCOS?**

Increased risk of early onset of Type II diabetes mellitus

Increased risk of endometrial hyperplasia and endometrial cancer because of unopposed estrogen stimulation

**What is HAIR-AN syndrome?**

It is a variant of PCOS that leads to hyperandrogenism, insulin resistance, and acanthosis nigricans

SECTION III

# Topics in Obstetrics

CHAPTER 8

# General Obstetrics

## Maternal-Fetal Physiologic Adaptation to Pregnancy

### EMBRYOLOGY

**What are the developmental stages of early pregnancy?**

Fertilization and cleavage result in a **zygote** (an 8-cell mass) which then divides to form the **morula** (a 16-cell mass) 3 days after fertilization. A **blastocyst** develops and implantation occurs approximately 10 days after fertilization. An **embryonic disk** develops after the first week and a **yolk sac** after 5 weeks

**What are the placental membranes and uterine layers (fetal to maternal)?**

Amnion

Chorion (with villi composed of syncytial trophoblasts and cytotrophoblasts)

Decidua parietalis (endometrium)

Myometrium (undergoes hyperplasia early in pregnancy with subsequent hypertrophy and distension)

Serosa (See Fig. 8-1)

**How does the timing of division affect the development of monozygotic twins?**

If division occurs <72 hours: two embryos, two amnions, two chorions ("di-di")

If division occurs between 4-7 days: two embryos, two amnions, one chorion ("mono-di")

If division occurs after 7 days: one shared amnion and chorion ("mono-mono")

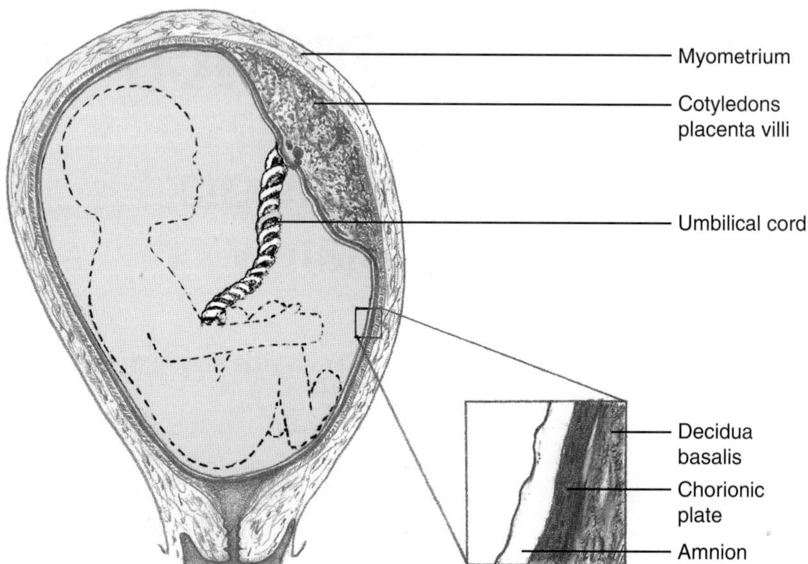


**Figure 8-1** Embryologic layers of the human fetus at 3 months.

If division occurs after the embryonic disk has developed, the twins will be conjoined

## FETAL CIRCULATION

**What are the major shunts involved with fetal circulation?**

Ductus venosus

Foramen ovale

Ductus arteriosus

**What are the patterns of fetal blood flow (starting from the umbilical vein)?**

1. Umbilical vein → ductus venosus → inferior vena cava → right atrium → foramen ovale → left atrium → left ventricle → cephalic/systemic circulation
2. superior vena cava → right atrium → right ventricle → fetal lungs → pulmonary artery → ductus arteriosus → aorta → hypogastric arteries → umbilical arteries (See Fig. 8-2)

**Do each of the following vessels carry oxygenated or deoxygenated blood?**

**Umbilical artery**

Deoxygenated

**Umbilical vein**

Oxygenated

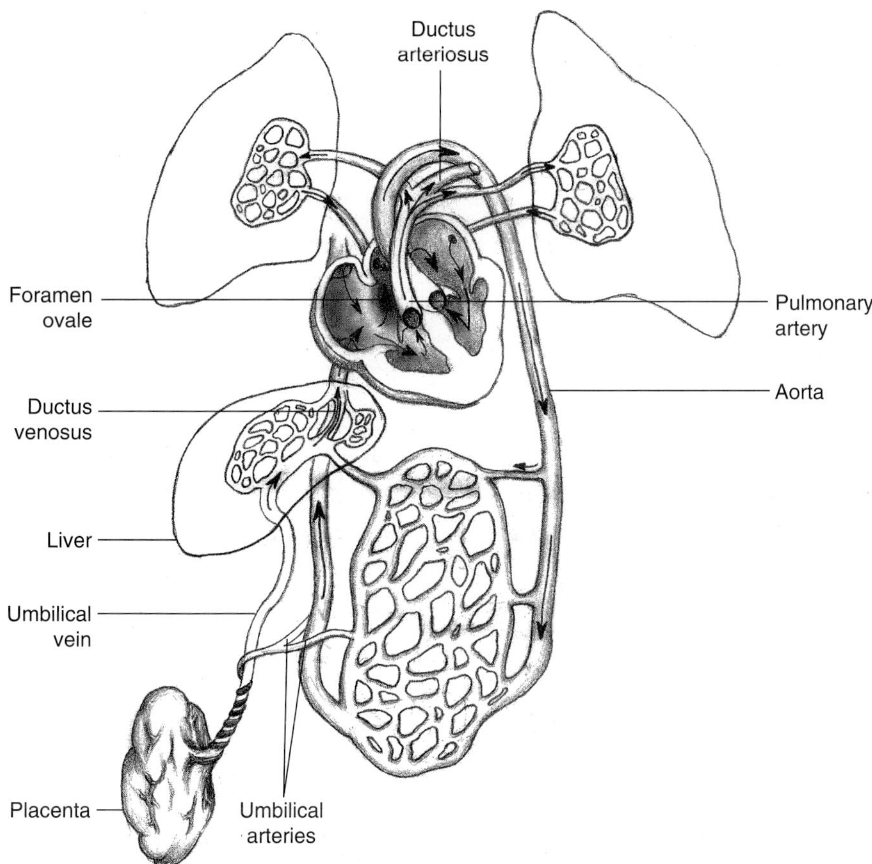


**Figure 8-2** Fetal circulation.

**What are the embryologic remnants associated with each of the following?**

| | |
|---|---|
| **Umbilical vein** | Ligamentum hepatis |
| **Ductus venosus** | Ligamentum venosum |
| **Ductus arteriosus** | Ligamentum arteriosum |
| **Umbilical arteries** | Medial umbilical ligaments |

## CARDIOVASCULAR

**How does pregnancy affect cardiac output (CO), blood volume, and blood pressure (BP)?**

**CO increases** up to 50% (1.8 L/min)

**Blood volume increases** by 50%

**BP decreases**

| | |
|---|---|
| | These changes **peak during the second trimester** and remain relatively constant until delivery; they are mediated by hormones (aldosterone, progesterone, human chorion gonadotrophin (HCG), relaxin, nitric oxide [NO]) |
| **Pregnancy affects which components of CO?** | Remember, CO = SV × HR. Both stroke volume (SV) and heart rate (HR) increase; however, SV increases more than HR |
| **How does pregnancy affect SV?** | Preload is increased with an increase in blood volume; afterload is reduced by the low-resistance uteroplacental circulation and by peripheral vasodilatation |
| **When do HR and SV peak during pregnancy?** | HR peaks around term; SV peaks during the second trimester |
| **What percentage of CO goes to the uterus during pregnancy?** | Up to 20% at term (compared to <1% in the nonpregnant state). Most of this goes to the placenta |
| **How does the cardiac examination change during pregnancy?** | Heart sounds are **louder** and **split**, there is often a **systolic murmur** and an **S3**. This manifests as a slight left axis deviation on EKG and as mild cardiomegaly on chest x-ray (CXR)<br><br>(A **diastolic murmur is never normal** and should be evaluated) |
| **Why does the cardiac examination change?** | All four cardiac chambers and valve diameters are increased and hyperdynamic. This may lead to mild pulmonic, tricuspid, and/or mitral regurgitation or a small pericardial effusion |
| **How does the gravid uterus affect CO?** | In the supine position the inferior vena cava is compressed, which may decrease CO by up to 30%. Maximum venous return and CO is maintained in the left lateral decubitus (LLD) position |
| **Describe the hematologic changes of pregnancy** | Red blood cell mass **increases** by 15–30% (because of increased erythropoietin)<br><br>Plasma volume **increases** by 30–50% (because of increased aldosterone) |

Hct and Hb **decrease**, causing the physiologic "anemia of pregnancy" (because of increased plasma volume)

***An Hb <11 is never normal and must be evaluated** for iron/folate deficiency or a hemoglobinopathy

**When does the anemia of pregnancy reach its nadir?**

Around 24 weeks

**What is the effect of pregnancy on BP?**

**BP decreases in the first trimester**, nadirs at approximately 24 weeks, and then almost normalizes by term. Diastolic is affected more than systolic

## RESPIRATORY

**How does pregnancy affect** pulmonary **function tests (PFTs)?**

**Tidal volume increases** by 40%

**Minute ventilation increases** by 50%

**Functional residual capacity decreases** by 20%

Total lung capacity slightly decreases

Expiratory reserve volume and total lung capacity decrease

Forced expiratory volume (FEV1) does not change

**Respiratory rate does not change**

**What hormone mediates these effects and how does it act?**

**Progesterone**. It acts centrally (through direct stimulation of the medulla and respiratory centers) as well as peripherally (through pulmonary vasodilation)

**How do these respiratory changes affect the blood gas levels?**

Alveolar and arterial oxygen levels increase

Arterial carbon dioxide levels decrease

**How is the acid base equilibrium affected during pregnancy?**

**Respiratory alkalosis** with metabolic compensation (pH between 7.40 and 7.45)

**What is the effect of pregnancy on oxygen consumption?**

Increases by over 20% owing to the placenta, fetus, and maternal organs

**How does the gravid uterus affect respiratory function?**

The thorax becomes more barrel-chested and dyspnea is a common symptom in advanced pregnancy because of the pressure of the gravid uterus and the central effects of progesterone

## RENAL/URINARY

| | |
|---|---|
| **What is the effect of pregnancy on renal function?** | Glomerular filtration rate (GFR) **increases** by 50% (because of the increase in glomerular plasma flow)<br>Renal blood flow **increases**<br>Plasma creatinine, BUN, and uric acid levels **decrease** (because of the increased GFR)<br>[*Normalization of Cr, BUN, or UA may indicate underlying pathology (preeclampsia, renal insufficiency)] |
| **Why is the pregnant woman at increased risk for urinary tract infections?** | **Progesterone** reduces ureteral tone and peristalsis, and relaxes the bladder wall allowing reflux through the incompetent vesico-ureteral valves. This results in stasis of urine, dilated ureters, increased pressure in the renal pelvis, and bacterial proliferation |
| **What are the common causes of bacteriuria in pregnancy?** | *Escherichia coli* >> *Klebsiella* > *Proteus* > *Group B streptococcus* (GBS) > Enterococci > Staphylococci |
| **What is a complication of pyelonephritis during pregnancy?** | Preterm labor |
| **Where does hydronephrosis in pregnancy most commonly occur?** | On the **right** side (because of right uterine dextrorotation and right ureter compression) |
| **What happens to plasma osmolality during pregnancy?** | It falls because of increased levels of relaxin (stimulated by HCG) and antidiuretic hormone (ADH). These lead to an increase in intravascular fluid which then decreases plasma osmolality |
| **What is the clinical affect of this change in plasma osmolality?** | **Pitting edema** in gravity-dependent areas |
| **What is the significance of trace protein or glucose in the second or third trimester?** | It is **normal**, because of increased GFR. In 24 hours protein may increase to 200 mg (normal is less than 100 mg/24 hours). However, higher values suggest renal pathology or preeclampsia |

## GASTROINTESTINAL

**When does morning sickness occur?**

During the **first trimester**, as levels of hCG double every 2 days. After hCG levels peak (~10 weeks), morning sickness decreases

**What is hyperemesis gravidarum?**

An idiopathic, noninfectious, **severe nausea and vomiting** that causes **dehydration, ketone formation, weight loss, and metabolic acidosis**

**How does progesterone affect the GI tract?**

**Lower esophageal sphincter tone decreases** (can lead to GERD)

**Small bowel and colon transit decreases** (can lead to bloating and constipation)

**Venous congestion** (can lead to hemorrhoids)

**Biliary tract peristalsis decreases** (increases risk of cholelithiasis and cholecystitis)

**What impact does estrogen have on hepatic metabolism?**

It increases the production of hormone-binding globulins (sex hormone-binding globulin [SHBG], thyroxine-binding globulin [TBG], ceruloplasmin [copper], transferrin total iron-binding capacity [TIBC], increases up to 100% and coagulation factors)

**How do liver function tests (LFTs) change in pregnancy?**

**Alkaline phosphatase is increased** (because of placental production). Other enzymes are within normal limits

[*Abnormalities may suggest pathology: hepatitis, HELLP, acute fatty liver of pregnancy, cholestasis of pregnancy, or other pathologies]

**How does pregnancy affect the risk of pancreatitis?**

Increases the risk (because of increased risks of cholelithiasis and hyperlipidemia)

**Why is the mortality associated with appendicitis higher in pregnancy?**

Because of the gravid uterus, the appendix is pushed higher leading to a delay in the diagnosis

## HEMATOLOGIC

**How is the coagulation system affected by pregnancy?**

Decreased protein S
Resistance to protein C

Increased factor I (fibrinogen), II, V, VII, VIII, X, and XII

Because of these, **pregnancy is a hypercoagulable state**

**What are the potential complications of this hypercoagulable state?**

**Venous thrombosis** (occurs 0.7 per 1000 women in pregnancy) and subsequent **pulmonary embolism**. Both occur predominantly in the **third trimester**

**What is the effect of pregnancy on immunity?**

Cell-mediated immunity is weakened but humoral immunity is strengthened

## ENDOCRINE

**What is hCG and where is it formed?**

Human chorionic gonadotropin; in the **syncytiotrophoblast** of the placenta

**hCG is structurally related to what other glycoprotein hormones?**

Luteinizing hormone (**LH**), follicle-stimulating hormone (**FSH**), and thyroid-stimulating hormone (**TSH**) (they all have the same $\alpha$ subunit but different $\beta$ subunits)

**How does hCG promote pregnancy?**

1. **Maintains the corpus luteum** for first trimester
2. Causes sexual differentiation in the male fetus
3. Ensures adequate $T_3$ and $T_4$ production
4. Increases relaxin secretion by the corpus luteum (leading to decreased vascular resistance)

**What are the three major types of estrogen are they predominately produced?**

**Estrone: adrenals** (dehydroepiandrosterone [DHEA] is the precursor)

**Estriol** (least bioactive): **placenta**

**Estradiol** (most bioactive): **ovaries**

**What happens to the adrenal hormones during pregnancy?**

Adrenocorticotropic hormone (ACTH), corticotropin-releasing hormone (CRH), and cortisol all increase

**What is oxytocin?**

A hormone produced by the supraoptic and paraventricular nuclei of the hypothalamus and released by the posterior pituitary. Concentrations rise throughout gestation, during labor, and with lactation or nipple stimulation

**What are the major actions of oxytocin?**

**Contraction of uterine myometrium**, ductal myoepithelial contraction (milk expression), orgasm, and bonding

**What peptide is similar to oxytocin and what are the clinical consequences?**

Antidiuretic hormone (ADH). Induction/augmentation of labor with oxytocin may cause severe fluid retention and pulmonary edema

**What happens to thyroid hormone levels during pregnancy?**

**TBG increases**
Total $T_3$ and $T_4$ levels increase but **free $T_3$ and $T_4$ levels** (and thus thyroid function) **remain unchanged**
TSH does not change

**What mediates these thyroid hormone changes?**

hCG stimulates TSH receptors to increase total $T_4$ and $T_3$ levels. Estrogen increases the hepatic production of TBG

**What is hPL and where is it formed?**

Human placental lactogen; in the **syncytiotrophoblast** of the placenta

**What is the function of hPL?**

It **antagonizes insulin** and **increases lypolysis** to ensure adequate glucose delivery to the fetus

**How does maternal glucose metabolism change during pregnancy?**

hPL causes maternal insulin resistance

**Why does gestational diabetes mellitus (GDM) occur?**

There is insufficient maternal insulin to counter the hyperglycemic effects of placental hPL. It occurs most commonly in the third trimester, when hPL levels are highest

## DERMATOLOGY

**What are striae distensae or striae gravidarum?**

Stretch marks; caused from a diminution of elastin fibers and fibrillin microfibrils

**What other skin changes occur during pregnancy?**

**Chloasma** or **melasma** ("mask of pregnancy," hyperpigmentation of the face)

**Linea nigra** (darkening of the linea alba from the pubic symphysis to the xiphoid process)

**Hyperpigmentation** of the axilla, genitalia, perineum, anus, inner thighs, neck, scars, nevi, and lentigo

**Palmar erythema** and **telangiectasias**

**Hirsutism** and **acne**

## REPRODUCTIVE

**What is Chadwick sign?**

**Bluish color** of vulvar and vaginal membranes because of venous congestion; a normal finding in pregnancy

**What other vaginal changes occur in pregnancy?**

Increased vascularity and distensibility; increased vaginal discharge (because of increased capillary permeability and desquamation)

**What changes occur to the cervix and uterus during pregnancy?**

**Hegar sign (softening of the lower uterine segment** that occurs in early pregnancy)

Increased eversion of the cervical columnar epithelium

**What breast changes occur in pregnancy?**

Enlargement, increase in cystic components, darkening of areolae, hypertrophy of sebaceous glands, colostrum production (in late pregnancy)

# Prenatal Care

## DIAGNOSIS AND TERMINOLOGY

**When should prenatal care begin?**

Preconception or as soon as pregnancy is suspected

**What are the major goals of preconceptive counseling?**

Minimize unplanned pregnancies

Optimize chronic medical disorders (diabetes mellitus [DM], epilepsy, hypothyroid, cardiovascular disorders)

Promote healthy behaviors

Counsel regarding adequate diet, exercise, and nutritional supplements (folic acid and iron)

Offer appropriate vaccinations (rubella, diphtheria, hepatitis B virus)

Screen for genetic or chromosomal abnormalities

Improve patient's readiness for pregnancy and parenting

**What are the major goals of prenatal care?**

Prevention, ensure a healthy mother, ensure a healthy baby

**What are some important medical conditions that adversely impact pregnancy?**

DM, hypertension (HTN), cardiovascular disease, autoimmune disorders, kidney disease/UTIs, pulmonary disease (asthma or TB), seizures or other neurologic disorders, psychiatric disorders, hepatitis, phlebitis, thyroid abnormalities, blood transfusions, hemophilia or blood disorders (thalassemia or sickle cell)

**What does folic acid supplementation help prevent?**

Neural tube (NT) defects

**Who should take folic acid supplementation?**

All women of reproductive age; the NT closes 26 days after fertilization (often before a woman is aware of pregnancy)

**How much folic acid should women of reproductive age consume?**

A balanced diet plus 0.4 mg daily

**What are the early signs and symptoms of pregnancy?**

Amenorrhea or irregular bleeding

Fatigue

Nausea/vomiting

Breast tenderness

Urinary frequency

Chadwick sign (bluish discoloration of the vagina)

Hegar sign (softening of the cervix)

**How is pregnancy diagnosed?**

**β-hCG**

**When does β-hCG become positive?**
Serum tests become positive following implantation (about 10 days after fertilization); urine tests become positive 2–3 weeks after fertilization or around on the first day of a missed period

**Where is hCG formed?**
In the **placental trophoblasts**

**What is the primary function of hCG?**
To **maintain the corpus luteum** and **progesterone production** (it is "pro-pregnancy")

**Why is the β subunit of hCG measured?**
β subunit of hCG differentiates it from LH, FSH, and TSH, which all share the same α subunit

**What are some reasons that β-hCG may be abnormally elevated?**
Multiple gestations
Trophoblastic disease
Molar pregnancy
Choriocarcinoma

**At what rate does serum β-hCG increase?**
Serum concentrations **double every 48 hours during the first trimester** and peak at 100,000 IU/L; levels then regress to 30,000 IU/L from the 20th week until term

**A woman with a positive pregnancy test presents to the ER with vaginal bleeding. She has been trying to become pregnant and cannot remember her last menstrual period (LMP). Her serum β-hCG is 200 IU/L and no gestational sac is visualized on transvaginal ultrasound. What is your next step in management?**
Ask the patient to return in 2 days to recheck the β-hCG. If it is not doubling appropriately she may have an ectopic pregnancy or a spontaneous abortion (SAB). A gestational sac should be visualized with a β-hCG > 1000 IU/L

**What is the estimated gestational age (EGA)?**
Duration of the pregnancy **dated from first day of the LMP**. The EGA of a normal pregnancy at term is 40 weeks

**What is the developmental age (DA) of a pregnancy?**
Duration of the pregnancy **dated from fertilization**; typically 14 days less than the EGA (such that the DA of a normal pregnancy at term is 38 weeks)

**What is the estimated date of confinement (EDC)?**
The "due date" when the pregnancy is full term

**What is Nügele rule?**
For women with a regular 28-day menstrual cycle:

**EDC = LMP – 3 months + 7 days + 1 year**

**What gestational ages are defined by the following terms:**

**First trimester:** <14 weeks

**Second trimester:** 14–28 weeks

**Third trimester:** >28 weeks

**Viability:** 24 weeks

**Prematurity:** 24–36 weeks

**Term:** 37–42 weeks

**Post dates:** >40 weeks

**Post term:** >42 weeks increased risk of perinatal morbidity and mortality

**What ages are defined by the following terms:**

**Neonate:** birth to 28 days of life
**Infant:** birth until 1 year of life

**What are the patient's Gs and Ps?**

**Gravidity**: total number of pregnancies

**Parity**: all viable and nonviable pregnancies, including spontaneous, therapeutic, and voluntary abortions

**What are the four numbers that follow parity?**

First: deliveries >37 weeks EGA
Second: viable deliveries before 37 weeks

Third: abortions and ectopic pregnancies

Fourth: living children (including twins or adoptions)

**What are the Gs and Ps for a mother of three with a history of an normal spontaneous vaginal delivery (NSVD) at term, preterm twins, a fetal demise at 23 weeks, and an ectopic pregnancy at 6 weeks?**

G4 P1213

**How is pregnancy dating confirmed?**

**Ultrasound** (most accurate in the first trimester) and **fundal height** on physical examination

**What size-date discrepancy* would require further evaluation?**

1. Ultrasound should be within 1 week of the EGA during the first trimester, within 2 weeks during the second trimester, and within 3 weeks in the third trimester
2. FH should be within 3 weeks of the EGA (determined by LMP)

*A size-date discrepancy suggests either underlying pathology or an error in dating (requiring the EDC to be changed)

**To what EGA does each fundal height correspond?**

**Symphysis pubis:** 12 weeks EGA
**Umbilicus:** 20 weeks EGA

**Xiphoid process:** 36 weeks EGA

Fundal height in centimeters above the symphysis pubis corresponds to EGA after 20 weeks

**What fetal parameter is most important in assessing viability?**

Fetal cardiac activity

**With each of the following tools, when can fetal cardiac activity be detected?**

**Transvaginal ultrasound**

6 weeks EGA

**Abdominal ultrasound**

10 weeks EGA

**Doppler fetal heart monitor**

12 weeks EGA

**Ascultation**

20 weeks EGA

**What fetal parameters are measured on ultrasound to assess EGA?**

First trimester: crown-rump length

Second/third trimesters: femur length; abdominal circumference; biparietal diameter; head circumference

**Why is dating important?**

Monitoring growth, appropriate timing of screening markers (quad screen, gestational diabetes mellitus [GDM]), delivery planning (fetal lung maturity, postdates)

**A woman presents to the emergency room with abdominal pain. Her period is 1 week late and her serum β-hCG measures 1000 IU/L. Transvaginal ultrasound (TVUS) visualizes thickened endometrial tissue and fluid in the cul-de-sac. What is the greatest concern?**

Ruptured ectopic pregnancy (with possible hemorrhage and shock) TVUS can visualize a gestational sac at 5 weeks EGA, which corresponds to a serum β-hCG level of 1000–1500 IU/L

## MANAGEMENT

**What information should be incorporated in a patient's prenatal care (PNC) records and the labor admission note?**

Age, Gs & Ps, LMP, EDC (determined by LMP and ultrasound)

Chief complaint or presenting issue (routine prenatal care, SOB, CP)

Four cardinal questions (ctx, LOF, vaginal bleed, fetal movements)

Prenatal care: doctor's name, number of visits

Complications during this pregnancy: GDM, AMA, IUGR, teenage pregnancy, and so on

Prenatal labs (PNL)

**Ultrasound:** date/placental location/amniotic fluid volume (AFV)/estimated fetal weight (EFW)/abnormalities/presentation

Past obstetric history (ObHx), past gynecologic history (GynHx), past medical history (PMHx), psychiatric history, past surgical history (PSHx), meds, allergies, family history (FHx), social history (SHx)

**Physical examination: vital signs:** BP, P, T, R, FS (diabetic), urine dip (for everyone if possible, *must* for preeclampsia)

**General, cardiac, lungs, abdomen:** typically soft, NT, gravid, **Leopold**: vertex, left lateral lie, EFW

**Extremities:** Homans +/−, no calf tenderness

**Electronic fetal monitoring (EFM):** baseline, +/− accelerations, +/− decelerations, minimal/moderate/ marked long-term variability

**Tocolysis history (TOCO):** contractions q minutes

**SSE:** normal EFG (external female genitalia), discharge, bleeding, fluid, lesions

**Vaginal examination (VE):** cervical (cx) dilation/ effacement/station of the presenting fetus, cx consistency (firm, soft), cx position (posterior, anterior), clinical pelvimetry

**Assessment and plan:** age (y/o) GxPxxxx @(EGA) weeks with (diagnosis . . . early labor, active labor, SROM, PROM, induction of labor (IOL) secondary to ______) admit to labor and delivery

- Antibiotic prophylaxis (Pphx) if GBS+
- CBC/Type and Screen (T&S)
- NPO except ice chips
- Intravenous fluid (IVF): lactate ringers (LR) @ 120 cc/h
- Plan for pain management
- Fetal heart rate (FHR) tracing reactive/reassuring/ concerning. Continue EFM/TOCO
- Any additional issues that will need to be addressed postpartum

**What are relevant aspects of a patient's past obstetrical history (ObHx)?**

For each prior pregnancy: date of delivery, mode of delivery or outcome, gestational age and weight at delivery (weeks), anesthesia complications, (maternal and fetal)

History of infertility

Type of uterine incision with prior C-sections

Year and EGA of all abortions and procedures (spontaneous abortion [SAB], elective termination of pregnancy [ETOP] or voluntary termination of pregnancy [VTOP], intrauterine demise [IUD] c dilation and curettage [D&C], dilation and evacuation [D&E])

**What are relevant aspects of a patient's past gynecologic history (GynHx)?**

Gyn triad: age of menarche/cycle length/duration of menstruation

History of cysts, fibroids, abnormal Pap smears, gyn surgeries

STIs

Prior use of contraception

**What are relevant aspects of a patient's social history (SH)?**

Domestic violence
Social support

Occupation

Highest level of education

Nutrition

Tobacco, alcohol, drug use

**What are relevant aspects of a patient's genetic & family history (FHx)?**

Relatives with pregnancy-related disorders (e.g., pregnancy losses)

Family history of chronic medical conditions (diabetes, thyroid disorders, hemoglobinopathies)

Consanguinity

Twins

Congenital, chromosomal, or metabolic abnormalities (blood disorders, mental retardation)

Ethnicity of the mother and father (for possible screening tests)

**How much weight should a woman be advised to gain in pregnancy?**

Average women should gain **between 25–35 lbs** (underweight women should gain more and overweight women should gain less)

**When does a fetus experience the most rapid weight gain?**

In the third trimester; the fetus gains approximately $\frac{1}{2}$ lbs/week

**What is the recommended daily nutritional intake during pregnancy?**

Calories: an **additional 300 kcal/day** for each fetus

Protein: increase daily intake by 5–6 g

Iron: requirements double to 30 mg/day

Calcium: increases by 1000 mg in the third trimester during fetal bone calcification

Daily intakes of copper (2 mg), folate (0.4 mg), vitamin C (50 mg), vitamin D (10 mcg or 400 IU), and vitamin $B_{12}$ (2 mcg) should continue

**Which substances and foods should be limited or avoided?**

Tobacco, alcohol, street drugs

Herbal medications

Caffeine > 500 mg or > 4 cups a day (can cause SAB or small for gestational age [SGA])

Iodine (can cause fetal goiter)

Large amounts of vitamins A, D, E, and K

Unpasteurized dairy

Methylmercury (in raw fish, shark, swordfish, king mackerel, and tilefish)

**Should exercise and sexual behaviors change during pregnancy?**

Activity can be maintained at the same intensity prior to pregnancy, in the absence of obstetric or medical complications. If a patient does not, she should be encouraged to begin light exercise

**Should pregnant women continue to wear seat belts?**

**Yes!** All patients should be encouraged to continue to wear seat belts during pregnancy. The lap belt can be placed below the uterus

**How often are prenatal care visits scheduled?**

Every 4 weeks during the first and second trimesters

Every 2 weeks in the third trimester (28–36 weeks)

Once a week near term (36–40 weeks)

Postdates will require more involved monitoring

(Adequate prenatal care requires more than nine visits, with the first visit during the first trimester)

**What are the four cardinal questions asked during each prenatal care visit?**

Presence of:

**Contractions; leakage of fluid; vaginal bleeding; fetal movement (after 20 weeks)**

**What are important parameters in evaluating the pelvic shape?**

Pelvic inlet (diagonal conjugate = distance from the pubic symphysis to the sacral promontory)

Prominence of ischial spines

Pelvic sidewalls (convergent vs parallel)

Shape of sacrum

**What measurements are taken during each standard prenatal care visit?**

Weight

Blood pressure

Urine dip (protein, glucose, leukocytes)

Fundal height

Abdominal doppler fetal heart rate (after 12 weeks)

**Which vaccines should be offered to pregnant women?**

Any required inactivated vaccines and the **influenza vaccine** (in the second or third trimester)

Note: **Do not give vaccines that contain active viral components** (measles, mumps, oral polio vaccine [OPV], or rubella)

**What is advanced maternal age (AMA)?**

**>35 years of age** at the time of delivery (with a singleton pregnancy)

**What symptoms must a patient be educated about? What do each signify?**

**Vaginal bleeding** (SAB in first trimester, placental abruption/previa in second or third trimester)

**Edema, headache, black spots, blurry vision, right upper quadrant pain, epigastric pain** (preeclampsia)

**Dysuria, fever, chills** (pylonephritis)

**What are the signs and symptoms of preterm labor?**

Any of the following symptoms between 20 and 37 weeks EGA:

Abdominal, vaginal, or lower back pain or pressure that does not improve after hydration/rest

Uterine contractions every 10 minutes for more than 1 hour

A sudden thinning or increase in vaginal discharge

Bleeding from the vagina

**What should a patient be advised to do if she experiences these symptoms?**

Contact her health care provider and present to the clinic or hospital for further evaluation

**What is the prevalence of domestic violence (DV) among pregnant women?**

DV is more prevalent among pregnant than nonpregnant women; it affects approximately 1 in 6 women

## SCREENING

**What are routine intake prenatal labs?**

**Hematology**: blood type and screen,

Hemoglobin and hematocrit

**Immunity and infectious:** rubella status (immune or nonimmune)

HIV

HBV (HBsAg & HBsAb)

Syphilis (RPR or VDRL)

*Chlamydia* and gonorrhea cervical cultures

tuberculosis (PPD)

urine culture

**Cytology**: Pap smear

**What are some appropriate screening tests for the following groups?**

**Mediterranean descent** MCV or Hgb electrophoresis for thalassemia (defect in the α or β chain)

**African descent** Hgb electrophoresis for sickle cell

**Ashkenazi Jews descent** Hexosaminidase A leukocyte assay for Tay-Sachs

DNA analysis for: Canavan disease, Bloom syndrome, cystic fibrosis, familial dysautonomia, Fanconi anemia, Gaucher disease, mucolipidosis Type IV, Niemann-Pick disease, or Tay-Sachs disease

**Caucasian descent** Delta F 508 mutations for cystic fibrosis (autosomal recessive)

Serum phenylalanine level for phenylketonuria

**In an Rh(–) pregnant woman with an Rh(+) father of the baby, would her first or second child be at greatest risk?**

Her **second child**, because of isoimmunization and the development of anti-Rh antibodies. The first Rh(+) fetus will only be mildly affected, if at all

**What is the major complication associated with isoimmunization?**

**Hemolytic disease of the newborn** (with possible hydrops, anasarca, or death)

**How is Rh isoimmunization prevented?**

With Rh immune globulin (RhoGAM)—an antibody to the D antigen

**Who is given RhoGAM?**

All Rh(–) mothers with a possible Rh(+) fetus

**When is RhoGAM given?**

At 28 weeks EGA

At delivery

Within 72 hours of an abortion or vaginal bleeding at any gestational age

Following all invasive procedures (CVS or amniocentesis)

**Maternal isoimmunization to which antibodies affect fetal outcome?**

Blood cell antigens: C, D (Duffy), E, K (Kell), and Rh

"Duffy dies, Kelly kills, Lewis lives" (L antigen does not have a significant deleterious affect on the fetus)

**Name some additional screening and diagnostic tests. At what EGA are these routinely completed?**

Nuchal translucency screen (with serum free β-hCG and PAPP-A) 11–13 weeks

Quad or triple screen 15–18 weeks

Anatomic survey with ultrasound (to assess for fetal anomalies) 18–20 weeks

Glucose challenge test (GCT) 24–28 weeks

Streptococcus group B (perineal and rectal culture) 36 weeks

Hgb, Hct, and syphillis >28 weeks (third trimester)

**In appropriate patients what tests should be repeated? At what EGA?**

Gonorrhea, *Chlamydia*, and HIV >28 weeks (third trimester)

Antibody testing in unsensitized Rh(D[−])women 28–30 weeks

**What is the nuchal translucency?**

A cystic space dorsal to the cervical spine measured by ultrasound at 11–13 weeks. It is a **sensitive indicator of chromosomal abnormalities**; a larger diameter signifies a greater risk of aneuploidy and poor fetal outcome

**What other tests enhance the sensitivity of a nuchal translucency?**

Maternal serum free **β-hCG** and plasma protein A (**PAPP-A**) measurements

**What is measured in the triple screen? In the quadruple screen?**

**Triple screen**: **α-fetoprotein (AFP)**, **β-hCG**, and **estriol (E3)**

**Quad screen**: all of above plus **inhibin A**

**When are these tests employed and what do they assess?**

Between 16–20 weeks
Abnormal values correlate with various chromosomal, genetic, and developmental disorders

**How should an abnormal triple/quad screen be followed-up?**

With a detailed ultrasound and possibly an amniocentesis

**What do the following triple screen results suggest?**

**↓ AFP, ↑ hCG, ↓ E3:** Trisomy 21

**↓ AFP, ↓ hCG, ↓ E3:** Trisomy 18

**An elevated AFP may indicate what fetal conditions?**

**Neural tube defects**

**Gastroschisis** (abdominal wall defect, often lateral to the rectus on the right)

| | |
|---|---|
| | **Omphalocele** (midline umbilical hernia covered by peritoneum) |
| **A decreased AFP may indicate what fetal condition?** | Down syndrome |
| **What are the most common neural tube defects (NTDs)?** | Anencephaly and spina bifida |
| **Acetylcholinesterase is a specific marker for NTD when it is increased or decreased in the amniotic fluid?** | Increased |
| **What is a Glucose tolerance test (GCT)?** | A screening test for gestational diabetes. The patient drinks 50 g of glucose and her blood sugar is tested 1 hour later |
| **What is the cutoff for the GCT?** | Serum glucose >130–135mg/dL |
| **What should be done if a patient has an abnormal GCT?** | A diagnostic test called the glucose tolerance test (GTT) |
| **What is a Glucose tolerance test (GTT)?** | After an overnight fast, blood sugar is tested. 100 g glucose is then given and blood sugar is checked every hour for 3 hours |
| **What are the normal values for a GTT?** | Fasting <95 mg/dL<br>1 hour <180 mg/dL<br>2 hours <155 mg/dL<br>3 hours <140 mg/dL |
| **When is gestational diabetes diagnosed?** | If there are two or more abnormal values on the GTT |
| **What is chorionic villus sampling (CVS)?** | A diagnostic procedure for chromosomal and genetic anomalies that involves transvaginal or trans-abdominal aspiration of placental cells at 9–12 weeks EGA |
| **What is the risk of CVS?** | There is a 1/200 risk of adverse fetal outcome or demise |
| **What is an amniocentesis?** | A diagnostic procedure done at **>15 weeks** that can detect chromosomal/genetic abnormalities, amniotic infection, inflammation, and fetal lung maturity. It involves trans-abdominal aspiration of the amniotic fluid from the uterine cavity |
| **What is the risk of amniocentesis?** | There is a 1/300 risk of adverse fetal outcome or demise |

## PRENATAL TESTING AND MONITORING OF THE FETUS

**What is quickening and when does it occur?**

The mother's first **perception of fetal movement (FM)**; it usually occurs **between 16–20 weeks** (may be earlier in a multipara)

**What is a "kick count"?**

After 26–32 weeks, fetal well-being can be assessed by asking the mother to count FM, "kick counts," which should occur eight times every 2 hours

**What are the commonly used tests of fetal well-being and when are they used?**

Non-stress test (**NST**) and biophysical profile (**BPP**)

They are used most commonly for: **decreased fetal movements, diabetic mother, post-dates, chronic HTN,** intrauterine growth restriction (**IUGR**)

**What is an NST?**

Placement of an EFM to trace the fetal heart variability (which rises with fetal movement). A tocodynamometer monitor is also placed to assess for uterine contractions (See Fig. 8-3)

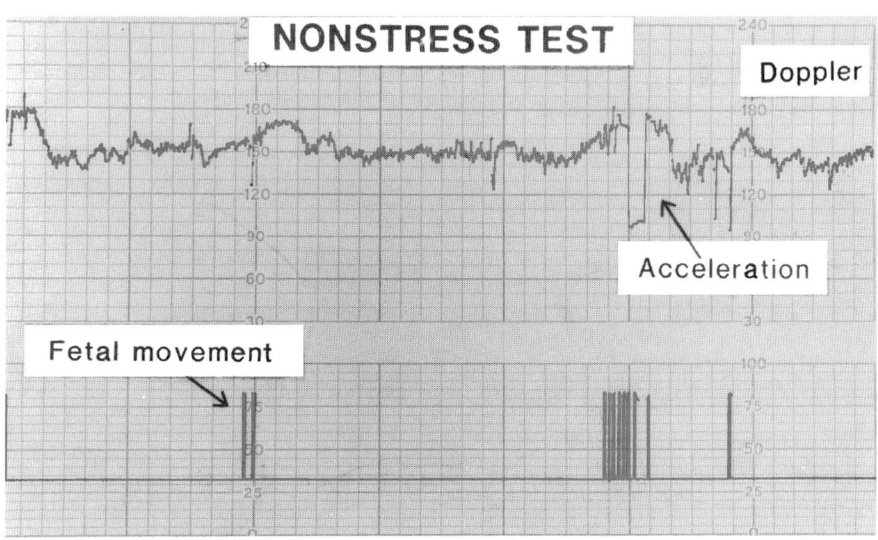


**Figure 8-3** Reactive nonstress test. (Reproduced with permission, from Cunningham FG et al: *Williams Obstetrics,* 22nd ed. New York. McGraw-Hill, 2005:279.)

**What is a reactive NST?**

**Two accelerations** above the baseline of **15 beats per minute (bpm) for 15 seconds** within 20 minutes

**What does a reactive NST indicate?**

Good vagal tone and reassuring fetal status

**What is fetal tachycardia?**

A baseline FHR > 160 bpm

**What is the most common cause of fetal tachycardia?**

Maternal tachycardia

**What are some other causes of fetal tachycardia?**

Maternal fever

Anemia

Asphyxia

Infection

Autoimmune disorders

Adrenergic medications

Cardiac anomalies (e.g., SVT)

**What is fetal bradycardia?**

A baseline FHR < 110 bpm

**What are some causes of fetal bradycardia?**

Physiologic (short episodes because of transient compression of the fetal head/umbilical cord)

Maternal hypotension

Local anesthesia (e.g., paracervical block)

Uteroplacental insufficiency (e.g., placental abruption, uterine rupture, cord prolapse)

Cardiac anomalies

**How is fetal heart rate variability assessed?**

10 minutes of fetal heart tracing is reviewed to assess peak-to-trough long-term variability. Variability may be:

**absent**

**minimal (<5 bpm)**

**moderate (normal = 6–25 bpm)**

**marked (>25 bpm)**

**What is suggested by a sinusoidal pattern on EFM?**

Severe fetal anemia, hypoxia, or exposure to sedative hypnotics

**What are the five components of the bio-physical profile BPP?**

1. **Breathing**: 30 seconds after 30 minutes of observation
2. **Movement**: three gross body movements in 30 minutes

3. **Tone**: extension and flexion of an extremity
4. **Amniotic fluid**: vertical pocket > 2 cm
5. **Reactive NST**

Each is worth 2 points for 10 possible points. The fetus is given 30 minutes to demonstrate each variable

**What do each of the following BPP scores signify?**

**8–10** Reassuring fetal status with an intact CNS

**6** Equivocal test; repeat in a few hours

**4** High risk of fetal hypoxia; consider delivery

**0–2** Fetal hypoxia; delivery immediately regardless of EGA

**Other than fetal hypoxia, what are some other causes of a low BPP?**

Fetal sleep cycle

Transplacental sedatives

Corticosteroids

**Which of the BPP elements are lost first as the fetus becomes progressively more hypoxic?**

Breathing is lost early, then FHR accelerations, movement, and finally tone

**How is chronic fetal stress manifested?**

**Oligohydramnios** (AFI <5 cm or vertical pocket <2 cm), because of several days of decreased renal perfusion

**During hypoxic stress, where is fetal blood preferentially shunted?**

Brain, heart, adrenals, and placenta

**How is fetal perfusion assessed with doppler ultrasound?**

Systolic versus end diastolic flow velocity (**S/D flow**) in the umbilical vessels, middle cerebral artery, and ductus venosus

**What is a normal S/D ratio?**

Less than three (because of low placental resistance) in the third trimester; however, this ratio is dependent on gestational age

**What is a high S/D ratio associated with?**

PEC and IUGR. Reversed diastolic flow suggests a poor fetal outcome

**Before the development of NST/BPP, what test was performed to assess uteroplacental insufficiency?**

A **contraction stress test** (CST). Nipple stimulation or oxytocin was administered to induce three contractions (ctx) every 10 minutes with concurrent FHM. A normal test

| | |
|---|---|
| | has no late decelerations. This is rarely performed today |
| **What are the three types of decelerations?** | Early, late, and variable |
| **Describe early decelerations.** | A gradual decrease from baseline that mirrors a contraction |
| **What do early decelerations signify?** | A vagal response from **compression of the fetal head** during uterine ctx; they are **normal** |
| **Describe variable decelerations.** | A **rapid decline** of more than 15 beats from the baseline that is **unrelated to uterine ctx** |
| **What do variable decelerations signify?** | Usually **cord compression** (can be relieved by changing the mother's position) |
| **Describe late decelerations.** | A gradual decrease from baseline that **starts at the peak of the contraction** and persists until the ctx is finished |
| **What do late decelerations signify?** | **Uteroplacental insufficiency** |
| **Fetal metabolic acidosis and hypoxia are suggested by what findings on a fetal heart tracing?** | Recurrent (>three), prolonged (>3 minute), **late decelerations**<br>Minimal (>5 bpm), **decreased or absent long-term variability**<br>**Tachycardia** (>160 bpm), which may also be associated with infection or maternal fever |
| **What is the significance of irregular contractions in the third trimester?** | If the fetal status is reassuring, there is no cervical change (patient remains closed/long/high), and ctxs are less than 4 per hour (they are likely insignificant **Braxton Hicks contractions**.) If the contractions are painful, the patient may be in latent labor |
| **What is fetal fibronectin?** | A glycoprotein that is normally present in maternal circulation and amniotic fluid. If it is present in the cervicovaginal secretions (>50 ng/mL), it suggests that the **cervix is undergoing structural change** and the patient may go into labor in the next 2 weeks |
| **How is fetal fibronectin used clinically?** | It has a high negative predictive value, so it is used to rule out preterm labor |

# Labor and Delivery

## DIAGNOSIS AND DEFINITIONS

**What percentage of deliveries at U.S. hospitals are** normal spontaneous vaginal deliverys **(NSVDs) with no intervention?**

Approximately 50%

**How is labor defined?**

**Regular uterine contractions** that result in **cervical effacement** and **dilation** and eventual **expulsion of the fetus** and **placenta**

**How is labor diagnosed?**

With **tocodynamometry** and **serial cervical examinations**

**What are some of the signs of labor?**

**Painful contractions**

**Bloody show**

**Spontaneous rupture of membranes** (SROM)

**What is bloody show?**

Vaginal passage of blood-tinged mucus

**What are the four characteristics of cervical change?**

Change in **consistency** (from firm to soft)

Change in **position** (from posterior to anterior)

Progressive **effacement** (cervix becomes shorter and thinner)

**Dilation** of the internal and external os (from 0 to 10 cm)

**The following terms refer to rupture of fetal membranes (ROM) under what conditions?**

**PROM;** premature rupture of membranes; at least 1 hour before the onset of labor

**PPROM;** preterm, premature rupture of membranes; EGA <37 weeks with rupture at least 1 hour before the onset of labor

**Prolonged PROM;** rupture of membranes >18 hours without the onset of labor

**What are the four signs and symptoms of spontaneous rupture of membranes?**

Initial gush with **continued loss of fluid**

**Pooling** of vaginal fluid on sterile speculum examination

Positive **nitrazine** blue test (indicating that the vaginal fluid is alkaline, with a pH greater than 6)

**Ferning** of dried fluid under low power magnification (because of fetal urine salt crystals in the amniotic fluid [AF])

**What can cause a false-positive nitrazine blue test?**

Anything that causes the vagina to become more alkaline, such as:

Sperm

Blood

Infection

Douching

**What is the pH of amniotic fluid?**

7.0

**Describe the following terms:**

**Nulligravida;** a woman who never conceived a fetus

**Nullipara;** a woman who never carried a fetus to viability

**Primipara;** a woman who has delivered a viable fetus in the past, regardless of the outcome of the fetus

**Multigravida;** a woman who has carried more than one fetus to viability, regardless of the outcome of the fetus

**Grand multiparity;** given birth five or more times

**What is the term for a difficult delivery, protracted labor, or arrest of labor?**

**Labor dystocia**

**How do labor forces and the passage of the fetal head through the birth canal affect the fetal head (in cephalic presentations)?**

The fetal calvarium undergoes **molding**, where the bones of the skull shift to minimize the diameter that must pass through the bony pelvis

**On vaginal examination, the presenting fetal vertex is noted to be soft without any identifiable sutures or fontaneles. What is the term for this fetal finding (which often occurs in prolonged labors with slow cervical dilation)?**

**Caput succedaneum**; the tissues overlying the fetal calvarium become edematous and swollen

**How is cardiac output (CO) affected during labor?**

There is a 50% increase in CO during the second stage (preload increases as blood from the uterine sinusoids enters systemic circulation)

**How much does maternal blood pressure increase during labor?**

Systolic blood pressure increases up to 25% and diastolic blood increases up to 15%. It is increased during uterine contractions, with pain or anxiety, and with maternal positions that affect venous return. The pressure in the amniotic fluid, cerebrospinal fluid, and dural compartments also increase with labor

**Why are women in labor predisposed to gastric aspiration?**

Increased intra-abdominal pressure

Relaxation of the lower esophageal sphincter

Recumbent laboring position

**What are some of the consequences of gastric aspiration?**

Pneumonia

Bronchospasm

Adult respiratory distress syndrome (ARDS)

**What precaution is taken in labor to minimize this risk?**

Oral intake is restricted to occasional ice chips

**What is a pudendal block?**

A method of administering local anesthesia to the pudendal nerve (sacral nerve roots 2, 3, and 4), with subsequent decreased vulvar sensation

**How is a pudendal block administered?**

Transvaginally; the anesthetic is injected medial and inferior to the ischial spines through the sacrospinous ligaments bilaterally

**Where is an epidural catheter placed?**

A guide needle is used at the interspinous space between the fourth and fifth lumbar vertebra. The ligamentum flavum is penetrated and the catheter is threaded into the potential epidural space, which is comprised of lymphatics and venous plexuses. An epidural injection enters the extradural or peridural space; it does not penetrate the dura mater

**Where is a spinal block placed?**

It enters the dura and then the subarachnoid space, bathed by cerebral spinal fluid. Only the pia mater separates the cord from the injected substance

**What are the risks associated with epidurals and spinal blocks?**

Spinal headache

Hypotension

Infection

Hematoma

High spinal blockade

Cord compression (a surgical emergency)

**What advantages does a spinal block offer?**

A faster onset and requires a lower dose of anesthetics

**What risks are increased with a spinal block?**

Hypotension (sympathectomy causing peripheral vasodilatation)

Nausea

Compromised placental perfusion

Ascending respiratory paralysis (because of anesthesia reaching the cervical nerve roots 3, 4, & 5)

**Does regional, local, or general anesthesia increase the rate of cesarean delivery?**

No

## FETAL POSITION

**What is the fetal lie?**

The **crown-rump axis** of the fetus **in relation to the longitudinal axis of the uterus**

**What types of fetal lie are there?**

Longitudinal

Transverse

Oblique

**What is the fetal presentation?**

The **fetal part closest to the cervix and pelvic inlet**

**What is the most common fetal presentation?**

Cephalic, followed by breech

**What are the other types of fetal presentation? Describe them.**

**Types of cephalic presentation:**

Vertex

Brow

Mentum

Face (depending on which part is leading through the cervix)

**Types of breech presentation:**

Frank breech (flexed hips and extended knees)

Complete breech (flexed hips and knees)

Footling breech (one knee flexed, one knee extended) (See Fig. 8-4)

**Other:**

Hand

Shoulder

Funic

Compound (involves more than one fetal part leading) e.g., cord and head or hand and head)

**What is the incidence of mal-presentation (any presentation not cephalic) at the onset of labor?**

Less than 4%

**Fetal attitude or posture describes what characteristic?**

The **degree of flexion of the fetal neck, back, and joints** of the limbs

**Describe the fetal postures from most flexed to most extended**

**Vertex → Military → Brow (forehead) → Face**

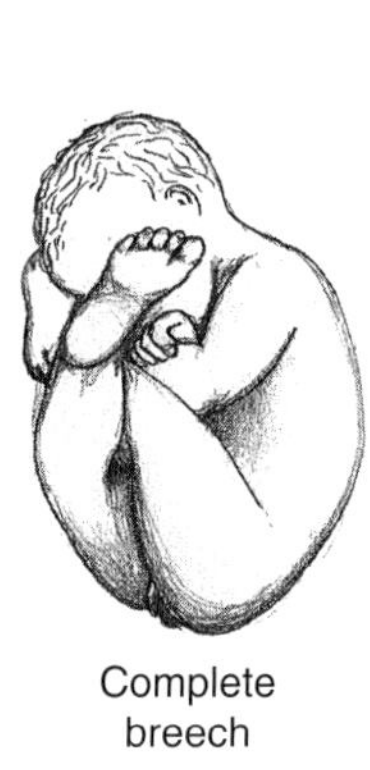


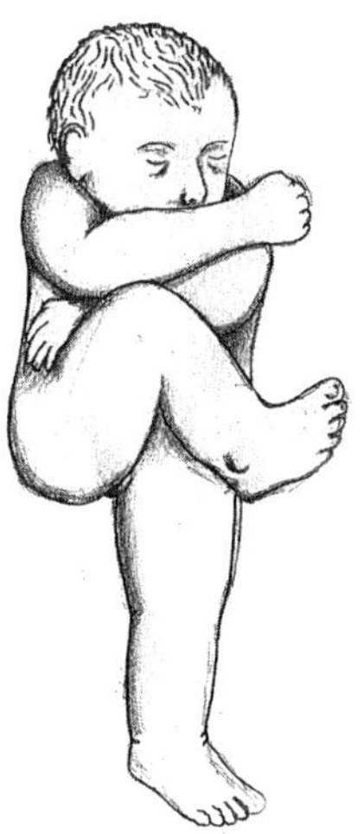


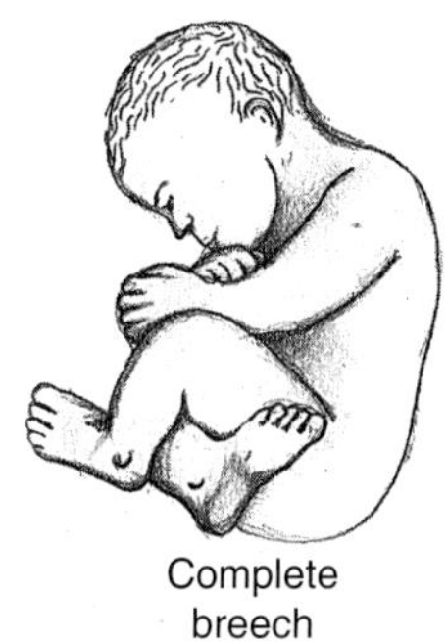


**Figure 8-4** Breech presentation.

**What are the risks associated with an extended neck?**

The fetus requires a larger leading diameter and thus has less ability to negotiate the birth canal. This can lead to **labor dystocia**

**What are the shapes of the two fetal fontanels and when do they close?**

The **anterior** or frontal fontanel is **diamond shaped** and closes late in infancy (near 13 months). The **posterior** or occipital fontanel is **triangle shaped** and closes early in infancy (near 2 months)

**During labor how are the fetal fontanels examined? What is the significance of this examination?**

The fetal scalp is examined through the dilating cervix on sterile vaginal examination (SVE). The **location of the posterior fontanel** is noted with regard to **maternal left/right** and **anterior/ posterior/transverse orientation**. This describes the specific **position** of the presenting fetal head. (See Fig. 8-5)

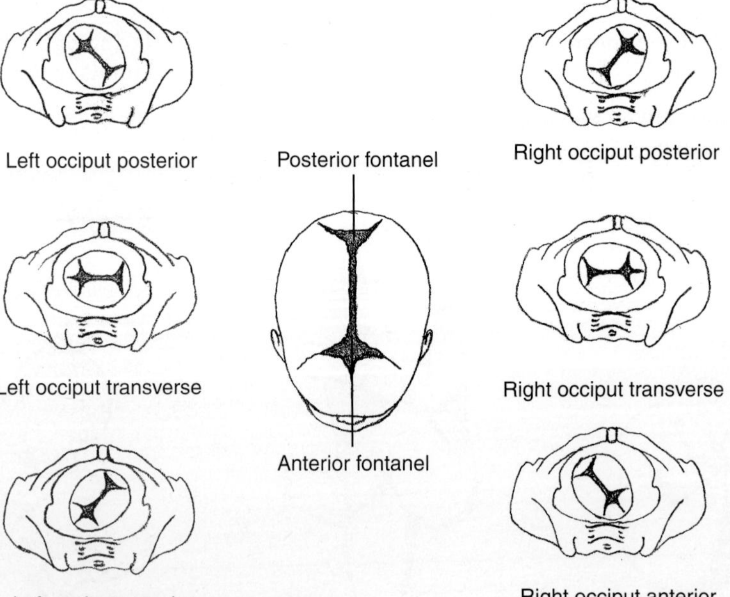


**Figure 8-5** Vertex presentations.

**Why does the occiput posterior (OP) position frequently cause labor dystocia?**

Because the fetal head must be more flexed and rotate more extensively (135 degrees instead of 90 degrees) to pass under the symphysis pubis. Additionally, this position is often associated with brow or face presentations

**What is a normal synclitism?**

When the leading sagittal suture is parallel to the pelvic outlet

**What is anterior asynclitism?**

When the **sagittal suture is deflected toward the sacrum**, allowing more of the parietal bone to be palpated anteriorly

**What is posterior asynclitism?**

**Deflection of the fetal sagittal suture toward the maternal symphysis pubis**. It is normal unless the tilt is severe

**How is the position of a fetus described in a face or breech presentation?**

The relationship of the fetal mentum (chin) or sacrum are described in relation to maternal right, left, anterior, and posterior

**Leopold maneuvers convey what information about the fetus?**

Estimated fetal weight (EFW)

Fetal presenting part

Fetal lie

Engagement

**What are the four Leopold maneuvers?**

**First position:** hands are placed at the cephalic margins of the fundus, to determine the nonpresenting part that occupies the fundus, and the fetal lie

**Second position:** hands are placed at the right and left margins of the fundus, to feel for small fetal parts, to confirm fetal position

**Third position:** thumb and finger are placed just above the symphysis pubis to assess engagement of the presenting part

**Fourth position:** facing the patient's feet, the examiner's fingers trace the fundus toward the pelvic inlet to identify the anterior shoulder with cephalic presentation and to assess the degree of descent of the presenting part (See Fig. 8-6)

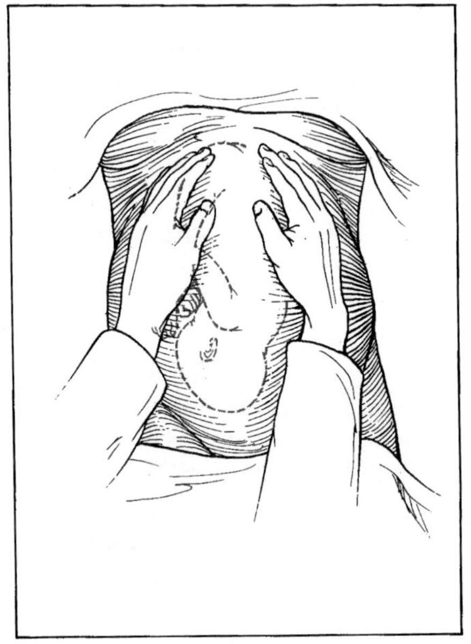

First maneuver

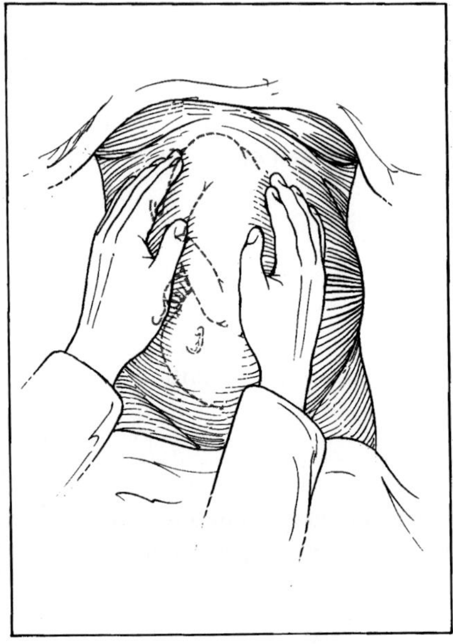

Second maneuver

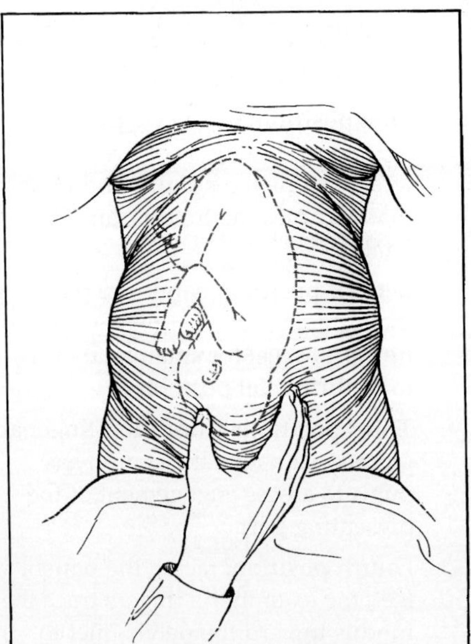

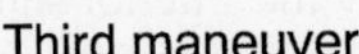

Third maneuver

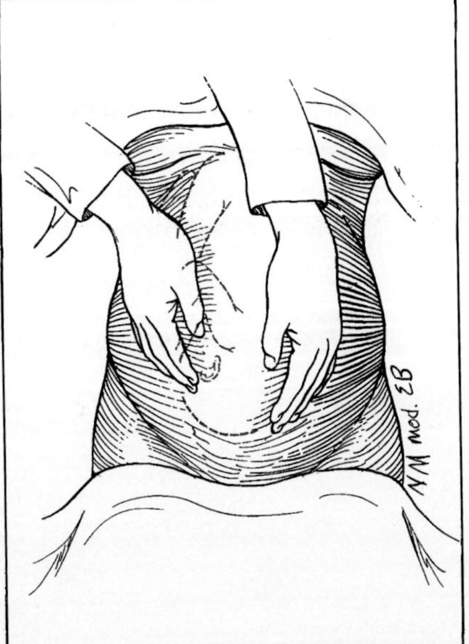

Fourth maneuver

**Figure 8-6** Leopold maneuvers. (Reproduced with permission, from Cunningham FG et al.: *William Obstetrics,* 22nd ed. New York: McGraw-Hill, 2005:416.)

## PELVIMETRY AND VAGINAL EXAMINATION

**The pelvis is composed of what eight bones?**

Ilium (× 2), ischium (× 2), pubis (× 2), sacrum, coccyx

**When is an SVE indicated?**

During PNC visits at term

Upon presentation to labor and delivery with symptoms of labor

Periodically throughout the course of labor (approximately every 2 hours) to assess progress

**When should a manual pelvic examination *not* be performed?**

When there is **bright red blood per vagina** (because of risk of increased trauma with vasa previa or placenta previa), ultrasound should be performed first to confirm no previa

**What information is gathered during a manual pelvic examination?**

Fetal position

Cervical dilation/cervical effacement/station of the presenting fetus

Cervical consistency (firm, soft)

Cervical position (posterior, anterior)

Clinical pelvimetry (diagonal conjugate, pelvic sidewalls, interspinous diameter, and a wide pubic arch)

**What is the interspinous diameter and what is its significance?**

It is the distance between the ischial spines and is used to estimate the station of the presenting fetal part

**What station is associated with each of the following positions?**

**A leading edge that is –3 cm above the ischial spines** (–3 station)

**A leading edge that is at the level of the spines** (0 station)

**A leading edge that is 3 cm past the spines** (+3 station)

**What is zero station (determined on SVE)?**

When the **leading fetal edge is at the level of the maternal ischial spines**

**What is its obstetrical significance of zero station?**

It represents the **most narrow sagittal obstetric diameter** and so signifies that the largest fetal diameter has engaged the bony pelvis

**What modalities can be used for pelvimetry?**

X-ray, computed tomography, magnetic resonance imaging, and physical examination

**What is the significance of pelvic classification and clinical pelvimetry?**

Clinical pelvimetry seeks to describe the pelvic inlets, angles, and diameters. However, pelvic type and pelvimetry are not reliable predictors of vaginal delivery, labor dystocia, or cesarean section and so they are rarely employed in contemporary obstetrics

**What is the best indicator of pelvic adequacy?**

Prior vaginal delivery, prior progress of labor, or family history of cephalopelvic disproportion (CPD)

**From what reference point are all three anterior posterior (AP) pelvic diameters measured?**

From the sacral promontory

**List the following from narrowest to widest: true, obstetric, and diagonal conjugates**

Obstetric < true < diagonal

**Which conjugate can be directly measured on physical examination?**

The **diagonal conjugate** (or transverse diameter)

**How is the diagonal conjugate measured?**

From the inferior margin of the pubic bone to the sacral promontory (average diameter 12.5 cm)

**How is the diagonal conjugate used?**

To indirectly assess the obstetric conjugate (which is 2 cm shorter and cannot be measured by clinical examination)

**What is the obstetric conjugate? What is its significance?**

Measured from the middle of the pubic bone to the sacral promontory, it is the **shortest AP diameter** of the bony pelvis (average diameter 10.5 cm)

**What is the true conjugate?**

Also known as the anteroposterior diameter or conjugate vera, it is the **diameter at the inlet of the true bony pelvis** (average diameter 11 cm). It is measured from the superior margin of the symphysis pubis to the sacral promontory

## STAGES OF LABOR

**What is the biggest difference between the labor of nulliparous and multiparous women?**

**Labor tends to be longer in nulliparous women**, who are also more likely to experience a failure to progress

**What defines the first stage of labor?**

The onset of **consistent painful contractions** until the cervix is

| | |
|---|---|
| | **completely dilated** (10 cm) and **100% effaced** |
| **The first stage of labor is considered to be abnormal when it exceeds what length?** | Over **24.7 hours in nulliparas**; over **18.8 hours in multiparas** ***(based on Friedman data)*** |
| **How is the first stage of labor further subdivided?** | Into **latent** and **active phase** (See Fig. 8-7) |

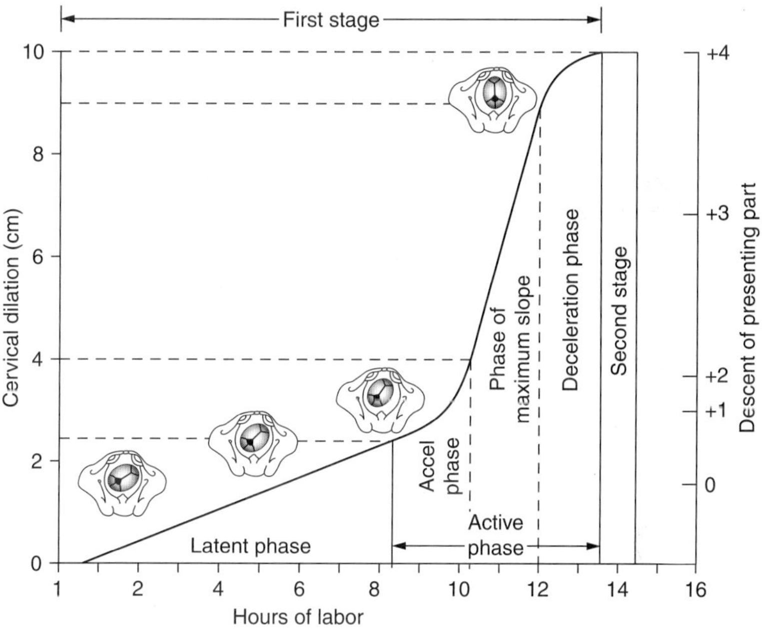


**Figure 8-7** Schematic illustration of progress of cervical dilation against time in the successive stages of labor.

| | |
|---|---|
| **Describe the latent phase** | **Regular painful contractions** every 5–10 minutes that result in **cervical dilation up to 3–5 cm** |
| **Describe the active phase** | A **faster rate of cervical dilation** which typically begins after 3–5 cm dilation in the presence of regular uterine contractions that **continues through full cervical dilation of 10 cm** |
| **What are minimum adequate rates of cervical dilation during the active phase?** | For **multiparas**: at least **1.5 cm/h**<br>For **nulliparas**: at least **1.2 cm/h** |

**What are some conditions that slow the active phase?**

Uterine dysfunction

Fetal malposition

CPD

**How is the active phase of the first stage of labor further subdivided?**

**Acceleration phase**: an increasing rate of dilation from 3-5 cm cervical dilatation to 8 cm

**Deceleration phase**: a slower rate of cervical dilation after 8 cm until full dilation

**How is arrest of dilation defined?**

**>2 hours with no cervical change in the presence of adequate contractions**

**What are adequate contractions?**

More than 200 Montevideo units (MU) as calculated by internal fetal monitoring

**What is the average duration of the active phase in nulliparous patients?**

3.3 hours

**What is the second stage of labor?**

From a **fully dilated** and **fully effaced** cervix **until delivery** of the fetus

**What is the average duration of the second stage of labor?**

In **nulliparas**: **54 minutes** (but can be up to 146 minutes)

In **multiparas**: **18 minutes** (but can be up to 64 minutes)

**What is a protracted labor?**

When there continues to be some cervical change or descent of the fetus; however, it is **progressing slower than would be expected for the parity**

**Define protraction of the second stage in terms of fetal descent**

In **nulliparas**: fetal head descent **<1 cm/h**

In **multiparas**: fetal head descent **<2 cm/h**

**Define protraction of the second stage in terms of length of labor (without anesthesia)**

In **nulliparas**: **>118 minutes (or 2 hours)**

In **multiparas**: **>47 minutes (or 1 hour)**

**What is arrest of labor?**

**Complete cessation of dilation** (no change for 2 hours) **or descent** (no change for 1 hour) despite adequate contractions

**What are the causes of secondary arrest of labor?**

The three "P"s:

**Power** (inadequate uterine contractions)

**Passage** (pelvic disproportion)

**Passenger** (malpresentation or hydrocephalus)

**Define arrest of descent**

**More than 2 hours** in a nullipara or **>1 hour** in a multipara with no descent of the fetus despite adequate contractions

If the patient has had an epidural or regional anesthesia she is given 1 additional hour

**When should a woman begin pushing to aid in the descent and delivery of the fetus?**

During the **second stage** (after full cervical dilatation)

**Why is pushing avoided in the first stage of labor?**

To prevent cervical lacerations and maternal exhaustion

**A nulliparous patient at term has dilated from 6 to 7 cm over 2 hours. Is this adequate change, protracted dilation, or arrest of dilation during the active phase of labor?**

Protracted dilation (a nullipara should dilate at least 1.2 cm/h during the active phase of the first stage of labor)

**In the above patient, what should be done?**

Her contraction pattern should be evaluated and, in the setting of reassuring fetal status, her labor can be augmented if her contractions do not appear to be adequate

**A rate of cervical dilation >5 cm/h in a nulliparous or 10 cm/h in a multiparous patient is considered what type of labor?**

Precipitous labor

**What risks are associated with precipitous labor?**

An increased risk of fetal hypoxia, brain injury, and maternal morbidity such as hemorrhage and vaginal/cervical lacerations

**A multiparous patient progressed from 3 cm on admission to 10 cm in 30 minutes, and pushed for 2 hours to deliver a viable baby girl. How would you describe the first and second stage of her labor?**

A precipitous first stage with a significantly protracted second stage of labor. Greater than 20 minutes for multiparas is considered a prolonged second stage

**How is the third stage of labor defined?**

It begins **after delivery** of the fetus and continues **until the placenta is delivered**

**What is the acceptable duration of the third stage of labor?**

Less than 30 minutes (although some clinicians will wait up to 60 minutes)

**What are the three Gs that indicate the placenta has separated and is ready to be delivered?**

Globular uterus

Growing cord

Gush of blood

**What is the fourth stage of labor?**

The acute maternal **hemodynamic adjustment to the fluid shifts** associated with labor that lasts 1–2 hours after delivery of the placenta

**Why is the woman at increased risk for in the fourth stage of labor?**

Postpartum hemorrhage

## CARDINAL MOVEMENTS OF LABOR

**What are the seven cardinal movements of labor?**

The positions that describe the behavior of the fetal head during the second stage of labor. They include **engagement, descent, flexion, internal rotation, extension, external rotation** (or restitution), and **expulsion**
(See Fig. 8-8)

**Fetal engagement occurs at what station?**

0 station (when the leading fetal edge has reached the ischial spines)

**What is considered to be inadequate downward passage of the fetus during the second stage of labor?**

Less than 1 cm/h in a nulliparous patient and less than 2 cm/h in a multiparous woman

**Why does a fetus flex and rotate during labor?**

To negotiate the 90 degree concave curvature of the pelvic passage (the curve of Carus)

**The fetus presents the smallest diameter of its head (suboccipito-bregmatic diameter) by engaging what position?**

Tight anterior **flexion** of the head (the inability to flex the head may lead to a dystocia)

**How does the fetal head undergo internal rotation?**

The fetus rotates so as to turn the saggital suture from a transverse to an anteroposterior position, it is a passive movement

**When does the fetal head undergo extension?**

As the fetus is crowning at the introitus and the head has passed under the symphysis pubis

**What cardinal movements occur while the fetal head is at the introitus?**

Extension and external rotation

**After the fetal head is delivered what subsequent steps should the clinician take?**

1. Check for nuchal cord (umbilical cord around the neck)
2. Apply gentle downward pressure to assist the delivery of the anterior shoulder

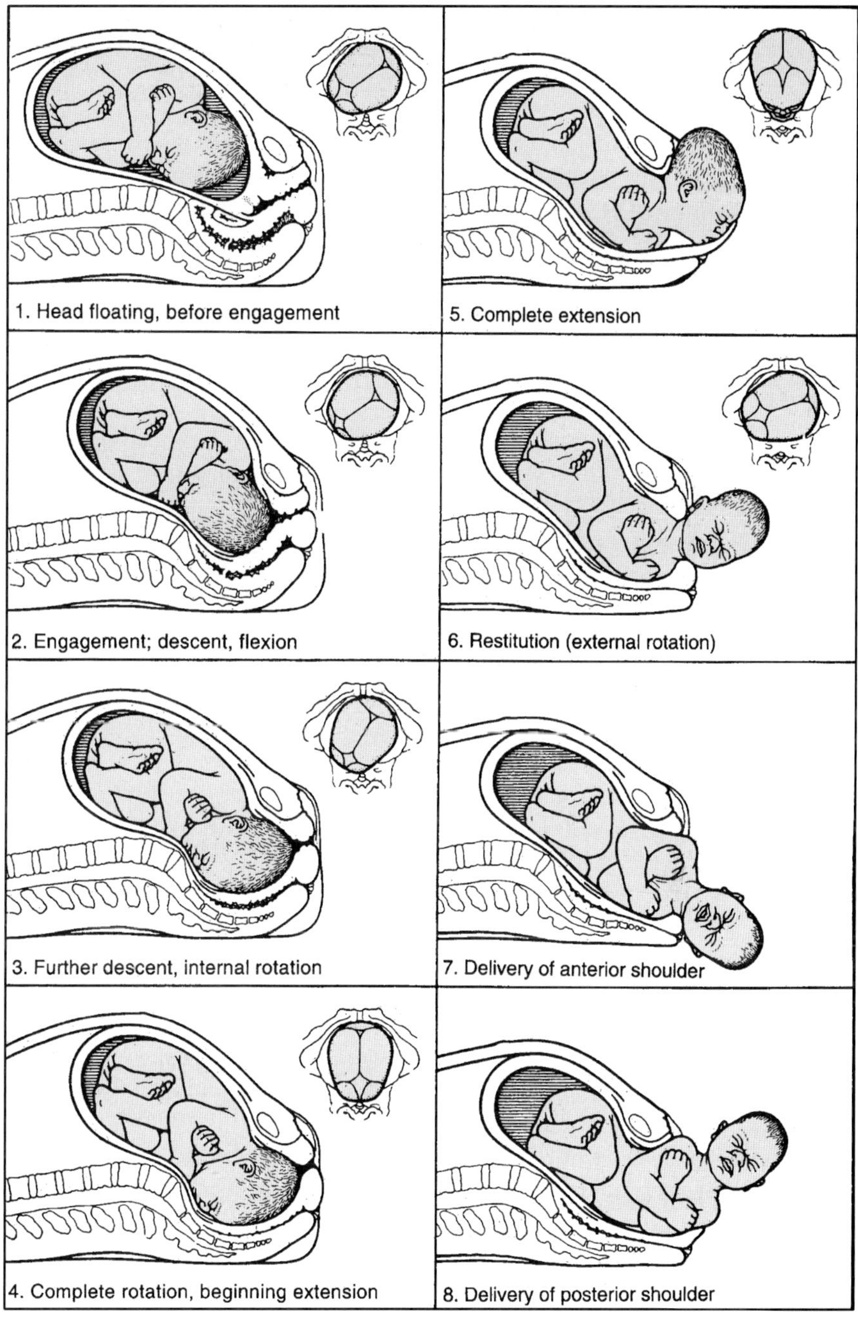


**Figure 8-8** Cardinal movements of labor. (Reproduced with permission, from Cunningham FG et al: *Williams Obstetrics,* 22nd ed. McGraw-Hill, 2005:418.)

3. Gentle upward pressure for the posterior shoulder
4. Support the subsequent delivery of the fetus's body

## INDUCTION OF LABOR

**What are some indications for induction of labor (IOL)?**

Prolonged pregnancy (postterm)

Diabetes mellitus

Rh alloimmunization

Preeclampsia

ROM at term

Placental insufficiency

Non-reassuring fetal status

Oligohydramnios

Intrauterine growth restriction

**What are some contraindications to IOL?**

Previous cesarean with a classical uterine incision

Prior uterine surgery involving the myometrium

EFW >4500 g

Severe fetal hydrocephalus

Malpresentation (breech)

Cervical cancer

Active genital herpes

Placenta or vasa previa

**What is the Bishop score?**

A rating system that evaluates a woman's cervix on SVE to **predict the likelihood that she will be able to complete a vaginal delivery following IOL**; a score of 5 or greater is favorable

**What are the five cervical components of the Bishop score?**

**Consistency**: firm 0, medium 1, soft 2

**Position**: posterior 0, middle 1, anterior 2

**Effacement**: 0–100% (0–3)

**Dilation**: 0–10 cm (0–3)

**Station**: –3 to +2 (0–3)

Mnemonic: "see peds" CPEDS

| | |
|---|---|
| **What Bishop scores correspond to the following probabilities of failed IOL?** | **Less than 50%:** 0–4<br>**Less than 10%:** 5–9<br>**Less than 1%:** 10–13 |
| **Preinduction cervical ripening can be achieved with what medications?** | Prostaglandin PGE1: **misoprostol** (tablets)<br>PGE2 or dinoprostone: **prepidil** (cervical gel) and **cervadil** (vaginal insert) |
| **What mechanical techniques are used to ripen the cervix for IOL?** | Hygroscopic cervical dilators (laminaria)—seaweed sticks that absorb water and expand<br>Balloon; tipped transcervical catheter or Foley bulb<br>Membrane stripping or rupture to increase endogenous prostaglandins |

## INTRAPARTUM ASSESSMENT AND MONITORING

| | |
|---|---|
| **Labor depends on the coordination of what three variables?** | Passage, powers, and passenger |
| **What are the components of the maternal pelvis (passage)?** | Soft tissues (cervix, vagina, pelvic floor muscles)<br>Bony pelvis (ilium, ischium, pubis, sacrum, coccyx) |
| **What is defined as adequate uterine contractions (power)?** | 3–5 contractions every 10 minutes (or 5–7 q 15 minutes) |
| **What techniques can be used to count the number of contractions?** | Palpation<br>External tocodynamometry<br>Intrauterine pressure catheter (IUPC) |
| **Which of these devices is able to assess the force of the contractions?** | Only **IUPC** |
| **What are Montevideo units?** | Quantifications of intrauterine pressure (IUP) as determined by IUPC. They are calculated by **multiplying the average peak strength** of the contraction **by the number of contractions** over 10 minutes |
| **At what target MU are contractions considered adequate?** | >200 |
| **What is uterine tachysystole?** | More than five contractions in 10 minutes with a non-reassuring fetal heart tracing |

**What is uterine hyperstimulation?**

More than five contractions in 10 minutes with a non-reassuring fetal heart tracing

**What is a tonic contraction?**

A contraction that lasts more than 3 minutes (in the context of a non-reassuring fetal tracing or fetal decelerations)

**Why does uterine hyperstimulation/ tonic contraction compromise placental blood flow?**

The pressure in the placental sinuses exceeds maternal systolic BP, resulting in insufficient perfusion and fetal hypoxia

**What aspects of the fetus can impact labor (passenger)?**

Size (macrosomic >4000 g)

Lie, presentation, attitude, position, asynclitism

Number of fetuses

Anatomic anomalies (sacrococcygeal teratoma)

**What are the ideal fetal characteristics for negotiating the maternal pelvis?**

A small fetus, longitudinal lie, flexed OA at 0 station

**What is the average EFW at term?**

3000–4000 g

**Fetal scalp electrode (FSE) monitoring offers what benefits to electronic fetal monitoring (EFM)?**

Continuous monitoring of the fetal heart rate in an obese patient or difficult to monitor fetus

Precise beat-to-beat assessment of variability and decelerations

**How is the FSE applied?**

Placental membranes must be ruptured and the electrode is adhered to the fetal calvarium

**In what clinical setting is fetal blood sampling (fetal scalp pH) performed?**

To acutely assess hypoxemia in the setting of non-reassuring FHR tracing, meconium, or other signs of fetal distress

**What is suggested by the following range of fetal scalp pHs?**

**pH >7.25** reassuring; a low probability of hypoxic-ischemic encephalopathy

**pH 7.24-7.20** indeterminate; should be repeated in 30 minutes

**pH <7.20** a non-reassuring pH; delivery should be expedited with operative intervention

**What other clinical information can be utilized to improve the predictive value of a low scalp pH?**

FHR variability

## MANAGEMENT

**What is the active management of labor?**

The proactive utilization of various techniques and augmenting interventions, with the goal of shortening the duration of labor and reducing cesarean deliveries

**What can be used to augment latent labor or prolonged early labor?**

Cervical ripening agents (prostaglandins)

Cervical dilators (laminaria or a Foley)

Intravenous oxytocin

An amniotomy

**Within what time frame following ROM is it recommended to administer antibiotic prophylaxis to GBS(+) patients?**

Within 6 hours of ROM or at the onset of labor

**What is the effect of oxytocin (Pitocin) on labor?**

It **increases the frequency** and **force** of **uterine contractions**

**What is the half-life of oxytocin?**

3–5 minutes

**A nulliparous patient is receiving 15 mU/min of intravenous oxytocin to augment her labor. Mother and fetus are tolerating labor well. There is no evidence of CPD, and an IUPC indicates 180 MU. What is the next step in management?**

Increase the oxytocin (up to 30–50 mU/min); the goal is to achieve >200 MU

**What are the risks involved with prolonged high-dose oxytocin administration?**

Maternal SIADH and excessive fluid retention (pulmonary edema)

Hyperstimulation of the uterus

Postpartum atony and hemorrhage

Hyperbilirubinemia of the infant

**Why is an amniotomy or assisted rupture of membranes (AROM) performed?**

To induce or augment labor

To assess for meconium in the amniotic fluid

To place an IUPC or FSE

**If the fetal head is not engaged in the pelvis or well applied to the cervix why is an amniotomy contraindicated?**

Because of the risk of **umbilical cord prolapse**, compression by the presenting fetal part, and subsequent fetal hypoxia

**A woman at 37 weeks EGA presents with painful uterine contractions, reassuring fetal status, no signs or symptoms of ROM,**

Braxton Hicks contractions (prodromal or false labor)

**and an unchanged SVE after 3 hours. The cervix remains long, closed, and high. Irregular contractions occur at 15–20 minute intervals, what is your diagnosis?**

**How should the above woman be managed?**

She should be **hydrated**, scheduled for **close clinical follow-up**, and advised to **go home** with labor precautions

**In the presence of a non-reassuring fetal heart rate what initial interventions should be tried?**

Position the mother in left lateral decubitus position with flexed knees

Supplemental oxygen with a face mask

Refrain from active pushing

Turn off the oxytocin and consider tocolytics

**What is tocolysis?**

Relaxation of the uterine smooth muscle in the context of persistent fetal distress

**What substances are commonly used for tocolysis?**

Terbutaline, magnesium sulfate, nifedipine, indomethacin

**What are the risks of applying traction on the cord during the third stage of labor?**

**Avulsion of the cord or placenta** and **uterine inversion**

**How can this risk be reduced?**

By **applying suprapubic pressure** when applying gentle traction to the cord (fundal pressure should not be applied). The placenta and uterus should be examined, to ensure that no membranes or accessory lobes are retained

**After delivery of the placenta what is given to prevent postpartum hemorrhage?**

20 units (2 mL) of **oxytocin** in 1 L of lactate ringers

**What are the four classifications of vaginal and perineal lacerations?**

**First degree** limited to vaginal mucosa and skin of the introitus

**Second degree** extends to the fascia and muscles of the perineal body

**Third degree** trauma involves the anal sphincter

**Fourth degree** extends into the rectal lumen, through the rectal mucosa

**What are the indications for an episiotomy?**

To expedite delivery in the setting of non-reassuring fetal heart tracing or maternal exhaustion

| | |
|---|---|
| | Shoulder dystocia (to facilitate operator maneuvers)<br>Breech delivery<br>Operative vaginal delivery (forceps or vacuum)<br>OP positions |
| **Why is an episiotomy only performed with clear indication?** | Third and fourth degree lacerations and anal incontinence of stool or flatus are more common with an episiotomy than with a spontaneous laceration |
| **What are advantages of midline episiotomies when compared with mediolateral episiotomies?** | They are associated with fewer infections, faster healing, less pain, less blood loss, less dyspareunia, and better anatomical results |
| **What is the one advantage of the mediolateral episiotomy?** | Decreased risk of extension to a third or fourth degree laceration |
| **What muscles are affected by second degree lacerations?** | Bulbocavernous and ischiocavernous laterally<br>Superficial transverse perineal muscle |

## OPERATIVE VAGINAL DELIVERY

| | |
|---|---|
| **What are the two major types of operative vaginal delivery?** | Forceps and vacuum |
| **What is required for operative vaginal delivery?** | Fully dilated cervix<br>Ruptured membranes<br>Engaged fetal head (at or below zero station)<br>Known absence of CPD<br>Known position of the fetal head<br>Experienced operator<br>The capability to perform an emergency cesarean delivery if necessary |
| **What are the various types of forceps deliveries?** | **Outlet:** fetal scalp is visible at the introitus and rotation does not exceed 45 degrees<br>**Low:** +2 station and may require more than 45 degrees of rotation to AP orientation |

**Mid-pelvic:** head is engaged at or below 0 station (but above +2 station), rotation is often required to mimic the cardinal movements of labor

**High:** above 0 station

**Operative vaginal delivery is appropriate or indicated in what context?**

Maternal or fetal distress (e.g., infection, heart, or lung disease, exhaustion, prolonged second stage)

**What are the most common maternal morbidities involved with forceps delivery?**

Increased perineal trauma (third and fourth degree extensions)

Increased need for blood transfusion (these risks are increased with more rotation or at a higher station)

**Vacuum delivery confers what advantages over forceps?**

Can be achieved with minimal analgesia

**What are some contraindications to vacuum-assisted delivery?**

Low birth weight fetus (estimated fetal weight <2500 g)

Prematurity <34 weeks

Suspected fetal coagulopathy

Recent scalp blood sampling

Face or breech presentation

An inability for the mother to engage in expulsive efforts

Cessation of contractions (vacuum traction must be coordinated with maternal effort)

**What are the most common fetal morbidities involved with forceps and vacuum delivery?**

Scalp lacerations, bruising, subgaleal hematomas, cephalohematomas, intracranial hemorrhage, neonatal jaundice, subconjunctival hemorrhage, clavicular fracture, shoulder dystocia, facial nerve injury, Erb palsy, retinal hemorrhage, and fetal death

**Which operative vaginal delivery is associated with more trauma to the fetus?**

Vacuum delivery—there is an increased risk of cephalohematoma and retinal hemorrhage when compared with forceps delivery

**Which operative vaginal delivery method is associated with more maternal trauma to the perineum?**

Forceps (except when electively applied to facilitate outlet delivery of the fetus)

## CESAREAN DELIVERY

**What are some indications for scheduled cesarean delivery?**

Previous classical uterine incision

Prior uterine surgery that involved the myometrium

EFW >4500 g

Severe fetal hydrocephalus

Malpresentation (breech)

Cervical cancer

Active genital herpes

Placenta previa

**What percentage of deliveries in the United States are emergent or scheduled cesarean deliveries?**

Over 20%

**What is the risk of a trial of labor in a woman with a prior classical uterine incision?**

A 12% risk of **uterine rupture**, which is associated with fetal death, maternal shock, and a 10% maternal mortality rate

**What is the risk of uterine rupture in a laboring patient with a prior lower uterine segment incision?**

<1%

**At what EGA is a cesarean section scheduled?**

**After 39 weeks in a patient with accurate dating of her pregnancy**. Fetal lung maturity tests should be performed if delivery is planned earlier or if the dating method is not adequate

**What is the lower uterine segment? What are the advantages of using this in a C-section?**

The region of the uterus just superior to the cervix. The myometrium is **significantly thinner** than the uterine fundus (especially during labor) and is associated with a **lower risk of uterine rupture**

**What are the layers (from exterior to interior) that are incised with a Pfannenstiel or low transverse abdominal incision?**

Skin → subcutaneous fat → superficial fascia (Camper) → deep fascia (Scarpa) → anterior rectus sheath → rectus abdominus muscle → preperitoneal fat → parietal peritoneum (with bladder flap) → visceral peritoneum → uterus

**What percentage of VBACs (vaginal births after cesarean) are successful?**

60–80% are successful (depending on the indication for prior cesarean)

**What term describes a pathologically thin lower uterine segment through which fetal membranes or fetal parts can be visualized prior to uterine incision?**

A **uterine window**

**What risk may be associated with a uterine window?**

Imminent risk of uterine rupture and expulsion of the fetus into the peritoneum

**What are some indications for a vertical lower uterine incision?**

Premature breech fetus

Poorly developed lower uterine segment

Extensive fibrosis of lower uterine segment (following multiple cesareans)

**Can the type of previous uterine incision be determined from the skin incision?**

No

# Postpartum Care

## PUERPERIUM MANAGEMENT

**What is the duration of the postpartum period, also known as the puerperium?**

6–8 weeks following delivery, when maternal physiology returns to the pre-pregnancy state

**What is uterine involution?**

The contraction of interlacing myometrium bundles, with subsequent atrophy, so as to constrict vessels and prevent hemorrhage, as well as gradually returning the uterus to its prepregnancy size

**What are common uterotonics and their contraindications?**

**Oxytocin (Pitocin):** pulmonary edema

**Carboprost (Hemabate):** asthma

**Methylergonovine (Methergine):** preeclampsia, pregnancy-induced HTN or HTN

**Misoprostol (Cytotec)**

**When is a pregnant woman at highest risk of developing venous thrombosis?**

During the immediate puerperium period because of vessel trauma, immobility, increased fibrinogen, factor VII, VIII, IX, X, and platelets. Approximately 0.7 per 1000 women experience a venous thrombosis during pregnancy or postpartum

**Stool softeners, intermittent strait catheterization (to relieve urinary retention), and ice packs are commonly employed to treat which complications of vaginal delivery?**

Peri-urethral, third or fourth degree lacerations, which are also associated with dyspareunia and bowel incontinence. Additionally, ice packs and nonsteroidal anti-inflammatory drugs (NSAIDs) decrease swelling and induration from the inflammatory reaction to suture used to repair lacerations

**Which nerve can be injured during delivery, with subsequent urinary retention?**

The pudendal nerve; the neuropathy normally resolves within 2 months

**Following a 300-minute second stage of labor, a G1P1 is unable to flex her hips against tension and has difficulty walking. What type of neuropathy is likely responsible?**

Femoral nerve compression, secondary to hyperflexion of the hips during a prolonged second stage

**Which episiotomy is associated with perineal or pelvic hematoma?**

Mediolateral episiotomies

**How soon should an Rh(D–) mother be given Rhogam (anti-D immune globulin), following delivery of an Rh+ fetus?**

Within 72 hours of delivery

**Where is the fundus during the postpartum period?**

**Immediately after delivery:** near the umbilicus

**After 24 hours** below the umbilicus

**1 week** near the symphysis pubis

**2 weeks** in the pelvis

**6–8 weeks** it has assumed its nonpregnant size

**What is lochia?**

A combination of blood, serous exudate, erythrocytes, leukocytes, necrotic decidua, epithelial cells, and bacteria

**What is the progression of the various types of lochia?**

Lochia **rubra** (red), is followed by lochia **serosa** (brown), and ultimately lochia **alba** (yellow white). Lochia rubra consists of primarily blood from the placental bed, mixed with tissue, lasting 3–5 days. Lochia serosa consists of smaller amounts of older blood mixed with serous drainage, leukocytes, and cervical mucus, ending by the 10th day after delivery. Lochia alba lasts from the second to sixth week after delivery and has a small amount of blood, combined with leukocytes, epithelial cells, cholesterol, fat, and mucus

**How long does a woman shed lochia?**

4–6 weeks however, it should not be red for more than 2 weeks

**What is suggested if a woman continues to have lochia rubra for over 2 weeks?**

Retained products of conception (POC) must be considered and her uterus, cervix, and vagina should be examined with possible dilation and curettage

**How much lochia is shed during the puerperium?**

Initially it may be as heavy as a period and should subside; the total amount lost is approximately 500 mL

**What is the management of wound dehiscence?**

Dehiscence of a vaginal laceration repair should be evaluated for infection, irrigated, and debrided of necrotic tissue. Sitz baths should be used liberally. If discovered in the first 2–3 days after delivery, the wound can be resutured; however, if the tissue is friable or has evidence of infection, a secondary repair should be delayed for 6–8 weeks. Antibiotics should be utilized if infection is noted

**What are some signs and symptoms of endometritis?**

Elevated temperature (>100.4°F or >38°C) in the presence of uterine tenderness. Additionally, purulent vaginal discharge may be noted, as well as leukocytosis. It is usually noted within the first 3–5 days after delivery. It occurs in 4% of all vaginal deliveries and up to 10% of cesarean deliveries

**Who is at increased risk for endometritis?**

Risk factors include: prolonged ROM, prolonged labor, multiple internal examinations, internal monitoring (FSE or IUPC), retained POC, lower socioeconomic status, poor nutrition, maternal anemia, and concurrent genital tract infection

**What is the treatment for endometritis?**

**It is a polymicrobial infection, with a mixture of aerobic and anerobic bacteria found. Treatment usually**

**consists of gentamicin and clindamycin until the patient is afebrile for 24–36 hours**

**What are some common causes of puerperal fever (postpartum or post-cesarean-section fever)?**

Wind (atelectasis or aspiration PNA)
Water (cystitis or UTI)

Wound (surgical site infection or laceration)

Walking (PE or a DVT)

Wonder drugs (medication SE or adverse reaction)

Womb (endometritis)

Wet nurse (engorgement or mastitis: infection often with *S. aureus* or *Streptococcus*)

Phlebitis or septic pelvic thrombophlebitis

## BREASTFEEDING AND INFANT CARE

**What are the five components of the Apgar score at 1, 5, and 10 minutes?**

Appearance (blue, acrocyanosis, pink)

Pulse (absent, <100, >100)

Grimace (none, present, vigorous irritability)

Activity (flaccid, flexed, moving)

Respirations (absent, slow, crying)

Each component is given 0, 1, or 2 points

**Silver nitrate, erythromycin, or tetracycline ointments are applied to the newborn's eyes to prevent what ocular infection?**

*Chlamydia* and gonorrhea

**Why is it required to emergently assess an infant with ambiguous genitalia?**

**Congenital adrenal hyperplasia is a life-threatening condition requiring mineralocorticoid supplementation to prevent salt wasting (hypovolemic-hyponatremia). The most common form is 21-alpha-hydroxylase deficiency. Electrolytes, 17-alpha hydroxyprogesterone, and dehydroepiandrosterone sulfate should be checked**

**How does an infant benefit from skin-to-skin contact at birth?**

Better temperature and glucose control, as well as an increased likelihood of maternal breastfeeding

**Which vitamin is absent from human breast milk?**

Vitamin K. Infants are given a vitamin K shot at birth to prevent hemorrhagic disease of the newborn

**What is the effect of decreased dopamine production in the hypothalamus following nipple stimulation?**

Decreased prolactin-inhibiting factor, thereby increasing prolactin from the anterior pituitary

**How does prolactin impact breastfeeding?**

Stimulates milk production by the terminal exocrine glands

**Nipple stimulation also increases oxytocin release from the posterior pituitary, which impacts breastfeeding. How?**

Causing contraction of the myo-epithelial cells of the lactiferous ducts, allowing milk letdown

**How does breastfeeding prevent ovulation?**

Prolactin inhibits the pulsatile gonadotropin-releasing hormone from the hypothalamus

**What is colostrum?**

Thick yellow breast secretions that contain plasma exudates, immunoglobulins (IgA), lactoferrin, albumin, and electrolytes. It is secreted during the first 2 days postpartum

**Why is an ELISA or Western blot repeated at 6 months and 1 year following delivery of an infant to an HIV+ mother?**

Maternal transplacental IgG persists for several months in the infant's serum. The above tests check for antibodies to HIV, not the actual virus

**When does a breastfeeding woman's milk "come in"?**

3–5 days postpartum. It contains protein, lactose, water, fats, and immunoglobins (IgA)

**Are mothers who are seropositive for the following conditions advised to breastfeed?**

**Hepatitis A:** Yes

**Hepatitis B:** Yes, with vaccination and hepatitis B IgG administration to the infant at birth. The virus is present in breast milk, although the benefits outweigh the risk of transmission, which is minimized with treatment

**Hepatitis C:** Yes

**HIV:** No

**Cytomegalovirus (CMV):** No

|  |  |
|---|---|
| **Are mothers who are exposed to the following substances advised to breastfeed?** | |
| **Alcohol** | No |
| **Heroine and other analgesics** | No |
| **Tobacco** | Yes |
| **Hepatitis B vaccination** | Yes |
| **Rubella vaccination** | Yes |
| **Rubeola vaccination** | Yes |
| **Ibuprofen** | Yes |
| **Tetracyclines** | No |
| **Sulfa drugs** | No, because they displace bilirubin and increase risk of kernicterus |
| **Quinolones** | No |
| **Chemotherapy (antimitotic medications)** | No |
| **Radiation** | No |
| **Lithium or heavy metals** | No |
| **Is previous mammoplasty (reduction or implantation) a contraindication to breastfeeding?** | No. If the integrity of the nipple ducts are preserved, a woman can breastfeed; however, the surgical technique and subsequent scarring may make this difficult |
| **What is the caloric demand of lactation?** | 640 kcal/day |
| **How much should breastfeeding women increase their daily caloric intake?** | 300–500 kcal, so as to ensure that loss of gestational weight |
| **How much calcium should a breastfeeding woman consume?** | 1200 mg/day of calcium |
| **A mother does not want to breastfeed although her breasts are extremely tender 5 days postpartum. What is appropriate management?** | Tight brassiere, avoidance of nipple stimulation, cool compresses, acetaminophen or ibuprofen will offer comfort and suppress lactation. She is experiencing ductal, venous, and lymphatic engorgement |

## PHYSIOLOGIC CHANGES AND RESOLUTION

|  |  |
|---|---|
| **How is cardiac output (CO) affected during the first day postpartum?** | A 60–80% increase in CO occurs with the autotransfusion of uteroplacental blood to the intravascular space and decompression of the vena cava, during the fourth stage of labor |

| | |
|---|---|
| **A leukocytosis <25,000 and low-grade fevers <101 are considered normal or abnormal 24 hours postpartum?** | Normal |
| **Over what time period does the CO and systemic vascular resistance gradually return to nonpregnant levels?** | 3–4 months, with concurrent reduction in left ventricular size and contractility |
| **How does a pre-partum cervix (cx) differ from a parous cx?** | The pre-partum cervix is composed of fibrous connective tissue without muscle, and the cervical os can be described as a "pinpoint." Over several weeks following delivery, the cx slowly contracts, with the cervical os appearing as a transverse, stellate slit, which can be dilated with greater ease |
| **Why is a woman who has delivered vaginally at risk for pelvic relaxation, cytocele, rectocele, or incontinence?** | The musculature and female genitalia slowly contract; however, connective tissue and fascial stretching may not return to the pre-gravid state, resulting in persistent trauma or changes |
| **What is a persistent defect of the abdominal wall musculature caused by the gravid uterus known as?** | Diastasis recti |
| **How much weight is lost following delivery?** | Almost half of the gestational weight gain is lost following delivery (13 lbs), with the additional weight loss occurring over the next 6 months (15 lbs) |
| **Do women typically gain weight following pregnancy?** | Most women maintain 10% of their gestational weight following the postpartum period |
| **Why do some women note increased alopecia postpartum?** | Scalp hair shifts from the predominant anagen phase (growing) during pregnancy to a predominant telogen phase (resting). This **telogen effluvium** typically resolves within 5 months |
| **What is the condition in which a woman displays hypopituitarism following a delivery with postpartum hemorrhage?** | Sheehan's syndrome, because of infarction and necrosis of the pituitary |
| **What are some symptoms of central diabetes insipidus?** | Polydipsia, polyuria, hypernatremia (>140 mEq/L), normal serum osmolality (<280 mOsm/kg), and dilute urine osmolality (<380 mOsm/kg) |

**When does serum human chorionic gonadotropin (HCG) return to normal (nondetectable levels)?**

Within 4–6 weeks of delivery or abortion

**What is suggested by a rising HCG postpartum?**

Gestational trophoblastic disease

**Why do some women note vaginal atrophy in the puerperium?**

Prolactin inhibition of systemic estrogens

**How is the thyroid affected postpartum?**

Hormone levels are within normal limits by 4 weeks and the thyroid gland decreases to pre-pregnancy size over 3 months

## POSTPARTUM CLINICAL CARE

**What is postpartum thyroiditis?**

Acute hyperthyroidism and subsequent hypothyroidism, each lasting approximately 1 month in duration. Women typically recover spontaneously

**How many women with gestational diabetes mellitus (GDM) develop Type II diabetes later in life?**

Up to 50%. A woman with GDM should be screened for diabetes postpartum

**How common are postpartum blues?**

50–70% of women

**When do they occur?**

Within 2 weeks of delivery and typically resolve within 2 weeks; they are attributed to dramatic shift in hormones and decreased progesterone

**How common is postpartum depression?**

4–10%

**When does a woman present with postpartum depression?**

A majority of cases occur between 2 weeks and 4 months postpartum. Depression may last 3–14 months

**How is postpartum depression diagnosed?**

The criteria is similar to major depressive disorder; five of the following symptoms must be present for 2 weeks: SIGECAPS

*S*leep changes

Loss of *I*nterest (anhedonia)

*G*uilt

Decreased *E*nergy

Decreased ability to *C*oncentrate

| | |
|---|---|
| | *A*ppetite increase or decrease |
| | *P*sychomotor increase or decrease |
| | *S*uicidal ideation |
| **Who is at increased risk for postpartum depression?** | An older, primaparous woman, without social support, with an unplanned pregnancy, a history of psychiatric hospitalizations, suicide attempts, depression or other mood disorders, and a family history of suicide |
| **How common is postpartum psychosis?** | 0 .1–0.2%, it can last up to 2 months |

## FERTILITY AND CONTRACEPTION

| | |
|---|---|
| **When does ovulation and menstruation begin in a postpartum nonlactating woman?** | Ovulation typically resumes within 45 days, but it may occur within 4 weeks. Average duration to menstruation is 8 weeks postpartum |
| **When does ovulation and menstruation begin in a postpartum breastfeeding woman?** | A woman who is breastfeeding more than 5 times a day can remain anovulatory for the duration of breastfeeding. Amenorrhea, feeding schedules > 8 times daily, maximum of 6 hours between feeds, and minimal supplementation are key predictors of anovulation |
| **How long should the woman maintain "pelvic rest," by refraining from coitus or inserting anything in the vagina?** | 6 weeks postpartum, so as to decrease the risk of an infection ascending through the patent cervical os, and to reduce the risk of infection or trauma to healing lacerations |
| **What type of birth control will not affect breastfeeding?** | IUD, barrier methods, progestin only pills (mini pill), Depo-Provera |
| **Why do oral contraceptive pills (OCPs) and Norplant affect breastfeeding?** | Estrogen decreases breast milk production. It can be safely started 6 weeks after delivery if milk production is adequate |
| **Why do some clinicians recommend that women obtain an IUD 6 weeks postpartum instead of insertion at the time of delivery?** | Decreased risk of expulsion because of patent os and uterine cramping |

CHAPTER 9

# Complications of Pregnancy

## Early Complications

### CONGENITAL ANOMALIES

**What is the prevalence of major congenital anomalies in the United States?**

Between 2 and 4%

**What are the causes of congenital anomalies and what are their relative frequencies?**

**Single gene disorders** (15–20%)

**Chromosomal abnormalities** (5%)

**Teratogens** (either maternal illness, infection, drugs, or chemicals; 10%)

**Unknown** (60–70%)

**What is the overall incidence of chromosomal anomalies in the United States?**

0.7% of all live births; however, it is more common among abortuses and stillbirths (up to 50%)

**What happens to most fetuses with chromosomal abnormalities?**

Most do not survive to term.
If they do, they are often with congenital abnormalities (with multiple organ system involvement), growth deficiency, and mental retardation

**Do the same cytogenetic abnormalities produce the same phenotype in each fetus?**

No. While it will produce the same pattern of malformations, there is significant variability

**What are the genetic etiologies of chromosomal abnormalities?**

Nondisjunction

Unequal recombination

Inversion

Deletions/duplications

Translocations

**What is the most common etiology of chromosomal abnormality?**

**Nondisjunction**—the loss or gain of a chromosome resulting in trisomy or monosomy

**What is the major risk factor for nondisjunction?**

**Advanced maternal age**

**Describe the syndrome associated with trisomy 21**

Known as **Down syndrome**, it is the most common chromosomal abnormality found in live births. It is associated with mental retardation, hypotonia, a single palmar crease, early-onset Alzheimer, and other serious congenital features such as duodenal atresia, congenital heart disease, and leukemia

**What is the cytogenetic etiology of trisomy 21 and what are the relative frequencies?**

True trisomy (94%)

Robertsonian translocation (3–4%)

Trisomy mosaicism (2–3%)

**What are the risk factors for trisomy 21?**

Advanced maternal age

**Describe the syndrome associated with trisomy 18**

**Major features include:**

Severe mental retardation

Hypertonia

Prominent occiput

Micrognathia

Short sternum

Flexed fingers

Congenital heart disease

Ectopic pancreatic tissue

Small pelvis

Horseshoe kidney

Meckel diverticulum or malrotation

Half of trisomy 18 infants die within 1 week of life and the vast majority die within 1 year

**Describe the syndrome associated with trisomy 13**

It primarily includes malformations of the midface, eyes, and brain. However, omphalocele, genitourinary (GU) anomalies, hemangiomas, polydactyly, rocker-bottom feet, and congenital heart defects are also often found

80% die within the first month and the vast majority die within the first 6 months

**What is genomic imprinting?**

Differential expression of genetic information, depending on whether it is from the mother or father. It is the basis of diseases such as Prader-Willi syndrome and Angelman syndrome, which involve the same microdeletion on chromosome 15 but result in a different phenotype depending on which parent the deletion came from

**Describe the following sex chromosome abnormalities**

**Turner syndrome** (45, X) characterized by short stature, streak gonads, mild MR, and other abnormalities such as webbed neck, lymphedema, pigmented nevi, and congenital heart defects

**Klinefelter syndrome** (47, XXY) characterized by tall stature, microorchidism, and azospermia

**What is a teratogen?**

Any agent that can lead to abnormalities in a developing fetus. They can be from maternal illness, microbial infections, drugs, or other chemicals in the environment

**What types of birth defects are associated with the following maternal illnesses?**

**Insulin-dependent diabetes mellitus (IDDM):** congenital heart disease, spina bifida, caudal regression, focal femoral hypoplasia

**Phenylketonuria:** microcephaly, mental retardation, congenital heart disease

**Adrenal/ovarian tumors:** virilization of female fetuses if they secrete androgens

**Autoimmune disease:** a similar disease in fetus as in the mother if the antibodies cross the placenta, congenital heart block

**Obesity:** neural tube defects

**What are some of the sonographic signs that suggest fetal infection?**

Microcephaly: cardiac malformations

Cerebral calcifications: hepatosplenomegaly

Hepatic calcifications: limb hypoplasia

Intrauterine growth restriction: hydrocephalus

## SPONTANEOUS ABORTIONS

**What is a spontaneous abortion?**

Also called a **miscarriage**, it is a pregnancy that spontaneously ends **prior to 20 weeks of gestation** or **before the fetus has reached 500 g** resulting in expulsion of all or any part of the products of conception

**How common is spontaneous abortion?**

It occurs in 8–20% of known pregnancies under 20 weeks and in an even higher percentage of subclinical pregnancies

**When do most spontaneous abortions occur?**

80% occur prior to 12 weeks

**Chromosomal abnormalities (aneuploidy) are the most common cause of spontaneous abortion in the first trimester. What are the two most common genetic abnormalities that cause this?**

Autosomal trisomies

Monosomy X

**Are there any therapeutic interventions that prevent first trimester pregnancy loss?**

No, nothing has been proven in randomized controlled trials to prevent this

**What are some causes of second trimester spontaneous abortion?**

Maternal factors such as cervical insufficiency, infection, chromosomal or structural malformation, or maternal thrombophilia

**What increases the risk of spontaneous abortion?**

**Advanced maternal age**

**Prior spontaneous abortion**

| | |
|---|---|
| | **Heavy cigarette use** |
| | Short interpregnancy interval |
| | Maternal medical disease (e.g., celiac dz, IDDM) |
| | Heavy alcohol or caffeine intake |
| | Trauma |
| | Increased parity |
| | Advanced paternal age |
| **What are the three most common symptoms of a spontaneous abortion?** | History of amenorrhea, vaginal bleeding, pelvic pain |
| **Describe each of the following types of spontaneous abortions:** | **Complete abortion:** uterine bleeding with complete expulsion of the product of conception (POC) and closed cervical os |
| | **Inevitable abortion:** uterine bleeding with cervical dilation but without expulsion of any POC |
| | **Incomplete abortion:** uterine bleeding with cervical dilation but with incomplete expulsion of the POC |
| | **Missed abortion:** embryonic demise without expulsion of POC and with closed cervical os |
| | **Septic abortion:** embryonic demise with evidence of infected products of conception (e.g., fever, uterine tenderness) |
| | **Threatened abortion:** uterine bleeding with closed cervical os and normal cardiac activity |
| **What percentage of women exhibit signs of threatened abortion during their pregnancy? What percentage of these women will spontaneously abort?** | Approximately 25% and 50%, respectively |
| **What must be considered in the differential diagnosis of a threatened abortion?** | Ectopic pregnancy |
| | Cervical, vaginal, or uterine pathology |
| | Bleeding related to implantation |
| **What is the first diagnostic test you should perform in a woman with a known intrauterine pregnancy who presents with vaginal bleeding?** | Ultrasound |

**How is vaginal bleeding in the first trimester evaluated?**

Via history, physical examination, hCG levels, and ultrasound. The following algorithm (Fig. 9-1) can be used:

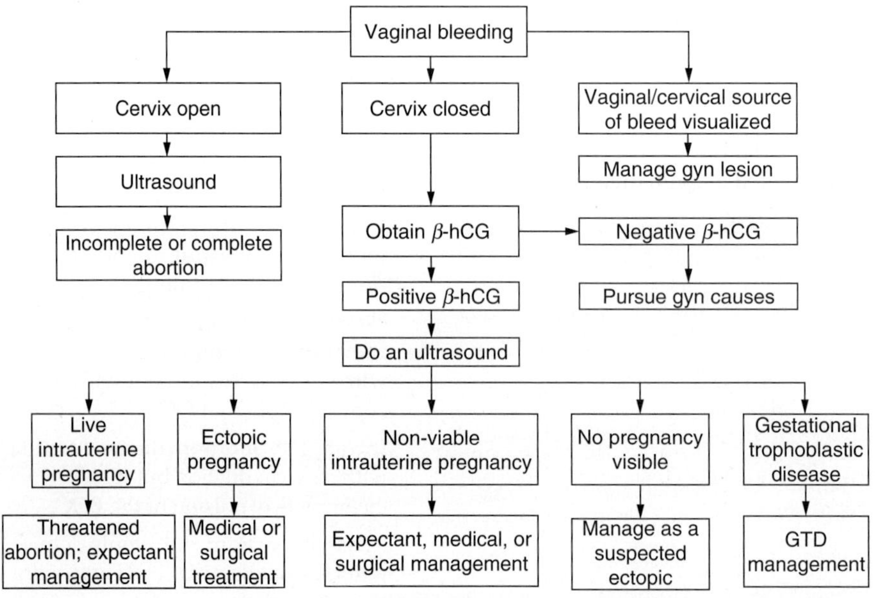


**Figure 9-1** Evaluation of vaginal bleeding in the first trimester. (Adapted, with permission, from uptodateonline.com *Clinical manifestations, diagnosis, and management of ectopic pregnancy* by Togas Tulandi).

**What are the ultrasonographic criteria for diagnosis of a nonviable intrauterine pregnancy?**

**Absence of fetal cardiac activity** in an embryo with a crown-rump length >5 mm

-or-

**Absence of a fetal pole** when the mean sac diameter >25 mm (transabdominally) or >18 mm (transvaginally)

**What are the treatment options for an incomplete, inevitable, or a missed abortion? What are the benefits of each?**

Surgical, medical, or expectant management

**What are the advantages and disadvantages surgical, medical, or expectant management?**

See Table 9-1

## Table 9-1 Treatment Options for Abortion

| | Advantages | Disadvantages |
|---|---|---|
| **Surgical Management** | Greatest efficacy; quickest evacuation | Invasive; procedural/ anesthesia risks |
| **Medical Management** | Less invasive; avoids anesthesia; patient can do it in the privacy of her own home | Requires more than two visits; less quick |
| **Expectant Management** | Least invasive | Timing is unpredictable; risk of needing an unplanned procedure |

| | |
|---|---|
| **Why is it imperative that spontaneous abortions be evacuated?** | Because after several weeks-months, the trophoblastic tissue might enter the maternal bloodstream, triggering the coagulation cascade and causing a **coagulopathy** |
| **What lab tests must be done after a spontaneous abortion?** | Type and screen (because Rh immunoglobulin must be given to Rh[–] women) |
| **Can a woman do anything to prevent a spontaneous abortion?** | Typically no, and so all women need to be reassured that it is not their fault |
| **Should a woman who has had a spontaneous abortion undergo an evaluation for the cause?** | No. These are fairly common and are often sporadic |
| **What is recurrent pregnancy loss (RPL)?** | **Three or more consecutive losses of** pregnancy prior to 20 weeks |
| **What is the incidence of RPL?** | Approximately 0.5–1% |
| **What is the risk of spontaneous abortion?** | **After one prior loss:** 10–20%<br>**After two consecutive losses:** 25–45% |
| **What does the diagnostic workup of RPL consist of?** | A complete medical, surgical, genetic, and family history<br>A physical examination with attention to signs of **endocrinopathies** or **pelvic organ anomalies**<br>Laboratory evaluation including: **uterine assessment** (sonohysterography)<br>**Anticardiolipin antibodies** and **lupus anticoagulant**<br>**Evaluation of ovarian reserve**<br>Possibly other tests (e.g., an evaluation for inherited thrombophilias, thyroid function tests [TFTs], and a karyotype) |

**What is the treatment for RPL?**

It is dependent on the etiology; however, it can include:

Surgery (for pelvic organ abnormalities)

Coumadin and aspirin (for antiphospholipid syndrome)

Synthroid (for hypothyroidism)

## ECTOPIC PREGNANCY

**What is an ectopic pregnancy (see Fig. 9-2)?**

Implantation of the pregnancy into a site outside of the endometrial lining of the uterine cavity

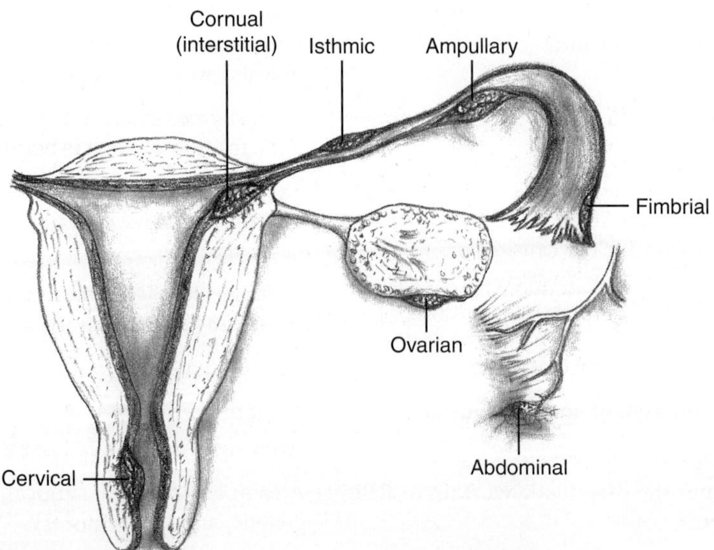


**Figure 9-2** Locations of ectopic pregnancies.

**What is the most common cause of pregnancy-related death in the first trimester?**

Rupture of an ectopic pregnancy

**What is the incidence of ectopic pregnancy?**

Approximately 2% of pregnancies in the United States are ectopic

**What is the mortality rate associated with an ectopic pregnancy?**

Approximately 3–4 deaths per 10,000 cases result in death

**What are the major risk factors for ectopic pregnancy?**

**History of pelvic inflammatory disease (PID),** (most common)

History of ectopic pregnancy

History of tubal surgery or pathology

Diethylstilbestrol (DES) exposure in utero

Current intrauterine device (IUD) use

Current oral contraceptive pill (OCP) use

Infertility

History of cervicitis

Multiple sexual partners

Cigarette smoking

**Describe the relationship between IUD use and ectopic pregnancy**

Women using an IUD are much less likely to conceive compared to women not using any form of birth control. However, in the unlikely event that they do conceive, there is a greater probability that it will be ectopic

**What are the major symptoms of ectopic pregnancy?**

Classic symptoms: **amenorrhea, abdominal/pelvic pain, vaginal bleeding**

Other symptoms: dizziness, nausea, vomiting, diarrhea

40% of cases present acutely and 60% of cases present as chronic symptoms. Many women are asymptomatic until rupture

**What are the signs on physical examination of ectopic pregnancy?**

Many women have a normal physical examination; however, the common signs are:

Adenexal mass and/or tenderness

Mild uterine enlargement

Cervical motion tenderness

Abdominal tenderness

Orthostatic hypotension, tachycardia, and rebound tenderness are all signs of rupture

**What is the differential diagnosis of these symptoms?**

Threatened abortion

Torsion

Ruptured corpus luteum cyst

Abnormal uterine bleeding

Tubo-ovarian abscess (TOA)
Molar pregnancy
PID
UTI or stones
Pyelonephritis
Diverticulitis
Appendicitis
Pancreatitis

**What diagnostic tests can be used to distinguish between these conditions?**

β-hCG
Transvaginal ultrasound

**What is the difference in β-hCG levels between an intrauterine and ectopic pregnancy?**

The rate of β-hCG rise is lower in most cases of ectopic pregnancy

**Where are ectopic pregnancies located and what are the relative frequencies of each (see Fig. 9-2)?**

**Fallopian tube** (95%; ampulla > isthmus > fimbria)

Ovarian (3.2%)

Interstitial or cornual (2.4%)

Abdominal (1.3%)

Cervix (rare)

Hysterotomy scar

**What are the causes of tubal implantation?**

Conditions that **delay transport** of the egg through the tube

Conditions in the embryo that lead to **premature implantation**

**What types of conditions cause a delay in transport of the egg through the tube?**

Chronic salpingitis
Salpingitis isthmica nodosa (SIN)

**What happens to the endometrium during an ectopic pregnancy?**

It still responds to pregnancy hormones and so often exhibits signs of decidual reaction or endometrial thickening

**What is a heterotopic ectopic pregnancy?**

A **concurrent intrauterine and extrauterine pregnancy**. While rare, it is more common in women pregnant through in vitro fertilization (IVF)

**What is the natural course of an ectopic pregnancy?**

Rupture, spontaneous regression, or tubal abortion

**What is a tubal abortion?**

The expulsion of the POC through the fimbria into the abdominal cavity. The POC can then either regress or reimplant in the abdominal cavity or in the ovary

**At what gestational age do the clinical manifestations of an ectopic pregnancy begin?**

At least **6–8 weeks** after the LMP

**Describe the algorithm for management of a suspected ecoptic pregnancy**

See Fig. 9-3

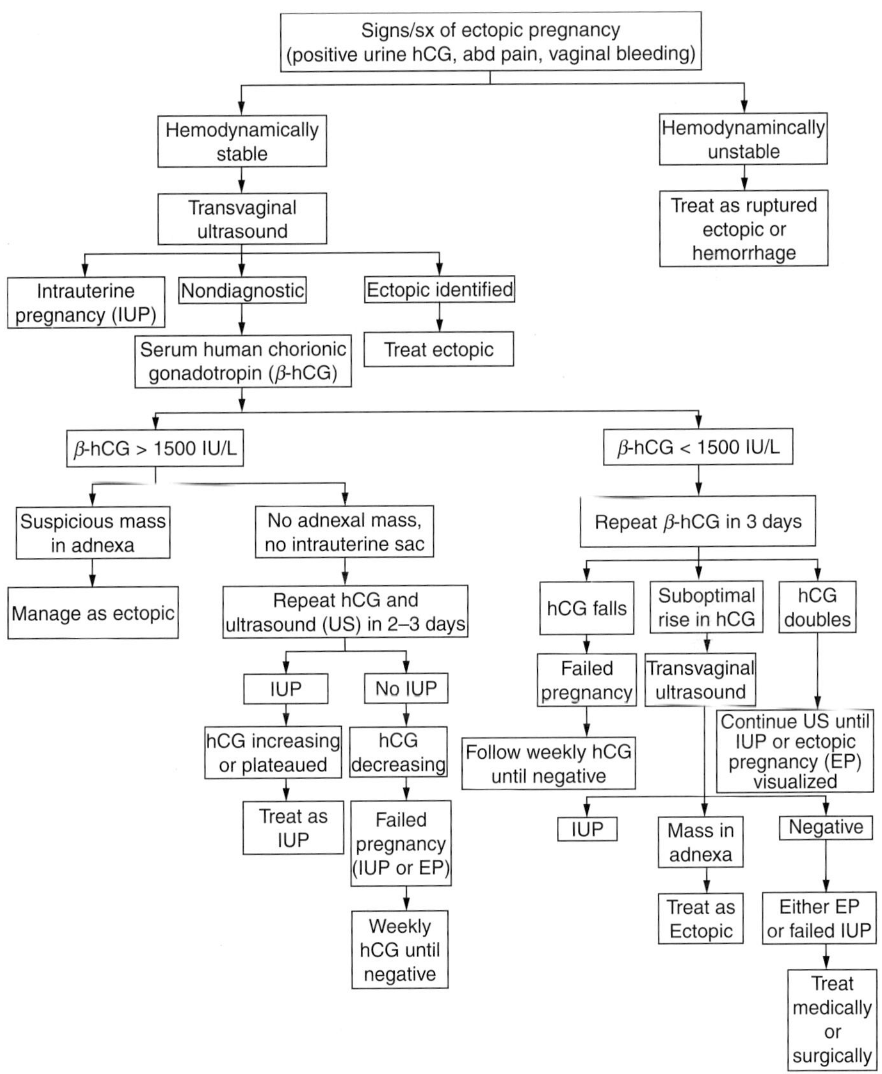


**Figure 9-3** Management of suspected ectopic pregnancy. (Adapted, with permission, from uptodateonline.com *Spontaneous abortion: Risk factors, etiology, clinical manifestations, and diagnostic evaluation* by Togas Tulandi and Haya M Al-Fozan)

| | |
|---|---|
| **What are the treatment options for an ectopic pregnancy?** | **Methotrexate** (for early, unruptured, ectopic pregnancies)<br>**Surgery** (laparoscopy with salpingostomy or salpingectomy) |
| **What are the contraindications of methotrexate used to treat an ectopic pregnancy?** | Active hemorrhage<br>Pregnancy larger than 4 cm<br>Breastfeeding<br>Alcoholism<br>Peptic ulcer disease<br>Liver or renal disease<br>Blood dyscrasias<br>Immunodeficiency<br>Active pulmonary disease |
| **What is methotrexate's failure rate?** | 5–10%, but higher in more advanced pregnancies |
| **What are the two methods of methotrexate administration for the treatment of an ectopic pregnancy?** | Give a single intramuscular (IM) dose of methotrexate and then follow β-hCG levels at days 4 and 7. hCG levels should decline by 15% between days 4 and 7.<br>Alternate day IM administration of methotrexate until β-hCG level decreases by 15% in 48 hours |
| **What are the differences between a salpingostomy and a salpingectomy?** | Salpingostomy: an incision is made on the antimesenteric part of the fallopian tube and the POCs are evacuated. The incision is closed by secondary intention<br>Salpingectomy: a tubal resection that involves partial removal of the oviduct, salvaging as much as possible |
| **What is the discriminatory zone?** | A **range of β-hCG levels** (1000–2000 IU/L) in which **a gestational sac should be seen** if there is an intrauterine pregnancy. If no sac is seen at β-hCG levels above the discriminatory zone, an ectopic pregnancy can be diagnosed in most cases |
| **How should a patient with a low β-hCG without a visible intrauterine pregnancy be managed?** | Both the ultrasound and the β-hCG should be repeated in 3 days. If the pregnancy is intrauterine and viable, |

| | |
|---|---|
| | the **β-hCG should double in 1.5–2 days** |
| **Does a negative pelvic ultrasound rule out the diagnosis of an ectopic pregnancy?** | No, an extrauterine pregnancy is visualized in only 50% of ectopic pregnancies |
| **What is the difference in progesterone levels between an intrauterine and an ectopic pregnancy?** | Serum progesterone levels are lower in ectopic pregnancies compared with viable intrauterine pregnancies. However, the sensitivity and specificity of progesterone levels are too low to make it a screening or diagnostic test for ectopic pregnancy |
| **What percentage of patients with an ectopic pregnancy experience tubal rupture?** | Approximately 18% |
| **In a patient with an ectopic pregnancy, what are the risk factors for tubal rupture?** | History of tubal damage/infertility<br>Induction of ovulation<br>Never having used contraception<br>High β-hCG |
| **How does the presence of an ectopic pregnancy affect subsequent pregnancies?** | It reduces the chance for a successful pregnancy. A repeat tubal pregnancy occurs in 12% of patients |

# GESTATIONAL TROPHOBLASTIC DISEASE

## Introduction

| | |
|---|---|
| **What is gestational trophoblastic disease (GTD)?** | A group of tumors that **arise from placental tissue** and **secrete β-hCG** |
| **What are the types of GTD?** | Hydatidiform mole<br>Persistent/invasive gestational trophoblastic neoplasia (GTN)<br>Choriocarcinoma<br>Placental site trophoblastic tumor (PSTT) |
| **Which of the types of GTD are benign and which are malignant?** | Hydatidiform moles are usually benign, whereas invasive GTN, choriocarcinoma, and PSTT are all malignant |

**What are the major risk factors for GTD?**

Extremes of maternal age

History of prior GTD

**When should GTD be suspected clinically?**

If there is unusual bleeding after a pregnancy or abortion

**What are the signs and symptoms of GTD?**

**First trimester bleeding**

**Uterine size/date discrepancy**

**Pelvic pressure or pain**

First trimester preeclampsia

Higher β-hCG than expected

Hyperemesis gravidarum

Hyperthyroidism

Passage of hydropic (grape-like) vesicles

**What is the differential diagnosis of GTD?**

Normal pregnancy

Spontaneous abortion

Preeclampsia

Placenta previa

Placental abruption

Endometriosis

Ectopic pregnancy

Ovarian tumor

Prolapsed fibroid

Cervical neoplasia

**How should post-pregnancy bleeding be investigated?**

Using curettage, serum hCG measurements, and a chest x-ray (CXR) (to assess if there are nodules associated with metastasis)

**What is the major sign that GTD disease is metastatic?**

hCG levels that do not decrease or that increase

**Describe the following stages of GTD:**

**Stage I**

Disease that is limited to uterus

**Stage II**

Disease that extends outside uterus but stays within pelvis or vagina

**Stage III**

Disease with pulmonary metastases

**Stage IV**

Disease spreads to other sites

**Where does metastatic GTD spread?**

In order from most likely to least likely:

Lung (80%)

Vagina (30%)
Brain (10%)
Liver (10%)
Other (bowel, kidney, spleen)

**What are the good prognostic indicators for GTD?**

Short duration between last pregnancy and disease (<4 months)
Low hCG level (<40,000 IU/L)
No metastatic disease to brain or liver
No prior chemotherapy

**What are the poor prognostic indicators for GTD?**

Long duration between last pregnancy and disease (>4 months)
High hCG level (>40,000 IU/L)
Brain or liver metastases
Prior chemotherapy
Development of disease after a term pregnancy

**What is the overall cure rate for GTD?**

Over 90%

**How does the diagnosis of GTD affect the prognosis for future pregnancies?**

It increases the risk of subsequent molar pregnancies; however, this risk is still low (1%)

## Hydatidiform Mole

**What is a hydatidiform mole?**

A localized, usually noninvasive **tumor of the placenta** that results from **aberrant fertilization** leading to proliferation of the trophoblastic tissue

**What is the incidence of a molar pregnancy?**

In the United States the incidence is 1 in 1500 pregnancies; however, it is much more common in the developing world

**What are the signs and symptoms of a hydatidiform mole?**

Amenorrhea
Positive β-hCG
Signs and symptoms consistent with early pregnancy
Pregnancy-induced hypertension early in pregnancy
Hyperthyroidism
Vaginal bleeding

**What is the difference between a complete and a partial hydatidiform mole?**

See Table 9-2

## Table 9-2 Difference Between Complete and Partial Mole

| | Complete Mole | Partial Mole |
|---|---|---|
| **Synonyms** | Classic or true mole | Incomplete mole |
| **Karyotype** | Diploid (46XX or 46XY) | Triploid (XXY or XYY) |
| **Fetal/embryonic tissue** | Absent | Present |
| **Uterine size** | Often large for dates | Often small for dates |
| **Appearance of trophoblast** | Diffuse hyperplasia, often atypia | Focal hyperplasia |
| **Appearance of villi** | Diffusely swollen | Focal swelling |
| **Theca lutein cysts** | Sometimes present | Never present |
| **hCG levels** | >50,000 IU/L | <50,000 IU/L |
| **Placental alkaline phosphate levels** | Normal | High |
| **Malignant potential** | 15–25% | 5–10% |

**Describe the pathogenesis of a complete mole**

An **"empty" egg** (caused by inactivated or absent maternal chromosomes) is **fertilized by a haploid sperm that then duplicates,** or occasionally by two sperm. This leads to a "normal" diploid karyotype with all chromosomes of paternal origin

**Describe the pathogenesis of a partial mole**

A haploid ovum is fertilized by two haploid sperm, leading to a triploid karyotype

**What is the typical sonographic appearance of a complete mole and a partial mole?**

A central heterogeneous mass without an embryo/fetus or any amniotic fluid but with theca lutein cysts; classically described as a **snowstorm pattern**

A growth-restricted fetus, reduced amniotic fluid, and a Swiss cheese pattern of chorionic villi; no theca lutein cysts

**What are the complications associated with a high hCG?**

Ovarian enlargement (with theca lutein cysts)

Hyperemesis gravidarum

Early preeclampsia

Hyperthyroidism (because hCG may stimulate TSH receptors)

**How is a molar pregnancy definitively diagnosed?**

It is suspected based on ultrasound and hCG levels; however, it must be confirmed with histologic studies of the tissue with analysis of the DNA content

**What is the treatment for a molar pregnancy?**

Dilation and curettage **(D&C**; suction curettage is preferred)

**Serum hCG levels must be followed** weekly until there are three consecutive normal values and then monthly for a total of 6 months of negative levels. During this time, effective contraception *must* be used to avoid misinterpretation of a rising hCG level

**What should be done before surgical evacuation of a complete molar pregnancy?**

A **CXR** to assess for metastatic disease

**When can another pregnancy be attempted after the diagnosis of GTN?**

The patient should wait for at least a year

**In what percentage of molar pregnancies will trophoblastic tissue persist after evacuation?**

19–28% of complete moles

2–4% of partial moles

**When is malignant disease suspected?**

After a molar pregnancy when hCG levels rise. This usually represents an invasive mole (75%), but can also represent choriocarcinoma (25%) or a placental site trophoblast tumor (rare)

After a nonmolar pregnancy when hCG levels rise. This usually represents choriocarcinoma, but can (rarely) represent a PSTT

**What are the risk factors for development of malignant disease?**

Theca lutein cysts >6 cm

Larger uterine size for dates

Advanced maternal age (>40 years)

History of GTD

Initial hCG >100,000 IU/L

Histologic findings of atypia or hyperplasia

**When does malignant disease develop?**

50% of cases follow a hydatidiform mole, 25% follow a normal pregnancy, and 25% follow an abortion

| | |
|---|---|
| **What is the major complication associated with malignant GTD?** | Hemorrhage—these lesions are highly vascular and often have AVMs which readily bleed |

## Invasive Gestational Trophoblastic Neoplasia

| | |
|---|---|
| **What is an invasive mole?** | A molar pregnancy whose chorionic villi invade into the myometrium |
| **Is an invasive mole more common after a complete mole or a partial mole?** | A complete mole |
| **What is the treatment of an invasive mole?** | **Methotrexate** and hCG follow-up as with a molar pregnancy (actinomycin-D or etoposide are alternative therapies) |
| **Can an invasive mole regress spontaneously?** | Yes |

## Choriocarcinoma

| | |
|---|---|
| **What is choriocarcinoma?** | A malignant carcinoma of the chorionic epithelium, usually after a molar pregnancy |
| **What is the incidence of choriocarcinoma after a normal gestation, an abortion, and a complete mole?** | 1 in 16,000; 1 in 15,000; 1 in 40 |
| **What are the common signs/symptoms of choriocarcinoma?** | **Irregular vaginal bleeding** (typically late postpartum bleeding, but it can present later)<br>Enlarged uterus with bilateral ovarian cysts |
| **What is the ultrasonographic appearance of choriocarcinoma?** | An enlarging, heterogeneous, hypervascular uterine mass with areas of hemorrhage and necrosis |
| **What is the histologic appearance of choriocarcinoma?** | Proliferation of cytotrophoblasts and syncytiotrophoblasts that penetrate the musculature and vasculature; no villi present |
| **What percentage of patients with choriocarcinoma develop metastases?** | Approximately 50% |
| **What is the treatment for choriocarcinoma?** | Chemotherapy (typically **methotrexate** or **actinomycin-D** for low-risk disease and a combination of **methotrexate, actinomycin-D,** |

**cyclophosphamide**, **etoposide**, and **vincristine** for high-risk disease)

Adjuvant hysterectomy decreases the dose of chemotherapy required for remission

**What is the recommended follow-up after treatment of an invasive mole?**

Serial hCG follow-up (weekly for 3 months, then monthly) is recommended for **at least a year**. If there are metastases outside of the lung, follow-up is recommended for 2 years

In both cases, the patient *must* use effective contraception in order to ensure appropriate interpretation of a rise in hCG

## Placental Site Trophoblastic Tumor

**What is a PSTT?**

A rare malignant tumor that arises from placental intermediate cytotrophoblastic cells

**What are the signs/symptoms of PSTT?**

**Irregular vaginal bleeding** (can be massive hemorrhage)

**An enlarging uterus**

**Amenorrhea**

Virilization

Nephrotic syndrome

Metastatic lesions

**Is PSTT always associated with high hCG levels?**

No, because there is no syncytiotrophoblast proliferation

**What is the ultrasonographic appearance of PSTT?**

A hyperechoic intrauterine mass that is invading the myometrial wall and has both cystic and solid areas

**What is the histological appearance of PSTT?**

Many mononuclear cells that invade the myometrium; proliferation of intermediate trophoblast cells (no cytotrophoblasts or syncytiotrophoblasts)

**What is the treatment for PSTT?**

**Hysterectomy** is the first-line therapy because chemotherapy is fairly ineffective and the tumor is usually confined to the uterus

# Late Complications

## HYPERTENSIVE DISORDERS OF PREGNANCY

**Hypertensive disorders in pregnancy are defined by blood pressures that are persistently elevated above what values?**

Systolic >140 mm Hg or diastolic >90 mm Hg

**What percentage of United States pregnancies are complicated by hypertensive disorders?**

10–20%

**What are the various hypertensive disorders observed during pregnancy?**

Chronic hypertension (cHTN), which affects 3% of all U.S. pregnancies

Pregnancy-induced hypertension (PIH) or gestational hypertension (GHTN), which affects 6% of all United States pregnancies

Preeclampsia (PEC), which affects 5–8% of all U.S. pregnancies

Eclampsia

**If a woman at 20 weeks estimated gestational age (EGA) presents with a systolic pressure ≥140 mm Hg or diastolic pressure 90 mm Hg, what is her probable diagnosis?**

Chronic hypertension (cHTN), because it was likely present and undiagnosed prior to pregnancy. She should be evaluated for a molar pregnancy

**A woman was noted to have multiple elevated blood pressures (BP) during the third trimester. At her IUD insertion 12 weeks postpartum, her BP is 140/90. Was her hypertension pregnancy induced?**

No, she meets criteria for cHTN because her elevated BPs persisted >12 weeks postpartum. cHTN was likely present prior to her pregnancy

**What antihypertensives are used to lower the BP of a pregnant woman?**

Methyldopa for management of cHTN. Hydralazine for the acute management of hypertension associated with PEC. Additional agents include nifedipine and labetalol

**How is GHTN diagnosed (dx)?**

The onset of two BPs >140/90, separated by 6 hours, after 20 weeks EGA

**What is the difference between GHTN and PEC?**

Proteinuria is present in PEC, and it is absent in GHTN

**Who are most at risk for PIH or toxemia?**

Adolescent primiparous women, multiparous women >35 years of age, women with a history of PIH (there is a 33% chance of recurrence), and women with a different partner between pregnancies

**What percentage of women with GHTN develop PEC?**

50%

**Does GHTN and PEC resolve postpartum?**

Yes, they typically resolve by 12 weeks postpartum

**How is PEC diagnosed?**

The new onset of hypertension (>140/90) and proteinuria (≥0.3 g protein in a 24-hour urine specimen or persistent 1+ on dipstick) after 20 weeks of gestation. The elevated blood pressure should be documented on two occasions at least 6 hours. Edema is no longer one of the criteria evaluated for diagnosis

**What is the cure for PEC?**

Delivery, though a woman remains at risk for the development of eclampsia postpartum

**What are other signs and symptoms of PEC?**

**Endothelial damage:**
Elevated uric acid, plasma urate level >5.5 mg/dL (327 mmol/L)

Sudden and rapid weight gain (>5 lbs/week)

Facial edema

**Uteroplacental insufficiency:**
Intrauterine growth restriction (IUGR)

Oligohydramnios (AFI <5)

Alkaline phosphates in maternal serum because of placental vascular stress

**Once PEC is suspected why is 24-hour urine collected to assess protein excretion?**

PEC is a dynamic process and single dipstick values do not correlate well with the degree of end-organ pathology present. 24-hour urine collection offers a more accurate reflection of the volume of protein lost by the kidneys. Proteinuria is defined as >300 mg/24 hours or >100 mg/dL

**What are risk factors for the development of PEC?**

Multiple gestations

Obesity

| | |
|---|---|
| | Personal or family history of PEC<br>Primigravid state<br>Pregestational diabetes<br>Existing hypertension (GHTN, cHTN)<br>Prolonged interval between pregnancies<br>Renal disease (focal glomerulosclerosis)<br>Advanced maternal age (greatest risk >40 years of age)<br>Collagen vascular disease<br>Antiphospholipid syndrome<br>Other coagulation abnormalities (protein C or S deficiency, factor V Leiden mutation, and hyperhomocysteinemia)<br>**Note: smoking is not a risk factor** |
| **In the setting of cHTN, how is PEC diagnosed?** | With the onset of proteinuria or other signs and symptoms of end-organ disease.<br>In hypertensive nephrosclerosis, protein excretion is typically <1 g/day.<br>In the setting of new onset PEC protienuria is typically >1+ on urine dip |
| **What are the two types of PECs?** | Mild and severe |
| **What percent of cases are mild in the United States?** | 75% |
| **How is severe PEC defined?** | PEC with any of the signs or symptoms of severe eclampsia, that are mentioned below |
| **What are the systemic and clinical features of severe PEC?** | **Endothelial damage**<br>Severe hypertension >160 mm Hg systolic or >100 mm Hg diastolic<br>Pulmonary edema because of capillary leak<br>**Liver abnormalities**<br>Elevated transaminases<br>Epigastric or right upper abdominal pain, because of hepatic congestion and pressure on the capsule |

**Hematologic abnormalities**

Hemoconcentration

Thrombocytopenia because of formation of microthrombi, platelets <100,000

Microangiopathic hemolysis, with schistocytes and helmet cells

Increased serum lactate dehydrogenase and bilirubin

**CNS manifestations**

Brisk deep tendon reflexes

Persistent headache, which does not resolve with medication, hydration, or rest

Visual changes (scotoma, blurring, cortical blindness)

**Renal dysfunction**

Nephritic range proteinuria (>5 g/day) because of the impaired integrity of the glomerular barrier

Glomerular capillary endotheliosis because of deposition of proteinaceous material

Oliguria <400 mL in 24 hours

**What percentage of women with a history of PEC have a recurrence in subsequent pregnancies?**

25–65% in severe PEC

5–7% in mild PEC

**What are considered to be maternal complications of PEC?**

Cerebral hemorrhage

Disseminated intravascular coagulation (DIC)

Eclamptic seizure

Pulmonary edema

Oliguria and renal failure

Rupture of the hepatic capsule

**What is considered to be the most severe manifestation of PEC, without the onset of eclampsia (without seizures)?**

HELLP syndrome (hemolysis, elevated liver function tests, low platelets), it is speculated that GHTN and eclampsia occupy a spectrum of hypertensive disorders that involve endothelial damage

**How many women with PEC develop HELLP?**

2% of patients

**Can a woman develop HELLP without a prior diagnosis of PEC?**

Yes, a small percentage of women do not exhibit hypertension or proteinuria

**What laboratory abnormalities are associated with HELLP?**

Lactate dehydrogenase >600 IU/mL

Bilirubin >1.2 mg/dL

Platelets <150

Elevated alanine and aspartate aminotransferase (AST and ALT)

**What is the appropriate management of severe PEC, HELLP, or eclampsia?**

Immediate delivery, through induction of labor or cesarean delivery (cxs), and anticonvulsant prophylaxis

**What is the difference between PEC and eclampsia?**

Grand mal or tonic-clonic seizures, which are not attributed to any other pathology. Eclampsia is associated with significant maternal and neonatal morbidity and mortality

**What is the most common symptom prior to the onset of seizures?**

Intense headache, which does not resolve with medication, hydration, or rest

**Do all women who develop eclampsia have proteinuria?**

No, 10% lack proteinuria; however, they typically have other clinical and histologic manifestations

**How often do women with mild or severe PEC progress to eclampsia?**

1 in 200 mild PEC patients and 2% of severe PEC patients seize if they are not treated with anticonvulsant prophylaxis. A woman is at increased risk for eclamptic seizures as she approaches delivery

**What percentage of seizures occur prior to the onset of labor, during delivery, and within 48 hours postpartum?**

25%, 50%, and 25% respectively

**What medication is used to treat eclamptic seizures, in addition to its use as an anticonvulsant prophylaxis?**

Magnesium sulfate ($MgSO_4$) is the primary treatment. Morphine, barbiturates, benzodiazepines (diazepam), and antiepileptics have also been used

**What are the signs and symptoms of magnesium toxicity?**

Decreased deep tendon reflexes at 8 mg/dL, they are lost at 10 mg/L

Lethargic and blunted mental status

Respiratory depression at 15 mg/dL

Pulmonary edema and shortness of breath

Chest pain and cardiac arrest at levels of 30 mg/L

**Why is urine output monitored during magnesium treatment?**

Magnesium is renally excreted and blood levels may quickly become toxic if the patient become oliguric, <0.5 cc/kg/h

**How is magnesium toxicity managed?**

Calcium gluconate IV, hydration, respiratory and cardiac support

## ABNORMAL PLACENTATION

**What is a velamentous insertion of the cord or a velamentous umbilical cord?**

Umbilical vessels that are surrounded only by fetal membranes, with no Wharton jelly. For this reason they extend to the maternal membranes, beyond the normal placental margin

**Is a velementous cord more common in twins?**

Yes, it occurs in 10% of twins and 1% of singleton gestations

**What is placenta previa?**

The edge of the placenta is in close proximity to or overlies the internal os of the cervix

**What is the incidence of placenta previa?**

4 per 1000 pregnancies and 1 in 200 births

**What are the various types of placenta previa?**

Complete previa placenta covers the internal os of the cervix; accounts for approximately 30% of all previas

Marginal previa <2 cm from the cervical os

Low-lying placenta >2 cm, has no significance

Vasa previa velamentous fetal vessels cross the internal os (see Fig. 9-4)

**Can placenta previa diagnosed early in pregnancy resolve during the course of the pregnancy?**

Yes, as the lower uterine segment enlarges and the placenta grows; 90% will resolve by term

**Rupture of membranes (ROM) or vaginal manipulation in vasa previa is associated with what risk?**

Fetal exsanguinations, with a concomitant finding of non-reassuring fetal heart rate (FHR) and a sinusoidal pattern

**What are risk factors for placenta previa?**

Endometrial scarring caused by increasing parity, increasing maternal age, prior cxs, prior curettages, increased maternal age

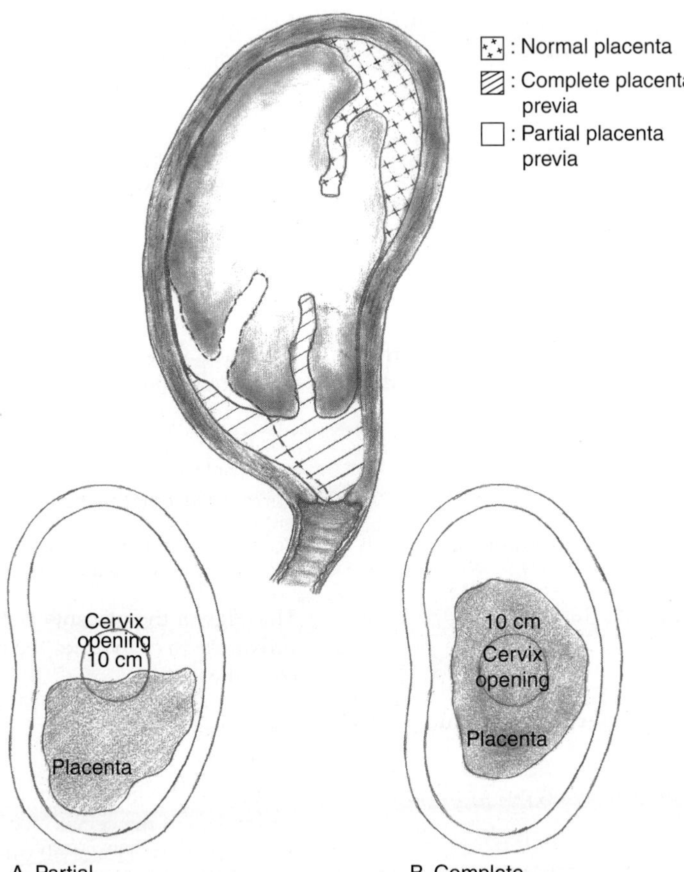


**Figure 9-4** Types of placenta previa.

| | |
|---|---|
| | Increased uteroplacental transport demand, which may be caused by maternal smoking, cocaine abuse, higher altitudes, or multiple gestations |
| | It is more common with male infants |
| **What are some of the complications of placenta previa?** | Hemorrhage, placenta accrete (10%), malpresentation, and preterm premature rupture of the membranes (PPROM) |
| **Are women with a history of placenta previa at risk for previa in subsequent pregnancies?** | Yes, the recurrence rate is 4–8% |
| **What type of delivery is indicated in previa?** | Cesarean delivery, amniocentesis is performed at 36 weeks to assess |

pulmonary maturity. If immature, it is repeated weekly until maturity is confirmed with subsequent delivery

**What are the other forms of abnormal placentation?**

**Bipartite placenta:** composed of two equal portions separated by membranes and exposed large vessels

**Battledore placenta:** involves a marginal insertion of the cord

**Fenestrated placenta:** involves a central defect

**Placenta diffusa (membranous):** all fetal surfaces are covered by villi

**Succenturiate placenta:** has a marginal accessory lobe(s) or cotyledon

**Circumvallata placenta:** is small and limited by an amniotic ring

**What abnormal placentation may cause retained products of conception and subsequent postpartum hemorrhage?**

Succenturiate placenta, examination of the delivered placenta will exhibit vessels that do not taper; instead they extend past the edge

**What abnormal placentation may cause increased risk of preterm delivery?**

Circumvallata placenta, which is more common in older, multiparous patients

## THIRD TRIMESTER BLEEDING

**What is the most common cause of bleeding in the second and third trimester?**

Bloody show associated with cervical insufficiency or labor (term and preterm)

**Antepartum hemorrhage refers to what type of bleeding?**

Vaginal bleeding after 20 weeks. EGA that is caused by some process other than labor and delivery. By definition this excludes preterm labor (PTL) and preterm delivery (PTD)

**What are the major causes of antepartum bleeding?**

Abruptio placentae 30%

Placenta previa 20%

Uterine rupture

Vasa previa

Other causes, such as, infections, trauma, polyps or neoplasia, and bloody show are associated with cervical changes because of insufficiency

**How often is antepartum hemorrhage observed in the third trimester?**

In 4% of pregnancies

**What is the initial management of painless blood per vagina in the third trimester?**

Transabdominal ultrasonography is used for initial placental localization and evaluation for abnormalities. A manual examination should *not* be performed until previa is ruled out

**Laboratory tests that identify the etiology of the vaginal bleeding (fetal vs. maternal) include:**

Ogita, Londersloot, Apt, or Kleihauer—Bentke tests identify fetal cells in maternal circulation

**What is the difference between a small marginal placental separation and placental abruption?**

EGA, or when the event occurs during pregnancy. The former is used to describe noncatastrophic placental hemorrhage before 20 weeks EGA. The latter refers to any placental separation after 20 weeks (see Fig. 9-5)

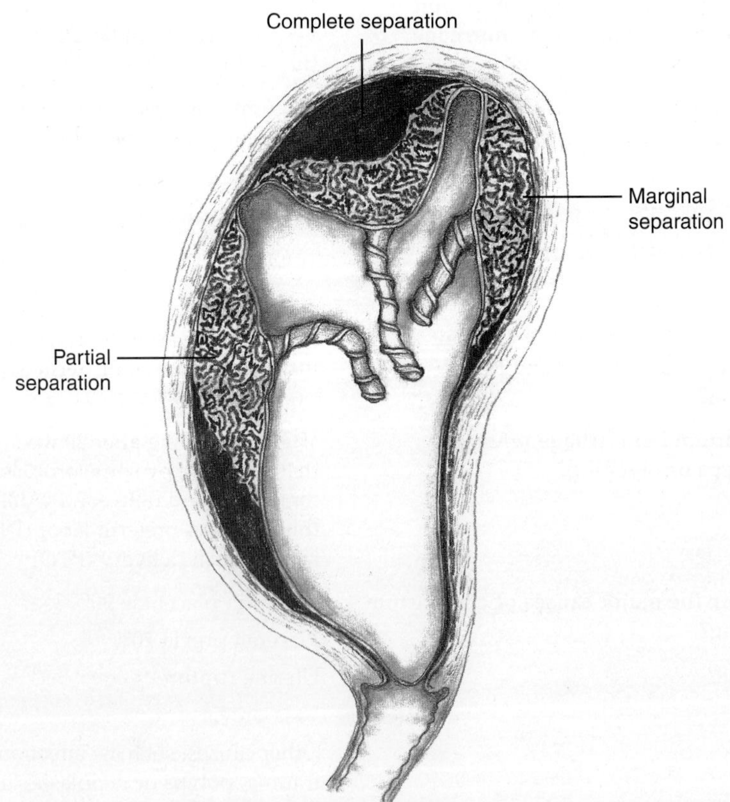


**Figure 9-5** Types of placental previa separation.

**What is the classic presentation of placenta previa?**

Painless blood per vagina after 20 weeks EGA, which may range from spotting to hemorrhagic. This presentation occurs in 70–80% of patients

**How often are painful uterine contractions reported in the setting of vaginal bleeding because of placenta previa?**

10% of presentations. However, vaginal bleeding and painful uterine contractions are more suggestive of abruption, especially in the setting of recent trauma

**Delivery should be expedited in which situations?**

Persistent non-reassuring FHR, hemodynamic instability because of refractory maternal hemorrhage, significant bleeding with known fetal pulmonary maturity (>34 weeks EGA), disseminated intravascular coagulopathy or other consumptive coagulation disorder

**In the context of intermittent contractions, third trimester bleeding, immature fetal lung maturity (FLM) results, and <32 weeks EGA, what conditions must be met to allow for 24 hours of corticosteroids with possible tocolysis?**

The mother must be hemodynamically stable and uninfected. The fetus should have a reassuring FHR. There are conflicting data regarding the benefit of steroids after 32 weeks EGA

## PROM AND PPROM

**A term patient reports a sudden gush of fluid with continued loss of fluid and no uterine contraction, what is the initial management?**

Ask her to come to the hospital for further evaluation, confirm membrane rupture, confirm the gestational age, and assess the fetal status

**What is the definition of premature rupture of membranes (PROM)?**

Rupture of placental membranes (ROM), or amniorrhexis, in a full-term pregnancy, with the absence of labor

**How prevalent is PROM?**

It occurs in 8% of U.S. pregnancies

**Pregnant women occasionally report leakage of fluid without ROM; this is because of what side effects of pregnancy?**

Sporadic urinary incontinence (stress incontinence), because of progesterone and increased pressure on the bladder by the gravid uterus. The patient should still be evaluated for possible ROM

**What physical findings support the diagnosis of ROM?**

Pooling of vaginal fluid or leakage with coughing on sterile speculum examination, positive nitrazine test of the vaginal fluid, ferning of dried fluid under low power magnification, ultrasound with decreased amniotic fluid (AF), amnio dye test (pigment is injected into the AF and a tampon is examined for leakage)

**What laboratory studies support the diagnosis of ROM?**

Placental alpha microglobulin-1, insulin-like growth factor binding protein-1 (IGFPB-1), alpha-fetoprotein (AFP), fetal fibronectin, creatinine, human chorionic gonadotropin, diamino-oxydase, prolactin, ceruloplasmin, and lactate are all substances found at higher concentrations in the AF

**Do women who present with PROM go into spontaneous labor?**

Yes, 70% will go into labor within 24 hours and 85% within 48 hours

**What is considered prolonged PROM?**

PROM for more than 18–24 hours, without the onset of labor

**In a patient with PROM, what is suggested by expectant management?**

The fetus and mother are monitored or closely followed, with the expectation that the patient is likely to go into spontaneous labor. No efforts are made to immediately induce delivery

**What are the benefits of immediate induction upon presentation to the hospital with PROM, instead of expectant management?**

Reduced fetal and maternal infections, such as chorioamnionitis, endometritis, neonatal sepsis, and intensive care unit admission

**What are the risks of induction with a poor Bishop score?**

Failed induction, cxs, protracted labor, cost of prolonged hospitalization, maternal or neonatal infection, uterine rupture because of hyperstimulation with tocolytics

**What is the definition of preterm premature rupture of membranes (PPROM)?**

ROM in the absence of labor at <37 weeks EGA

**How prevalent is PPROM?**

It affects 1–3% of U.S. pregnancies or 25% of PROM

**What is the most common risk factor for the development of PPROM?**

Genital tract infections and chorioamnionitis

**What are other risk factors for the development of PPROM?**

Placenta previa, smoking, cervical incompetence, multiple gestations, polyhydramnios, antepartum hemorrhage, personal history of PPROM

**What is the rate of PPROM recurrence in subsequent pregnancies?**

13.5%

**Is PPROM an indication for hospitalization?**

Yes, from the time of diagnosis until delivery

**Prior to delivery, what type of adverse outcomes are seen following PPROM?**

Intrauterine infection 13–60%

Placental abruption 4–12%

Umbilical cord prolapse 1–2%

Precipitous delivery

**What are the most severe adverse neonatal outcomes associated with PPROM?**

Hyaline membrane disease

Acute respiratory distress syndrome (ARDS)

Intraventricular hemorrhage (IVH)

Infection (sepsis, pneumonia, meningitis)

Necrotizing enterocolitis (NEC)

Other adverse events include: thermal instability, fluid and electrolyte disturbances (hypocalcemia, hypokalemia), hypoglycemia, hyperbilirubinemia, patent ductus arteriosus, irregularities in pulmonary and cardiac function (apnea and bradycardia), poor feeding

**In the setting of EGA ≥32 weeks, documented fetal lung maturity, and PPROM is it advisable to engage in immediate delivery or expectant management?**

In this context, immediate delivery has been shown to result in better outcomes, as long as expert neonatal care is available

**What are fetal lung maturity tests?**

Lecithin/sphingomyelin ratio (L/S) > 2–3.5

Acidic phospholipids phosphatidylinositol (PI) or foam stability index (TDX) >48

Phosphatidylglycerol (PG) present

Percent perceptible lecithin or fluorescence polarization >55 mg/g, optical density

Surfactant to albumin ratio (S/A)

Saturated phosphatidyl choline (SPC)

**What is surfactin?**

A phospholipid produced by type II pneumocytes at 29 weeks EGA, which decreases surface tension in

| | |
|---|---|
| | the alveoli. Insufficient surfactin production will result in ARDS |
| **When and why is betamethasone or dexamethasone used?** | They are corticosteroids that cross the placenta and stimulate production of surfactin and lung maturation in the 27–32-week EGA fetus. It is given in two doses 12 hours apart and is believed to attain its maximal impact after 12 hours |
| **In the context of immature fetal lung maturity results, <32 weeks EGA, and PPROM, delivery may be delayed 24 hours so as to offer what treatments?** | Two doses of corticosteroids, to hasten the production of surfactant in the type II pneumocytes. Antibiotics are often concurrently administered. There are conflicting data regarding the benefit of steroids after 32 weeks EGA, though several physicians will offer it to their patients through 34 weeks EGA |
| **What effect does prophylactic antibiotic administration have in the setting of PPROM?** | It reduces the rate of maternal and neonatal infection, and prolongs the latency period between the time of membrane rupture and the onset of labor. Ampicillin is often used with erythromycin |
| **What conditions would require immediate delivery of PPROM, regardless of lung maturity?** | The development of advanced labor, abruption placentae, maternal hemodynamic instability (likely because of hemorrhage), intrauterine infection, non-reassuring fetal testing, fetal compromise (severe oligohydramnios or cord prolapse) |
| **Corticosteroid administration increases the risk of:** | Chorioamnionitis |

## Preterm Labor and Preterm Delivery

| | |
|---|---|
| **What is the definition of preterm labor (PTL)?** | Labor (regular uterine contractions with cervical change) that starts between the 20th and 37th week of pregnancy |
| **What is the most significant risk factor for PTL?** | Previous history of preterm birth (PTB) or preterm delivery (PTD) |
| **What are other risk factors for PTL?** | Multiple gestations (the risk increases with increasing number of fetuses) |

Adolescent pregnancy (greatest risk <15 years of age)

Advanced maternal age (>35 years of age)

Cervical insufficiency

Maternal genital tract infections

Uterine malformations

Cigarette smoking

Maternal substance abuse (cocaine is the most common illicit substance associated with PTL)

A change in partners between pregnancies

Low socioeconomic status (education, occupation, and family income)

Race/ethnicity, with black women having the highest rates

**What is the definition of preterm birth (PTB) or preterm delivery (PTD)?**

Birth that occurs before 37 completed weeks (less than 259 days) of estimated gestation age (EGA). Less than 28 weeks of gestation is considered an extreme PTB

**What are the causes of PTD?**

20% Iatrogenic, for maternal or fetal indications

Intrauterine growth restriction

Severe PEC

Placenta previa with unstable hemorrhage

Non-reassuring fetal testing

30% Preterm premature rupture of the membranes (PPROM)

20–25% Intra-amniotic infection

25–30% Other pathology or idiopathic preterm labor

**What is the prevalence of PTD in the United States?**

12% of all deliveries, 2% occur before 32 weeks

**What is the impact of PTD on neonatal morbidity and mortality?**

In the United States, PTB accounts for 85% of all perinatal morbidity and mortality. Disability occurs in 60% of survivors of birth at 26 weeks EGA

**Hydration may decrease preterm uterine contractions based on dilution of what hormone?**

Antidiuretic hormone (ADH) is increased in the setting of dehydration and it may have some crossreactivity with uterine oxytocin receptors. Diluting ADH and decreasing the systemic production may decrease preterm uterine irritability

**What class of medications is used to prevent uterine contractions?**

Tocolytics, such as, magnesium sulfate (increases extracellular calcium), calcium channel blockers (nifedipine), beta adrenergic agonists (terbutaline, ritodrine)

**In what scenario is there a clear indication for tocolytics?**

To delay delivery 48 hours in PTL with EGA <32 weeks so as to administer 24 hours of corticosteroids and hasten the production of surfactant in the type II pneumocytes

**Why is it not advisable to use more than one tocolytic concurrently?**

Increased risk of pulmonary edema. The use of two tocolytics has not been show to benefit maternal or fetal outcomes

**What do contraindications to tocolysis include?**

Fetal distress, severe oligohydramnios, fetal demise, intrauterine infection

**Tocolysis with an antiprostaglandin, such as indomethacin, can prolong the interval to labor in a PTL patient; however, it carries what significant risk to the fetus?**

Premature closure of the ductus arteriosus, with subsequent pulmonary hypertension

**What type of patient has been shown to benefit from progesterone supplementation in randomized controlled trials?**

Patients with a history of spontaneous or idiopathic PTL. Progesterone injections are administered to asymptomatic patients as weekly injections 17 alpha-hydroxyprogesterone caproate (250 mg) or daily progesterone vaginal suppositories (100 mg) beginning in the second trimester and continuing through term

**Prophylactic progesterone injections reduce the rate of PTB by what percent?**

15–70%, but there is no significant impact on perinatal mortality, morbidity, or miscarriage

**A woman who presents with painless cervical dilation and bulging fetal membranes during the second trimester is consistent with what diagnosis?**

Cervical insufficiency, formerly known as cervical incompetence

**What sonographic findings are consistent with cervical insufficiency?**

Short cervical length, dilated internal cervical os, and funneling of the fetal membranes

**How prevalent is cervical insufficiency?**

2% of all U.S. pregnancies

**What treatment may be offered to patients with cervical insufficiency?**

Prophylactic or emergent cerclage, the efficacy of this intervention may be specific to certain subgroups; however, it has not been consistently demonstrated in trials

**What are risk factors for cervical insufficiency?**

History of cervical colonization, multiparity, history of cervical trauma

**What is considered a highly specific test for PTL?**

Fetal fibronectin (fFN) assay because of a false-positive rate of 3–4% or a low prevalence of positive results in asymptomatic low-risk women. Unfortunately, the sensitivity and positive predictive value (41%) are not as impressive

**What is fetal fibronectin?**

Fetal fibronectin is a glycoprotein present in maternal circulation and AF, if present in the cervicovaginal secretions >50 ng/mL; it suggests that the cervix is undergoing structural change and the patient may go into labor in the next 2 weeks. Positive predictive value is 41%

**Would fetal fibronectin be indicated in a 32-week EGA patient with painful uterine contractions?**

Yes. The test is more valuable for its negative predictive value of 96%. If the protein is low or absent there is a low probability that she will go into PTL in the next 2 weeks. The swab must be collected prior to any other vaginal cultures, examination, or procedure. It can be repeated in 2 weeks if she presents with signs or symptoms consistent with PTL

| | |
|---|---|
| **What common interventions have *not* proven to prevent PTL?** | Bed rest, home uterine monitoring, prophylactic broad-spectrum antibiotic therapy, abstinence from sex, hydration, long-term or prophylactic tocolytic therapy |

## Maternal and Fetal Pathology in Pregnancy

| | |
|---|---|
| **What is round ligament pain?** | As the gravid uterus increases rapidly during the second and third trimester, tension on the round ligament may cause sharp shooting inguinal and groin pain. Rest, warm compresses, and acetaminophen may relieve the pain |
| **In what circumstances is fundal height greater than dates?** | Twins, polyhydramnios, macrosomia, fibroids, hydatidiform mole (molar pregnancy) |
| **What conditions or anomalies are associated with polyhydramnios?** | Gestational diabetes mellitus (GDM), fetal anomalies of the nervous (anencephaly), or gastrointestinal system (tracheosophageal fistula or atresia) |
| **What conditions or anomalies are associated with olgohydramnios?** | Bilateral renal anomalies (Potter), posterior urethral valves in males, hypertensive disorders of pregnancy (gHTN, PEC, HELLP) |
| **What are amniotic bands?** | Placental membrane defects that result in fetal deformities or amputations; they are believed to be because of sclerosis and are associated with oligohydramnios |
| **How prevalent are birth defects of medical, surgical, or cosmetic significance?** | 2–4% of all viable infants, irrespective of ethnic background. Most birth defects are multifactorial |
| **What is the definition of a low birth weight infant?** | Less than 2500 g |
| **What are causes for infants born less than 2500 g?** | PTD, small for gestational age (SGA), intrauterine growth restriction (IUGR), infection (rubella or CMV), teratogen exposure, chromosomal or congenital anomalies. The smaller the infant the higher the mortality |

**When is a fetus considered small for gestational age?**

When the estimated fetal weight is less than the 10th percentile at a given EGA

**Is symmetric or asymmetric IUGR more prevalent?**

Asymmetric is observed in 80% of cases

**What type of insult or anomaly is believed to contribute to symmetric IUGR?**

A long-standing pathologic process, which began early in the pregnancy. Possible causes of IUGR include: first-trimester infections, fetal anomalies (severe cardiac defect), systemic maternal disease (DM type I, HTN), or chromosomal abnormalities (trisomy 13, 18, 21)

**What type of insult or anomaly is believed to contribute to asymmetric IUGR?**

Asymmetric IUGR is often attributed to a pathologic process occurring later in pregnancy such as: uteroplacental insufficiency because of PEC, twin transfusion syndromes, or teratogen exposure

**Following intrauterine fetal demise, what is the greatest maternal risk?**

Disseminated intravascular coagulation (DIC) because of increased thromboplastin release from the products of conception

**Why is a mother with multiple sclerosis likely to experience a flare postpartum?**

Pregnancy induces a state of weakened cell-mediated immunity. Th1, Il-2, and TNF are all decreased. For this reason certain autoimmune diseases seem to subside during pregnancy. However, humoral Th2 immunity is strengthened, with increased Il-4 and Il-10. This may result in lupus flares during pregnancy

**The following sonographic findings are characteristic of what fetal anomalies?**

Double-bubble duodenal atresia, the appearance is because of fluid collections in the stomach and truncated intestine

Banana sign communicating spina bifida, the appearance is because of the flattened cerebral hemispheres and cisterna magna

Lemon sign neural tube defects, the appearance is because of an indentation of the calvarium or scalloping of the frontal bones

**What is the incidence of stillbirth in the United States?**

6.4 per 1000 total deliveries

**What are the most common causes of stillbirth 24–27 weeks EGA?**

Infection

Abruption placentae

Anomalies

**What are the most common causes of stillbirth <28 weeks EGA?**

Unexplained

Fetal malnutrition

Abruption placentae

**What are the risk factors for stillbirth?**

Prepregnancy obesity

Advanced maternal age

Socioeconomic factors (low education attainment)

Hypertensive disorders

Diabetes

Systemic lupus erythematosus

Renal disease

Thyroid disorders

Thrombophilia

Cholestasis of pregnancy

Smoking >10 cigarettes per day

History of an SGA fetus

History of stillbirth

Multiple gestations

Race (black women have twice the risk)

**In North Americans what percentage of stillbirths are because of intrapartum asphyxia?**

Less than 1% of stillbirths. The rate was dramatically decreased by the implementation of intrapartum monitoring during the 1950s. Unfortunately, intrapartum monitoring has not reduced the rate of cerebral palsy

**What are the leading causes of traumatic maternal morbidity and mortality during pregnancy?**

Motor vehicle accidents (MVAs) account for 55–70% of injuries according to national hospital registries

Seat belt use was reported in less than half of these cases

Falls account for 10–20%

Interpersonal and domestic violence accounts for 12–31%

However, the CDC considers interpersonal violence to be the leading cause of traumatic maternal injury

**What percentage of U.S. pregnancies experience significant nonobstetrical trauma?**

6–7%, with the incidence of trauma increasing throughout the course of the pregnancy

**What is the risk of fetal death following abruption?**

42%

# Postpartum Complications

## POSTPARTUM HEMORRHAGE

**What is the significance of postpartum hemorrhage?**

It is the most significant cause of maternal death worldwide. There are approximately 140,000 deaths per year because of severe bleeding—otherwise estimated as 1 death every 4 minutes

**How is postpartum hemorrhage defined?**

It is excessive bleeding following delivery. Although uncomplicated vaginal deliveries may have an average blood loss of 700 mL, blood loss > 500 mL following a vaginal birth or a blood loss of > 1000 mL following cesarean birth qualifies as hemorrhage

**Postpartum hemorrhage is classified as primary or secondary. What is meant by each type?**

**Primary:** occurs within the first 24 hours of delivery and occurs in 4–6% of pregnancies

**Secondary:** occurs between 6–12 weeks postpartum in about 1% of pregnancies

**What are the etiologies for primary postpartum hemorrhage and secondary postpartum hemorrhage?**

**Primary: uterine atony (80%),** obstetric lacerations (episiotomy involving large arteries), retained placenta (i.e., placenta accreta), coagulation defects, uterine inversion

**Secondary: subinvolution of placental site, retained products of conception**, infection, inherited coagulation defects

**What are risk factors for postpartum hemorrhage?**

Prolonged labor, augmented labor, rapid labor, history of postpartum hemorrhage, overdistended uterus (macrosomia, twins, hydramnios), episiotomy, operative delivery, Asian or Hispanic ethnicity, chorioamnionitis

**Note: postpartum hemorrhage can often occur without warning**

**In addition to mortality, what major morbidities follow postpartum hemorrhage?**

Adult respiratory distress syndrome (ARDS), coagulopathy, shock, loss of fertility, and pituitary necrosis (Sheehan syndrome)

**How does Sheehan syndrome clinically manifest?**

Failure to lactate, amenorrhea, decreased breast size, loss of pubic and axillary hair, hypothyroidism, and adrenal insufficiency

**How should each of the following be evaluated as a cause of excessive bleeding immediately after placental separation? How is each etiology managed?**

**Uterine atony:** pelvic exam reveals a soft, poorly contracted ("boggy") uterus. Compression or massage of the uterus can diminish bleeding

**Obstetric-related lacerations:** careful visual assessment of the lower genital tract is necessary. Proper patient positioning, operative assistance, anesthesia, and proper repair of lacerations are indicated

**Genital tract hematomas:** patient complains of pelvic pressure and pain; mass enlargement may be visualized. The hematoma should be surgically drained. The bleeding vessels may also be embolized

**Retained products of conception:** ultrasound can help diagnose a retained placenta. This may be removed by forceps, guided by ultrasonography

**Coagulopathy:** patient and family history of clotting disorders, CBC, PT/PTT, fibrinogen levels. Type and cross should be ordered. Surgery and blood transfusion may be necessary

**What are proper supportive measures that should be instituted early in women suspected to have postpartum hemorrhage?**

IV access, type & cross, blood products requests from the blood bank, crystalloid infusions, communication with anesthesiologists, preparation of operating room

**How can uterine atony and subsequent bleeding be prevented?**

Administer uterotonic agents, such as oxytocin, immediately after delivery. If uterotonic agents fail to control the bleeding, packing or tamponade of the uterus may help

**If uterotonic agents with or without vaginal tamponade measures fail to control bleeding, what procedure is indicated next?**

Exploratory laparotomy

**What is the definitive measure to control postpartum hemorrhage?**

Hysterectomy

## PLACENTA ACCRETA

**Placenta accreta is one of the two most common reasons (the other being uterine atony) for postpartum hemorrhage and hysterectomy. Describe placenta accreta**

It is the abnormal attachment of the placenta to the inner uterine wall without an intervening decidual layer

**What is placenta increta and placenta percreta?**

**Placenta increta:** the placenta invades the myometrium

**Placenta percreta:** the placenta penetrates the full thickness of the myometrium

**What are risk factors for placenta accreta?**

**Placenta previa in current pregnancy**

**Previous cesarean delivery**

Previous myomectomy

Asherman syndrome

Submucous leiomyoma

Maternal age > 35 years

**Are there any tools that can diagnose placenta accreta?**

Though ultrasonography and color doppler studies may help in the diagnosis, they are not definitive for placenta accreta

**What is another consequence of placenta accreta that is life-threatening?**

Uterine rupture

**In what other situations can uterine rupture occur?**

History of a previous cesarean delivery

Excessive intrauterine manipulation

Congenital malformations of the uterus (small uterine horn)

Spontaneously

## UTERINE INVERSION

**What is uterine inversion?**

It is when the uterine corpus/fundus prolapses to (incomplete inversion) and sometimes through (complete inversion) the uterine cervix, so that it is in effect turned inside out. It is also associated with severe hemorrhage

**In addition to postpartum hemorrhage, what is the immediate morbidity associated with uterine inversion?**

Endomyometritis

**What are several conditions that predispose to uterine inversion?**

Fundal implantation of the placenta

Partial placenta accreta

Uterine anomalies

Weakness of the myometrium

Strong traction exerted on the umbilical cord

Fundal pressure

**What findings on physical examination suggest an inverted uterus?**

A bimanual examination may reveal a firm mass at or below the cervix, and an abdominal exam will reveal a depression in the location or the absence of the uterine fundus

**If uterine inversion occurs before placental separation, what should *not* be done?**

**Removal or detachment of the placenta should *not* be performed.** This will cause profound hemorrhage

**How should uterine inversion be managed?**

Either manual or surgical repositioning of the uterus

## POSTPARTUM AND PUERPERAL INFECTIONS

**How is puerperal infection and puerperal morbidity because of infection defined?**

**Puerperal infection** is used to describe any bacterial infection of the genital tract after delivery

**Puerperal morbidity because of infection** occurs when the patient develops a **temperature >38°C** (100.4°F) on **two separate occasions at least 24 hours apart following the first 24 hours of delivery**

**What are several risk factors for puerperal morbidity because of infection?**

Lower socioeconomic status

Cesarean delivery

Premature rupture of the membranes

Long labors

Multiple pelvic examinations

**What are several types of postpartum infections?**

**Uterine infection (endometritis)**

Respiratory Infections (ARDS, aspiration pneumonia, bacterial pneumonia)

Urinary tract infections (acute pyelonephritis)

Wound infections (cesarean delivery incision)

Mastitis

Thrombophlebitis

**Most postpartum infections are caused by organisms that are present in the female genital tract and which also normally cause female genital tract infections. What are these common bacterial agents?**

**Gram-positive cocci:** group A, B, and D streptococci, *Staphylococcus aureus*

**Gram-positive bacilli:** *Clostridium* species

**Aerobic gram-negative bacilli:** *Escherichia coli, Klebsiella, Proteus* species

**Anaerobic gram-negative bacilli:** *Bacteroides fragilis* group

**Other:** *Mycoplasma* species, *Chlamydia trachomatis, Neisseria gonorrhoeae*

## ENDOMETRITIS

**What does endometritis in the postpartum period refer to?**

It refers to infection of the decidua (i.e., pregnancy endometrium), and also the myometrium (endomyometritis) and parametrial tissues (parametritis)

**What is the most significant risk factor for endometritis?**

The route of delivery. The risk of infection is 5–10 times higher in cesarean delivery compared to vaginal delivery

**Which two bacterial agents have been found to be specific for endometritis?**

*Bacterial vaginosis and group B streptococcus*

**How is the diagnosis of endometritis determined?**

**Fever (> 100.4°F)**

Uterine tenderness

Foul lochia

Leukocytosis (increased neutrophil count with left shift)

Typically presents on postpartum day 2 or 3

**What is the "gold-standard" treatment?**

IV clindamycin and gentamycin q8h. Improvement is usually seen 48–72 hours after treatment has begun

**If the fever has not subsided after 72 hours of antibiotic administration or after a change in antibiotic therapy, what other sources of fever must be considered?**

Wound infection

Septic pelvic thrombophlebitis

Pelvic abscess

Drug-induced fever

**Are prophylactic antibiotics indicated in women undergoing cesarean delivery?**

Yes. Prophylaxis reduces the rate of endometritis by two-thirds to three-quarters. Single agents such as **ampicillin and first-generation cephalosporins** are ideal prophylactic antibiotics

**In what setting does chronic endometritis occur?**

It occurs when there are retained products of conception after spontaneous abortion, pregnancy termination, or delivery

**What are the clinical manifestations of chronic endometritis?**

Fever

Irregular vaginal bleeding

Pelvic pain

Malaise

A tender, boggy, and enlarged uterus with bloody and/or purulent discharge on physical examination

**What is the treatment of chronic endometritis?**

Curettage to remove the necrotic material

# Medical Conditions of Pregnancy

## ENDOCRINE DISORDERS

### Gestational Diabetes Mellitus

**What is pregestational diabetes mellitus (GDM) and how is it characterized?**

It is a **diagnosis of diabetes mellitus prior to pregnancy**. It occurs in 1% of all pregnancies and includes both Type I diabetes and Type II diabetes. Type II pregestational diabetes is more common and is characterized by onset later in life, obesity, peripheral insulin resistance, some insulin deficiency, and end-organ complications (renal, vascular, nervous). Type I pregestational diabetes is less common and occurs most often early in life. It is characterized by an autoimmune process that destroys the pancreatic β cells

**What is GDM and how is it characterized?**

It is a **diagnosis of diabetes mellitus defined as glucose intolerance with onset or first recognition during pregnancy**. 90% of diabetes cases encountered during pregnancy are GDM and more than one half of those patients at risk will end up developing pregestational diabetes later in life

**How may pregnancy predispose some women to GDM?**

Placental secretion of anti-insulin and diabetogenic hormones that contribute to the diabetic state include:

Growth hormone

Corticotropin-releasing hormone

Human placental lactogen

Prolactin

Progesterone

| | |
|---|---|
| | Tumor necrosis factor-α and leptin have also been implicated in creating the insulin-resistant state of pregnancy |
| **What are several risk factors for the development of GDM?** | Age >25<br>Obesity (BMI >30 in the nonpregnant state)<br>Prior history of GDM<br>Family history of diabetes (especially in a first-degree relative)<br>Previous stillbirth or child with a congenital malformation<br>Birth of a prior infant with weight >9 lbs (or history of macrosomia)<br>Polycystic ovary syndrome (contributes to the insulin resistance state)<br>$2^+$ glycosuria (debatable in the literature) |
| **In addition to diabetic retinopathy, nephropathy, and neuropathy, what are several obstetric-related maternal complications associated with GDM?** | **Preeclampsia**<br>Preterm birth<br>Macrosomia and birth trauma (especially shoulder dystocia)<br>Intrauterine growth restriction<br>Polyhydramnios<br>First trimester abortions and stillbirths<br>Asymptomatic bacteriuria<br>Higher incidence of cesarean section, vacuum, and forceps deliveries<br>Higher incidence of neonatal respiratory distress syndrome (delay in the fetal lung maturity) |
| **With what other endocrine disorders is Type I diabetes mellitus associated?** | There is a 5–8% incidence of hypothyroid disease as well as ~25% risk of developing postpartum thyroid dysfunction |
| **What are several adverse neonatal outcomes associated with hyperglycemia?** | **Congenital malformations**<br>Macrosomia<br>Intrauterine fetal demise<br>Hypoglycemia<br>Hypocalcemia<br>Respiratory distress syndrome |

Polycythemia

Organomegaly (cardiac)

Hyperbilirubinemia

**What congenital malformations are associated with maternal pregestational diabetes mellitus?**

Heart defects (**transposition of the great vessels**, ventricular septal defect [VSD], atrial septal defect [ASD])

Neural tube defects

**Caudal regression** (pathognomonic, but very rare)

Situs inversus

Anal/rectal atresia

Renal anomalies (duplex ureter)

**How does hyperglycemia cause congenital malformations?**

Hyperglycemia is teratogenic during the period of organogenesis (first 8 weeks of pregnancy); therefore, preconceptual glucose control and monitoring is crucial for normal development

**Glycosylated hemoglobin ($HbA_{1c}$) levels correlate directly with the frequency of congenital anomalies. What is this relationship?**

| $HbA_{1c}$ Levels (%) | Frequency of Anomalies (%) |
|---|---|
| 5–6 | 2–3 |
| 8.9–9.9 | 8.1 |
| 10 | 20–25 |

**How does GDM cause fetal macrosomia?**

Maternal glucose crosses the placenta and creates a hyperglycemic environment for the fetus. In response, the fetus produces more insulin. Insulin is a potent growth hormone and leads to increased somatic growth, macrosomia, central fat deposition, and enlargement of internal organs (i.e., heart)

**Which women should be screened for gestational diabetes?**

Though controversial, **universal screening of all pregnant women is recommended by ACOG**. However, low-risk women may be exempt from screening. These women should have all of the following characteristics:

Age <25 years

Normal weight or BMI before pregnancy

No first-degree relative with diabetes mellitus

No history of abnormal glucose tolerance test

No history of poor obstetric outcome, macrosoma, vacuum, forceps, shoulder dystocia (even with good outcome)

Member of an ethnic group with a low prevalence of GDM (i.e., patient is *not* Hispanic, African, Native American, South or East Asian, Pacific Islander)

**When should screening be performed?**

If there is a high suspicion of GDM, screening should be done at the first antenatal visit; otherwise, screening can be performed at 24–28 weeks of gestation. (If a high-risk patient has a negative screening test at the first antenatal visit, she should be rescreened at 24–28 weeks.)

**What screening test is recommended for GDM?**

A **50 g oral glucose challenge test (GCT)** is given. Plasma or serum glucose level is measured 1 hour later without regard to the time of the prior meal. A value 140 mg/dL (7.8 mmol/L) is the most commonly used parameter and is considered abnormal (some authors recommend using a cut-off as low as ≥130)

**If the screening test is positive, what are the next recommended tests for diagnosing gestational diabetes?**

A **100-g, 3-hour oral glucose tolerance test (GTT)** performed after an overnight fast. GDM is present if a diagnosis of two or more of the following are met or exceeded:

| Status | Plasma or Serum Glucose Level (mg/dL) | Plasma or Serum Glucose Level (mmol/L) |
|---|---|---|
| Fasting | 95–105 | 5.3 |
| 1 hour | 180 | 10.0 |
| 2 hours | 155–165 | 8.6 |
| 3 hours | 140 | 7.8 |

**What is the White Classification of Diabetes?**

The White Classification System initially attempted to predict perinatal risk according to the age of onset of diabetes, duration of diabetes, and type of end-organ damage. The American College of Obstetricians and Gynecologists has recommended a single diabetes classification system as follows:

| Class | Onset | Fasting Plasma Glucose | 2-Hour Postprandial Glucose | Therapy |
|---|---|---|---|---|
| $A_1$ | Gestational | <105 mg/dL | <120 mg/dL | Diet |
| $A_2$ | Gestational | >105 mg/dL | >120 mg/dL | Insulin |

| Class | Age of Onset (yr) | Duration (yr) | Vascular Disease | Therapy |
|---|---|---|---|---|
| B | >20 | <10 | None | Insulin |
| C | 10–19 | 10–19 | None | Insulin |
| D | ″10 | ≥20 | Benign retinopathy | Insulin |
| **EF** | Any | Any | Neph (**NEF**) ropathy | Insulin |
| **R** | Any | Any | Proliferative **r**etinopathy | Insulin |
| **H** | Any | Any | **H**eart disease | Insulin |
| **RT** | Any | Any | **R**enal **t**ransplant | Insulin |

**What are the main considerations in the management of GDM?**

1. Preconceptual counseling, achievement of normal hemoglobin $A_{1c}$ levels before pregnancy, glucose monitoring and control, diet and exercise adjustments, and insulin if necessary
2. In addition to a routine prenatal checkup, the patient should be assessed for glycosylated hemoglobin concentration; baseline renal function with serum creatine level and a 24-hour urine collection analysis; asymptomatic bacteriuria by urine culture; thyrotropin and free thyroxine; electrocardiogram; dilated and comprehensive eye examination by an

ophthalmologist; and first trimester ultrasound examination to confirm gestational age
3. Monitoring of and intervention for fetal or obstetrical complications

**What antepartum fetal assessment is appropriate in women with**

1. An ultrasound assessment for fetal growth and anatomy **pregestational diabetes?** (i.e., heart) and a fetal echocardiogram should be completed around 18–20 weeks
2. Testing for fetal malformations should also be performed in the first trimester (nuchal translucency and serum screening for neural tube defects and/or second trimester triple or quadruple screening)
3. At 32 weeks, a weekly nonstress test and/or biophysical profile, and amniotic fluid volume should be performed increasing to two times a week beginning at 36 weeks
4. Another ultrasound at 38 weeks of gestation to estimate fetal weight, reevaluate cardiac morphology, and assist with delivery plans

**How common is diabetic ketoacidosis (DKA) in women with pregnancy-related diabetes and what is the typical presentation?**

It is found in 5–10% of all pregnancies complicated with pregestational diabetes mellitus. It is more common in Type I pregestational diabetes mellitus. The typical presentation includes abdominal pain, nausea and vomiting, altered sensorium, low arterial pH, low serum bicarbonate, serum and urine ketones, and increased anion gap. Recurrent late decelerations may be seen on fetal heart monitoring (improves when maternal ketoacidosis is corrected) and are signs of fetal distress (academia)

**How is DKA managed in the pregnant woman?**

The same as in nonpregnant women. Aggressive hydration and IV insulin is mandatory. Glucose, potassium, and bicarbonate levels should be monitored closely and replenished appropriately. Admission to the hospital is mandatory and establishment of fetal well-being is crucial

**When is cesarean delivery indicated for women with gestational diabetes?**

If the expected fetal weight is greater than 4500 g, to prevent birth trauma from shoulder dystocia

## Thyroid in Pregnancy

**What are the two major changes in thyroid function during pregnancy?**

An increase in serum thyroxine-binding globulin (TBG) concentrations and stimulation of the thyrotropin (TSH) receptor

**What two hormones have thyroid-stimulating activity?**

Estrogen (increases serum TBG concentration); hCG

**How do thyroid function test results change in normal pregnancy, and in hyperthyroid and hypothyroid states?**

See Table below

| Maternal Status | TSH | $FT_4$ | $TT_4$ | $TT_3$ | $RT_3U$ |
|---|---|---|---|---|---|
| Normal | NC | NC | ↑ | ↑ | ↓ |
| Hyperthyroid | ↓ | ↑ | ↑ | ↑ or NC | ↑ |
| Hypothyroid | ↑ | ↓ | ↓ | ↓ or NC | ↓ |

TSH: thyroid stimulating hormone; FT4: free thyroxine; FTI: free thyroxine index; TT4: total thyroxine; TT3: total triiodothyronine; RT3U: resin T3 uptake; NC: no change

**Which of the thyroid-related hormones does *not* cross the placenta?**

TSH

**Which thyroid hormones or thyroid-related molecules can cross the placenta?**

Thyroid hormone, $T_3$, $T_4$, TRH, iodine, TSH receptor immunoglobulins

## Hyperthyroidism

**What are the clinical manifestations of hyperthyroidism?**

Nervousness, tachycardia, palpitations, hypertension, weight loss, tremors, flushing, frequent bowel movements, excessive sweating, and insomnia

**What are several pregnancy-related complications associated with poorly controlled hyperthyroidism?**

Spontaneous abortion or stillbirth

Preeclampsia

Preterm delivery

Placental abruption

Cardiac arrhythmias, congestive heart failure

Low birth weight

Thyroid storm

Hyperemesis gravidarum

**What are several etiologies of hyperthyroidism?**

**Graves' disease (90%)**

Toxic nodular goiters

Iatrogenic

Iodine induced

Subacute thyroiditis

hCG-mediated

**What three syndromes are associated with hCG-mediated hyperthyroidism?**

See Table below

| Syndrome | Description | Treatment |
|---|---|---|
| **Transient subclinical hyperthyroidism** | It occurs in 10–20% of normal pregnant women during the period of highest serum hCG concentrations. | None needed |
| **Hyperemesis gravidarum** | It is a syndrome that is characterized by nausea and vomiting with weight loss of more than 5% during early pregnancy. Women may have either subclinical or mild overt hyperthyroidism. | Includes IV fluids, IV vitamins, NPO to Clears, IV anti-nauseam, thiamine, and tx. of hyperthyroidism |
| **Trophoblastic hyperthyroidism** | It occurs in about 60% of women with a hydatidiform mole or choriocarcinoma | Removal of the mole or therapy directed against the choriocarcinoma (IV/IM methotrexate + repeat β-hCG until it trends to 0 |

**What additional clinical manifestations suggest Graves' disease?**

Exophthalmos; goiter; pretibial myxedema

**How is hyperthyroidism diagnosed?**

Elevated levels of serum FT4 or elevated FTI, and low serum TSH (<0.01 mU/L)

**What is the management and treatment for pregnant women with hyperthyroidism?**

The goal of treatment is to maintain the mother's serum free $T_4$ concentration in the high-normal range for nonpregnant women using the lowest drug dose

1. **Radioiodine is absolutely contraindicated**
2. **Iodine is contraindicated as it can cause fetal goiter**
3. Propylthiouracil (PTU) 50 mg bid or less is recommended for treatment of moderate to severe hyperthyroidism-complicating pregnancy. If treatment fails, consider methimazole
4. Beta blockers may be given to ameliorate the symptoms of moderate to severe hyperthyroidism in pregnant women (low-dose atenolol may be appropriate to begin)
5. Thyroidectomy during pregnancy may be necessary in women who cannot tolerate thionamides because of allergy or agranulocytosis (preferably during second trimester)

**What percent of neonates born to women with Graves' disease have hyperthyroidism because of transplacental transfer of TSH receptor-stimulating antibodies?**

1–5%

**What are the clinical manifestations of fetal hyperthyroidism?**

Fetal tachycardia (>160 beats/min)

Fetal goiter

Advanced bone age

Poor growth

Craniosynostosis

Cardiac failure

Fetal hydrops

**Though rare, what are several manifestations of fetal and neonatal thyrotoxicosis?**

Fetal tachycardia and intrauterine growth restriction are the most common signs

**What is a thyroid storm?**

It is an acute, life-threatening medical emergency characterized by a high metabolic state in patients with thyrotoxicosis

**What is a major consequence of thyroid storm?**

Maternal heart failure

**What are the clinical signs and symptoms of a thyroid storm?**

Fever, tachycardia out of proportion to the fever, changed mental status, confusion, nervousness, nausea and vomiting, seizures, diarrhea, and cardiac arrhythmias

(It can be initiated by infections, stress, surgery, labor, and/or delivery)

**How is a thyroid storm treated?**

Transfer to the ICU

PTU, 600–800 mg PO STAT, followed by 150–200 mg PO for 4–6 hours

IV sodium iodine or 2–5 drops of supersaturated solution of potassium iodide is given PO 1 hour after PTU

IV or IM dexamethasone

Propranolol IV or PO

Phenobarbital for restlessness (if needed)

Supportive measures ($O_2$, antipyretics, cooling blankets, IV hydration)

## Hypothyroidism

**How often do hypothyroidism-complicating pregnancies occur?**

Hypothyroidism-complicating pregnancy is rare (1:1000–1:1600 deliveries) because many women with hypothyroidism are anovulatory and infertile, and, in addition, the rate of first-trimester miscarriages is high

**What are the clinical manifestations of maternal hypothyroidism?**

Fatigue, constipation, intolerance to cold, dry skin, muscle cramps, hair loss, weight gain, myxedema, carpal tunnel syndrome, and prolonged relaxation of deep tendon reflexes

**What are the most common etiologies of hypothyroidism in pregnant or postpartum women?**

**Hashimoto disease (most common in developed countries)**

**Iron deficiency (worldwide)**

Subacute thyroiditis

Thyroidectomy

Radioactive iodine treatment

**What other endocrine disease is hypothyroidism associated with?**

Type I diabetes mellitus

**What are the several pregnancy-related complications associated with hypothyroidism?**

Preeclampsia

Preterm delivery

Low-birth weight

Placental abruption

Postpartum hemorrhage

**What is the management and treatment for pregnant women with hypothyroidism?**

**Levothyroxine**. TSH levels should be checked 4 weeks later. Levothyroxine doses should be adjusted at 4-week intervals until the TSH level is stable

**What is a significant impact of maternal hypothyroidism on the fetus and/or neonate?**

Congenital cretinism

Mental retardation

Intrauterine growth restriction

Small for gestational age

**What are the signs of congenital cretinism?**

Growth failure, mental retardation, floppy baby, macroglossia, other neuropsychologic deficits

**How common is congenital hypothyroidism in neonates?**

1:4000 births and only 5% of neonates are identified by clinical symptoms at birth

**What is the common cause of congenital hypothyroidism in neonates?**

75% of hypothyroid infants have some form of thyroid agenesis

**What are the clinical manifestations of hypothyroidism in neonates?**

Lethargy and slow movement

Hoarse cry

Feeding problems

Constipation

Macroglossia

Umbilical hernia

Large fontanels

Hypotonia

Dry skin
Hypothermia
Prolonged jaundice

**Which neonates should be screened for hypothyroidism?**

Screening of all newborns is now routine in all 50 states of the United States

## Other Thyroid Disorders

**How common is postpartum thyroiditis?**

It occurs in 5–10% of women during the first year of childbirth or pregnancy loss. It is directly related to increasing serum levels of thyroid autoantibodies

**What are the clinical phases and characterstics of postpartum thyroiditis?**

**Phase 1 is characterized by thyrotoxicosis**-like symptoms (small, painless goiter; fatigue; palpitations) between 1 and 4 months after delivery. Some women return back to a euthyroid state, while others go into **Phase 2—the development of transient hypothyroidism or permanent hypothyroidism** (4–8 months postpartum). See Table below.

### Phases and Characteristics of Postpartum Thyroiditis

| Clinical Phase | Onset | Incidence | Mechanism | Symptoms | Treatment | Sequelae |
|---|---|---|---|---|---|---|
| **Thyrotoxicosis** | 1–4 months postpartum | 4% | Destruction-induced hormone release | Painless goiter, fatigue, palpitations | β-blocker for symptoms | Return to euthyroid state or develop hypothyroidism |
| **Hypothyroidism** | 4–8 months postpartum | 2–5% | Thyroid insufficiency | Goiter, fatigue, depression | Thyroxine for 6–12 months | Transient or permanent hypothyroidism |

**What laboratory results help make the diagnosis of postpartum thyroiditis?**

New-onset abnormal values of TSH and T4 may be present. The presence of antimicrosomal and/or

| | |
|---|---|
| | thyroperoxidase—antithyroid peroxidase antibodies confirm the diagnosis |
| **Postpartum thyroid dysfunction is seen 25% of the time with what other endocrine disorder?** | Type I diabetes mellitus |
| **How is the presence of a thyroid nodule or thyroid cancer assessed and managed during pregnancy?** | The same as in a nonpregnant woman. Thyroid radionuclide scanning is contraindicated, and fine-needle-aspiration biopsy of the nodule should be done. Benign nodules are followed; if required, surgery is best performed in the second trimester |

## Other Endocrine Disorders of Pregnancy

| | |
|---|---|
| **What is Sheehan syndrome?** | It is partial or complete pituitary insufficiency because of postpartum necrosis of the anterior pituitary gland following severe intrapartum or early postpartum hemorrhage |
| **What are the characteristic signs and symptoms of Sheehan syndrome?** | Failure of lactation, amenorrhea, breast atrophy, loss of pubic and axillary hair, hypothyroidism, and adrenal cortical insufficiency |

# GASTROINTESTINAL DISORDERS

## Acute Fatty Liver of Pregnancy

| | |
|---|---|
| **What is acute fatty liver of pregnancy (AFLP)?** | It is a rare complication of pregnancy (1:5000 to 16,000) characterized by microvesicular fatty infiltration of hepatocytes |
| **In which trimester does this disease typically appear?** | Third trimester |
| **Deficiency of which enzyme has been associated in the pathogenesis of acute fatty liver of pregnancy?** | Long-chain 3-hydroxyacyl-CoA dehydrogenase (LCHAD) |
| **What are the common clinical manifestations of this disease?** | **Nausea and vomiting (most frequent symptoms; indicative of acute fatty liver of pregnancy if onset in third trimester)** |

Abdominal pain (commonly epigastric)
Malaise
Anorexia
Jaundice

**What laboratory findings may be seen in patients with acute fatty liver of pregnancy?**

Elevated AST and ALT
Elevated bilirubin
Prolonged prothrombin time
Elevated liver enzyme levels
Low platelets and fibrinogen
Elevated serum creatinine
Low glucose levels (30% of patients)

**What other major disorder with similar laboratory results must be ruled out and how is this condition characterized?**

HELLP syndrome. It is characterized by hemolysis, elevated liver enzymes, and low platelets

**What is the gold standard for diagnosis of acute fatty liver of pregnancy?**

**Liver biopsy** revealing microvesicular fatty infiltration of hepatocytes. However, this is rarely performed since it is an invasive procedure

**What is the management and treatment?**

Maternal stabilization (fluids, blood products, antibiotics)
Supportive care (mechanical ventilation, dialysis)
Prompt delivery of the fetus

**What test should be considered for newborns of mothers with acute fatty liver of pregnancy?**

Deficiency of LCHAD

**What is the rate of recurrence?**

It can recur in future pregnancies but the rate is unclear

## Intrahepatic Cholestasis of Pregnancy

**What is intrahepatic cholestasis of pregnancy (ICP)?**

It is a condition characterized by jaundice and pruritis secondary to the accumulation of bile acids in the liver and plasma

**In what trimesters does it usually occur?**

Onset is more common in the third trimester, but sometimes occurs in the second

**What genetic factors may be involved in the pathogenesis of ICP?**

Defects in either the ABCB4 (adenosine triphosphate-binding cassette, subfamily 4, member 4)

gene or multidrug resistance 3 (MDR3) gene (encoding for a canalicular phospholipid translocator) may be involved in ICP

**What hormonal factors may be involved in the pathogenesis of ICP?**

High concentrations of estrogen and excess progesterone may be risk factors for ICP

**What is the cardinal clinical manifestation of ICP that helps distinguish this disease from other liver conditions?**

**Severe pruritis** (especially on the palms and soles of the feet) (Jaundice is present 10% of the time; jaundice without pruritis warrants other causes of liver disease.)

**What do laboratory values reveal in patients with ICP?**

Increased serum total bile acids (chenodeoxycholic acid, deoxycholic acid, cholic acid)

Marked elevation of the cholic/ chenodeoxycholic acid ratio

Elevated alkaline phosphatase

Elevated total and direct bilirubin

Elevated AST and ALT

Normal prothrombin time (usually)

**What are the main liver conditions that must be ruled out?**

Hepatitis (autoimmune and viral)

Biliary tract disease

Acute fatty liver of pregnancy

HELLP syndrome

**What is the treatment of ICP?**

Treatment is focused on relieving symptoms and preventing maternal and fetal complications.

Ursodeoxycholic acid (500 mg bid until delivery) has been shown to alleviate pruritis and normalize bile acids and improve liver function test results. Early delivery (36–38 weeks) improves symptoms in majority of patients suffering from ICP

**Can oral contraceptives that contain estrogen be given postpartum?**

Yes. Oral contraceptives containing low-dose estrogen can be given after normalization of liver function tests. Women should be advised of a potential recurrence of pruritis

**What are several fetal complications of ICP?**

Fetal death

Spontaneous preterm birth

Postpartum hemorrhage

Neonatal respiratory syndrome

Meconium-stained amniotic fluid

**What is the rate of recurrence?**

It recurs 60–70% in future pregnancies, but may be milder in severity

## Hyperemesis Gravidarum

**What is hyperemesis gravidarum?**

It is persistent vomiting typically in the first trimester that is severe enough to cause weight loss, dehydration, acidosis from starvation, alkalosis from vomiting, and hypokalemia

**What hormones may be associated with hyperemesis?**

It may be related to high or rapidly rising levels of serum **estrogen or hCG, or both**

**What abnormalities are seen on laboratory tests?**

Elevated levels of hCG or serum thyroxine

Elevated levels of serum transaminases (typically <200 IU/L, and ALT > AST)

Elevated levels of bilirubin, amylase, lipase, and electrolytes

**What is the association between hyperthyroidism and hyperemesis gravidarum?**

Although there are biochemical signs of hyperthyroidism (elevated thyroxine levels), this is most likely the effect of hCG on the TSH receptor (seen in 60–70% of patients). Clinical symptoms of hyperthyroidism during hyperemesis gravidarum are not seen

**How is hyperemesis gravidarum treated?**

**First-line pharmacotherapy consists of vitamin $B_6$ or vitamin $B_6$ plus doxylamine.** Vitamin $B_1$ should also be administered to prevent Wernicke encephalopathy. Antiemetics, IV crystalloids, and IV fluids should be given until the vomiting is controlled

**What are several life-threatening complications of hyperemesis gravidarum?**

Mallory-Weiss tears

Esophageal rupture

Pneumothoraces

Pneumomediastinum

**What two vitamin deficiencies are a result of prolonged vomiting and can have severe consequences?**

Vitamin $B_1$ (thiamine) deficiency can cause Wernicke encephalopathy

Vitamin K deficiency can cause coagulopathy with epistaxis

**What is the effect of hyperemesis gravidarum on the fetus?**

IUGR and fetal death may occur in the setting of persistent vomiting and maternal weight loss

**What should mothers be advised regarding recurrence of hyperemesis gravidarum?**

It often recurs in subsequent pregnancies

# RENAL AND URINARY TRACT DISORDERS

## Urinary Tract Infections

UTI is the most common medical complication of pregnancy.

**Why is pregnancy considered a high-risk condition with asymptomatic bacteriuria?**

Both hormonal and mechanical changes predispose the pregnant woman with asymptomatic bacteriuria to develop acute pyelonephritis, which is associated with preterm birth and perinatal death. Pyelonephritis in pregnancy will lead to septicemia in 10–20% and ARDS in 2% of cases

**How prevalent is asymptomatic bacteriuria in pregnancy?**

It is estimated to occur in 4–7% of pregnant patients. If left untreated, up to 40% of cases will progress to pyelonephritis

**How is this condition detected?**

Screening for asymptomatic bacteriuria using urine culture is recommended at the first prenatal visit

**How is asymptomatic bacteriuria treated?**

Any FDA category B drug such as **cephalosporins, nitrofurantoin, or trimethoprim-sulfamethoxazole** can be used. Quinolones (FDA category C) are generally not used during pregnancy. Seven-day courses are recommended, along with a follow-up culture to document sterile urine. Persistent bacteriuria should be treated based on sensitivities. Suppressive antibiotics (most commonly nitrofurantoin) should then be considered in these patients. See the following table.

## Antimicrobial Used for Treatment of Pregnant Women with Asymptomatic Bacteriuria

| 7-Day Course (Recommended) | 3-Day Course |
|---|---|
| Amoxicillin, 3 g | Amoxicillin, 500 mg tid |
| Ampicillin, 2 g | Ampicillin, 250 mg qid |
| Cephalosporin, 2 g | Cephalosporin, 250 mg qid |
| Nitrofurantoin, 200 mg | Ciprofloxacin, 250 mg bid |
| Trimethoprim-sulfamethoxazole, 320/1600 mg | Levofloxacin, 250 mg daily |
| | Nitrofurantoin, 100 mg bid |

**How is symptomatic cystitis treated in pregnancy?**

Treatment and follow-up are similar to asymptomatic bacteriuria. Acute pyelonephritis should be treated with IV antibiotics and hospitalization. Suppressive antibiotics should be given following treatment to any pregnant patient treated for acute pyelonephritis

# NEUROLOGIC DISORDERS

## Epilepsy and Seizure Disorders

Seizure disorders are the most frequent major neurologic complications encountered in pregnancy and more than 95% of patients who have seizures during pregnancy have a history of epilepsy or have been receiving anticonvulsant therapy.

**What are the two major pregnancy-related threats to women with epilepsy?**

Increase in seizure frequency

Increased risk of congenital malformations in the fetus

**Increased seizure frequency is associated with subtherapeutic anticonvulsant levels and/or a lower seizure threshold. What are the several factors that cause these characteristics?**

Pregnancy-related changes such as nausea and vomiting, decreased gastrointestinal motility, increased intravascular volume, increased drug metabolism from induction of hepatic and placental enzymes, antacid use (reduces drug absorption because of abnormal protein binding), and increased glomerular filtration rate decrease anticonvulsant concentrations

Decreased seizure threshold can be affected by sleep deprivation, and hyperventilation and pain during labor

**What are the maternal and fetal side effects for the following traditional anticonvulsant medications?**

See the table below.

| Anticonvulsant | Maternal Side Effects | Fetal Side Effects |
|---|---|---|
| Phenytoin | Nystagmus, ataxia, hirsutism, gingival hyperplasia, megaloblastic anemia | **Fetal hydantoin syndrome:** craniofacial anomalies (upturned nose, mild midfacial hypoplasia, thin philtrum, facial clefts), fingernail hypoplasia, growth deficiency, developmental delay, cardiac defects |
| Carbamazepine | Drowsiness, leukopenia, ataxia, mild hepatotoxicity | Fetal hydantoin syndrome, spina bifida, fingernail hypoplasia, IUGR |
| Valproate | Ataxia, drowsiness, alopecia, hepatotoxicity, thrombocytopenia | Neural-tube defects, heart and kidney malformations, hypospadia, polydactyly |
| Phenobarbital | Drowsiness, ataxia | Clefts, cardiac anomalies, urinary tract malformations |
| Primidone | Drowsiness, ataxia, nausea | Possible teratogenesis, coagulopathy, neonatal depression |

**What is the association between anticonvulsants and folic acid deficiency?**

All anticonvulsants interfere with folic acid metabolism and patients on anticonvulsants may become folic acid deficient and develop macrocytic anemia. Folic acid deficiency has been associated with neural tube defects and other congenital malformations. Folic acid supplementation (4 mg/day) should be begun before pregnancy if possible

**What are the recommendations regarding management and therapy with anticonvulsants?**

1. Women with epilepsy should have preconception counseling regarding the optimal anticonvulsant during pregnancy, a switch to the least teratogenic drug and the least

number of medications prescribed, and the lowest dose needed
2. Blood levels of anticonvulsants should be measured every trimester and prior to delivery to maintain a therapeutic range
3. Patients should be screened for neural tube defects and other fetal anomalies associated with anticonvulsants

**What is the effect of anticonvulsants on vitamin K levels?**

Many of the anticonvulsants, particularly phenytoin, induce a deficiency of vitamin K-dependent clotting factors (II, VI, IX, X). This places the patient and her fetus at risk for hemorrhage. The patient should receive vitamin K supplementation (10 mg/day) from week 36 until delivery, and the newborn should also receive an IM injection of vitamin K after delivery

## HEMATOLOGIC DISORDERS

### Thromboembolism

**All the elements of Virchow triad, venous stasis, vascular damage, and hypercoagulability are present during venous thrombosis. How does pregnancy increase the risk for venous thromboembolism?**

Increased venous capacity, relaxation of vascular smooth muscle, and compression of the pelvic veins by the gravid uterus cause venous stasis. Increased risk for endothelial damage occurs during delivery, especially during cesarean delivery. Lastly, estrogen stimulation of coagulation factors and a decrease in fibrinolytic activity favors coagulation during pregnancy

**Thrombosis of the superficial veins of the saphenous system can occur during pregnancy. What are the clinical manifestations of patients with superficial thrombophlebitis?**

Tenderness, pain, or erythema along the vein

**What diagnostic test should be ordered?**

In order to rule out DVT, a compression **ultrasound** of the affected extremity should be performed

**What is the treatment for superficial thrombophlebitis?**

Treatment consists of compression stockings, ambulation, leg elevation, and analgesics

**Does deep venous thrombosis (DVT) commonly occur in the left or right lower extremity?**

Greater than 80% of DVTs occurs in the **left lower extremity**. This is because of compression of the left iliac vein by the right iliac vein as it branches off the aorta

**What are the clinical features of DVTs?**

Although the presentation is variable, signs include **lower extremity tenderness, erythema, swelling, and a palpable cord**. Homan sign may be present (pain on passive dorsiflexion of the foot).

**How is DVT diagnosed?**

Doppler ultrasound is the gold standard

**What is the treatment for DVT that occurs during pregnancy?**

Initial anticoagulation with IV unfractionated or low-molecular weight heparin for 5–7 days followed by subcutaneous adjusted-dose low-molecular weight heparin therapy for the remainder of the pregnancy. Warfarin should be started postpartum for 6–18 weeks. Bed rest, analgesia, and ambulation with compression stockings should be initiated

**What effects does Coumadin have on the fetus, thus making it a contraindication for DVTs during pregnancy?**

Fetal warfarin syndrome (FWS) is possible. This is characterized by hemorrhage and embryopathy, which includes ventral midline dysplasia, nasal hypoplasia, CNS abnormalities, cardiac and renal anomalies

**What is a major complication of DVTs?**

If untreated, 24% of DVTs will result in **pulmonary embolus**. This can occur in 0.5–3.0 per 1000 pregnancies

**What are the clinical manifestations of pulmonary embolism (PE)?**

Dyspnea, pleuritic chest pain, cough, syncope, hemoptysis, tachypnea, and tachycardia

**How is a pulmonary embolism evaluated and diagnosed in the pregnant woman?**

It usually consists of an ABG, chest x-ray, EKG, spiral CT pulmonary angiography, V/Q scan

**What is the treatment of pulmonary embolism?**

Anticoagulation with low molecular weight heparin for at least 4–6 months, including up to

6 weeks postpartum. Vena caval filter should be considered in those with recurrent embolization

**What is septic pelvic thrombophlebitis?**

It is thrombosis in the veins of the pelvis because of infection. About 90% of cases occur after a cesarean delivery; however, the incidence is low, affecting 1:2000 pregnancies. It is a diagnosis of exclusion for postpartum fever

**What is the most common vein at risk for septic thrombosis?**

The pelvic veins (most commonly the ovarian veins)

**When should septic pelvic thrombophlebitis be suspected?**

Continuous and wide-swinging fevers (from normal to 105.8°F) in the puerperium and which do not respond to antibiotics

**How is it diagnosed and treated?**

A pelvic examination is often not helpful for diagnosis. A chest x-ray may reveal multiple, small septic emboli. CT and MRI should be considered for diagnosis. Treatment includes a combination of antibiotics and heparin

**What are the most significant complications of septic pelvic thrombophlebitis?**

Septic pulmonary emboli

Extension of the venous clot in the pelvis

Renal vein thrombosis

Ureteral obstruction

Death

## Thrombophilias

**What are the most common inherited thrombophilias?**

Factor V Leiden mutation

Antithrombin deficiency

Prothrombin G20210 mutation

Protein C deficiency

Protein S deficiency

Hyperhomocysteinemia

Methylene-tetra-hydro-folate-reductase (MTHFR)

**What is antiphospholipid syndrome?**

It is an autoimmune disorder characterized by the presence of certain clinical features, including venous and arterial thromboembolism, and the presence of specified levels of circulating antiphospholipid antibodies

**What are the two most well-characterized antiphospholipid antibodies?**

Lupus anticoagulant and anticardiolipin antibodies

**What are the most common medical problems associated with antiphospholipid syndrome?**

The most common and most serious medical problems are venous and arterial thromboses, most commonly in the lower extremities. Autoimmune thrombocytopenia occurs 40–50% of the time

**What are several obstetrical complications associated with antiphospholipid syndrome?**

Recurrent spontaneous abortions (most common)

Preeclampsia and eclampsia

Intrauterine growth restriction

Uteroplacental insufficiency

Preterm delivery

Placental abruption

Infertility

Intrauterine fetal demise

**Who should be tested for antiphospholipid syndrome?**

Those who have a complicated obstetrical history characterized by recurrent spontaneous abortions or stillbirths, or preterm delivery resulting from eclampsia, preeclampsia, or uteroplacental insufficiency. Those who have a history of unexplained venous or arterial thromboses should also be evaluated for antiphospholipid syndrome

## Anemias and Hemoglobinopathies

**What is physiologic anemia of pregnancy?**

During the course of pregnancy, there is an expansion in plasma volume greater than that of the RBC mass. This reflects in a decrease in hematocrit during pregnancy; however, it is not a true anemia

**How is true anemia in pregnancy defined?**

It is generally defined as an Hct <30% or a hemoglobin <10 g/dL

**What are the effects of maternal anemia on pregnancy?**

Several associations with maternal anemia have been found, including preterm birth and fetal growth restriction

**What are the two most common causes of anemia during pregnancy?**

Iron deficiency anemia and anemia from acute blood loss

**What red cell indices, laboratory results, and characteristics on a peripheral blood smear indicate an iron deficiency anemia? What is the treatment for this anemia?**

Red cell indices include an mean cell volume (MCV) <80 f/L, and mean corpuscular hemoglobin concentration (MCHC) <30%. Serumiron is decreased (<50 mg/dL), total iron-binding capacity (TIBC) is increased, and serum ferritin is decreased (a level <15 ug/L is confirmatory of iron deficiency anemia). The classic findings on a blood smear include small, pale erythrocytes (microcytic and hypochromic). Treatment is iron therapy consisting of ferrous sulfate 325 mg bid PO

**What is the most common cause of macrocytic anemia in pregnancy? What red cell indices, laboratory results, and characteristics on a peripheral blood smear indicate this anemia?**

Folate acid deficiency. Red cell indices reveal an MCV >80 f/L. Serum folate levels <4 ng/mL and erythrocyte folate activity <20 ng/mL are diagnostic. A smear of peripheral blood demonstrates macrocytes, hypersegmentation of neutrophils, and peripheral nucleated erythrocytes

**What is the recommended folate level in pregnant women and what is the treatment for folate deficiency anemia?**

A recommended level of folate during pregnancy is 400 ug/day and treatment is 1 mg of folic acid PO once daily

**What is the significance of folic acid deficiency on the fetus?**

The development of neural tube defects

**What are examples of hereditary hemolytic anemias?**

Hereditary spherocytosis, glucose 6-phosphate dehydrogenase deficiency (G6PD), pyruvate-kinase deficiency

**What are the most common hemoglobinopathies?**

Sickle-cell anemia (SS disease), sickle-cell hemoglobin C disease (SC disease), sickle-cell α-thalassemia disease, β-thalassemia, and $\alpha_\beta$-thalassemia

**What other infections are patients with sickle-cell hemoglobinopathies at an increased risk for?**

Urinary tract infections. Diagnosis should be established in first trimester

**What is a significant pulmonary complication in patients with sickle-cell disease?**

**Acute chest syndrome**. It is characterized by pleuritic chest pain, fever, cough, lung infiltrates, and hypoxia which all lead to hypoxemia and acidosis. Pathology of this complication includes infection, vaso-occlusion and infarction, pulmonary sequestration, and fat embolization from bone marrow

**Which thalassemia is associated with fetal hydrops, intrauterine death, and preeclampsia?**

Hb Bart ($\alpha$-thalassemia major, absence of both $\alpha$-globin chains)

## PULMONARY DISORDERS

### Asthma

**What percentage of women experience worsening of their asthma during pregnancy?**

40%, while another 40% of women experience no change and 20% of them report improvement of their asthma

**What are the potential maternal complications of an acute exacerbation of asthma?**

Pneumonia, hyperemesis gravidarum, preeclampsia, vaginal bleeding, complicated labor, and cesarean delivery

**What are fetal complications of an acute exacerbation of asthma?**

Intrauterine growth restriction, low birth weight, preterm birth, neonatal hypoxia, and increased overall perinatal mortality

**How is acute asthma managed in a pregnant woman?**

It is similar to that of a nonpregnant woman

IV fluids and supplemental $O_2$ (keep $O_2$ saturation >95%)

$\alpha$-agonists and high-dose steroids (IV prednisone 40–60 mg q6h)

Continuous pulse oximetry and electronic fetal monitoring

**Which vaccine is recommended for all pregnant women, especially those with asthma?**

Influenza vaccination

**What medications can be used to treat pregnant asthmatics?**

Beta-2 agonists, terbutaline SQ, theophylline, corticosteroids

**Which medications should be avoided in pregnant asthmatics during labor and delivery?**

Analgesics, which cause histamine release, respiratory depression, and bronchospasm, should be avoided. Prostagladin $F_2$ can cause bronchospasm

### Aspiration Pneumonitis

**Why are pregnant women at risk for aspiration of gastric contents?**

Elevated intra-abdominal pressure, decreased gastroesophageal sphincter tone, delayed gastric emptying, and diminished laryngeal reflexes during pregnancy increases the risk of aspiration

**How common are maternal deaths related to aspiration?**

It accounts for 30–50% of maternal deaths related to anesthetic complications

**What are symptoms and signs of aspiration?**

Dyspnea, bronchospasm, tachycardia, cyanosis, hypoxia, hypercapnea, and acidemia. Respiratory arrest is possible

## CARDIOVASCULAR DISORDERS

Heart disease complicates approximately 1% of all pregnancies. Pregnant patients with functional Class III and IV heart disease (see the table below for the New York Heart Association classification of heart disease) have high event rates and succumb to heart failure, arrhythmias, and stroke.

**Which heart diseases are associated with the highest maternal morbidity during pregnancy?**

Patients with septal defects, PDA, and mild mitral and aortic valvular disorders are often in classes I and II and have minimal complications during pregnancy. Primary pulmonary hypertension, uncorrected tetrology of Fallot, Marfan syndrome, and Eisenmenger syndrome are associated with a worse prognosis, and patients are advised against becoming pregnant

### New York Heart Association Functional Classification of Heart Disease

| Class | Description |
|---|---|
| Class I | No signs or symptoms of cardiac decompensation |
| Class II | No symptoms at rest; minor limitation with mild to moderate activity |
| Class III | No symptoms at rest; marked limitation with less than ordinary activity |
| Class IV | Symptoms at rest; increased discomfort with any physical activity |

**What are the signs and symptoms indicative of significant cardiovascular disease?**

See the table below.

### Signs and Symptoms Indicative of Significant Cardiovascular Disease

| | |
|---|---|
| **Symptoms** | Progressively worsening shortness of breath<br>Cough with frothy pink sputum<br>Paroxysmal nocturnal dyspnea<br>Chest pain with exertion<br>Syncope preceded by palpitations or exertion<br>Hemoptysis |
| **Physical examination** | Abnormal venous pulsations<br>Rarely audible $S_1$<br>Single $S_2$ or paradoxically split $S_2$<br>Loud systolic murmurs, any diastolic murmur<br>Ejection clicks, late systolic clicks, opening snaps<br>Friction rub<br>Sustained right or left ventricular heave<br>Cyanosis or clubbing |
| **Electrocardiogram** | Significant arrhythmias<br>Heart blocks |
| **Chest radiograph** | Cardiomegaly<br>Pulmonary edema |

Reprinted, with permission, from DeCherney AH et al: *Current Obstetrics & Gynecologic Diagnosis Treatment,* 10th ed. New York: McGraw-Hill, 2007:362.

**What are the potential risks to the fetus of patients with functionally significant cardiac disease?**

They are at risk for low-birth weight and prematurity. Congenital heart disease in the fetus is more likely to occur in patients with congenital heart disease (1–5%)

**For the following heart diseases, what are their pregnancy-related complications, associated signs and symptoms, and treatment modalities?**

See the table on the following page.

## Table 9-3 Common Heart Diseases Occuring During Pregnancy

| Heart Disease | Signs/Symptoms during Decompensation | Complications | Treatment | Comment |
|---|---|---|---|---|
| Mitral regurgitation | Chest pain, palpitations, tachycardia, anxiety, late systolic murmur with a late systolic click | Generally, pregnancy is well-tolerated and unaffected | β-Blockers (propranol) may aid in control of associated symptoms | May occur in as many as 5% of pregnancies |
| Mitral stenosis | Dyspnea on exertion and at rest, hemoptysis, loud $S_1$, an opening snap, low diastolic rumble at the apex, right ventricular lift | Pulmonary hypertension, right heart failure, hemoptysis, low cardiac output, atrial fibrillation, CHF during labor | Medical management is first line: digitalis, quinidine, β-adrenergic blocking agents, anticoagulation with heparin. Severe mitral stenosis may warrant mitral valvotomy, mitral valve replacement, or balloon valvuloplasty | Most common valvular lesion found in pregnancy. Mitral stenosis with a-fibrillation has a high likelihood of congestive failure |
| Rheumatic heart disease | Dependent on the affected valve | Patients are at high risk for thromboembolic disease, SBE, cardiac failure, and pulmonary edema; fetal loss is also more common | Corrective surgical procedures, such as balloon valvuloplasty, surgical commissurotomy, and valve replacement | 90% of rheumatic heart disease patients have mitral stenosis |
| Peripartum cardiomyopathy | Dyspnea; other frequent symptoms include cough, orthopnea, paroxysmal nocturnal | Heart failure and death are potential complications | Combination of digoxin, diuretics and sodium, β-blockers, and after-load reducers. | Usually affects women in late pregnancy (>36 weeks) or early puerperium |

*(Continued)*

## Common Heart Diseases Occuring During Pregnancy *(Continued)*

| Heart Disease | Signs/Symptoms during Decompensation | Complications | Treatment | Comment |
|---|---|---|---|---|
| | dyspnea, and hemoptysis | | Anticoagulants, such as heparin should be considered | (in first 5 months). Etiology is unknown, though myocarditis is responsible sometimes |
| Marfan syndrome | Dyspnea, chest pain, aortic diastolic murmur, and midsystolic clink | Aortic aneurysm and possible rupture | Surgical intervention | 25–50% of maternal mortality and 50% chance that offspring will inherit the disease |

**Describe the classic patient at increased risk for peripartum cardiomyopathy**

A black, multiparous woman who is over the age of 30, and who has had a multifetal gestation in the past and/or preeclampsia

**Which cardiac medications are considered safe during pregnancy? Which are contraindicated during pregnancy?**

Acceptable cardiac medications: digoxin, loop diurectics, thiazides, hydralazine, β-adrenergic blockers, calcium-channel blockers

Contraindicated: nitrates, angiotensin-converting enzyme inhibitors, and angiotensin II receptor blockers

## ACUTE ABDOMEN AND ABDOMINAL TRAUMA

**List the differential diagnoses for the pregnant woman who presents with acute lower abdominal pain**

**Gynecologic etiologies:** ruptured corpus luteum cyst; adnexal torsion; ectopic pregnancy; abruptio placentae; early labor; salpingitis

**Nongynecologic etiologies:** pyelonephritis; cholecystitis; diverticulitis

**What is the most consistent clinical symptom encountered in pregnant women with appendicitis?**

Signs and symptoms of acute appendicitis are not dramatic in the pregnant woman and also not as specific compared to the nonpregnant woman. In pregnancy, the appendix is commonly upwardly displaced. Vague pain on the right side of the abdomen is the most consistent clinical symptom of acute appendicitis in the pregnant woman, and there should be a high index of suspicion for appendicitis for any abdominal pain

**What is the first-line imaging modality in pregnant women with suspected appendicitis?**

MRI. an appendiceal CT may be used if an MRI is not feasible; it is also more accurate than a graded compression ultrasonography

**What are potential consequences of a ruptured appendix?**

Preterm labor, maternal and fetal sepsis which may lead to fetal neurologic injury, and spontaneous abortion/fetal demise

**What is the treatment for nonperforated acute appendicitis in the pregnant woman?**

Appendectomy is the gold standard. Laparoscopic appendicitis is being used more frequently, especially in the first half of the pregnancy

**How does pregnancy lead to more gallstones in pregnant women?**

Increased estrogens cause an increase in cholesterol saturation, which, in addition to biliary stasis and decreased gallbladder contraction, lead to more gallstones

**What percentage of pregnancies is complicated by trauma?**

7%. Motor vehicle accidents account for 40%, falls account for 30%, direct assaults to the maternal abdomen (20%), and others (10%)

**What is the most common nonobstetric cause of maternal death during pregnancy?**

Automobile accidents

**What is the most common cause of fetal death?**

Death to the mother

**What is the second most common cause of fetal death?**

Abruptio placentae

**What is the management of pregnant women who experienced abdominal trauma?**

Admit for observation for at least 24 hours

Monitor mother; an fetal well-being should be obtained (nonstress test, BPP, FHR monitor)

If bleeding is present, obtain Rh status by using the Kleihauer-Betke test. For the woman who is

D-negative, administration of anti-D immunoglobulin should be considered

Monitor for contractions

# Obstetric Infections

## TORCH INFECTIONS

### Introduction

**What are the TORCH infections?**

A group of nonbacterial perinatal infections that lead to significant neonatal morbidity and mortality

T: ***Toxoplasma gondii***

O: **Other** (such as syphilis, VZV, HIV, hepatitis, parvovirus B19)

R: **Rubella**

C: **Cytomegalovirus**

H: **Herpes simplex virus**

**How does the fetus become infected with the TORCH diseases?**

Usually through **transplacental migration of the infection;** however, infection can also occur via ascending chorioamnionitis, maternal exposure intrapartum, external contamination intrapartum, or nosocomial neonatal exposure

**What modalities can be used to diagnose these infections?**

Direct isolation of the pathogen via amniocentesis with culture or PCR of amniotic fluid

Indirect tests—ultrasound for fetal manifestations, maternal antibody titers (IgM, IgG), or testing of fetal blood for IgM via cordocentesis

**What is the difference between IgG and IgM?**

**IgG:** rises slowly and often persists for long periods of time

A better marker for **overall exposure** to a disease

Crosses the placenta (starting at 16 weeks) to provide passive immunity

**IgM:** rises acutely and disappears from the circulation relatively soon after acute infection

A better marker for **recent infection**

Cannot cross the placenta

Synthesized by the fetus to provide primary immunity starting at 9–15 weeks

## Toxoplasmosis

**What is toxoplasmosis?**

Infection with the **protozoa** *T. gondii* that causes an asymptomatic infection in adults but congenital disease if the primary infection occurs during pregnancy

**What is the incidence of toxoplasmosis?**

0.01–0.1% in the United States

**What is the life cycle of *T. gondii*?**

The domestic cat is the host and it passes the eggs in its feces. Humans can become infected by exposure to the **cat feces, which can occur with gardening, handling a cat's litter box**. Alternatively, many animals consume the eggs which are found in soil and humans also become infected by handling or eating the raw or **undercooked meat** of infected animals

**What is the chance of fetal infection if primary infection occurs during pregnancy?**

Approximately 33%

**What is the difference between first and third trimester infection?**

**First trimester: low** (15%) **congenital infection rate**

Most of those infected have **severe symptoms** and 5% result in fetal demise

**Third trimester: high** (65%) **congenital infection rate**

Most infections are **mild**

**What are the symptoms of maternal toxoplasmosis?**

Usually none; however, many patients report a syndrome of fevers, fatigue, headache, muscle pains, and lymphadenopathy after exposure

**What is the classic triad of congenital toxoplasmosis?**

**Chorioretinitis, hydrocephalus**, and **intracranial calcifications**

**What are the possible clinical manifestations of toxoplasmosis?**

Most infants are asymptomatic at birth. However, if signs are present at birth, they can include:

Low birth weight

Fever

Maculopapular rash

Hepatosplenomegaly

Microcephaly

Seizures

Jaundice

Thrombocytopenia

Generalized lymphadenopathy

**What abnormalities can develop after birth in an infected and untreated infant?**

Chorioretinitis

Mental retardation

Deafness

Seizures

Spasticity

**Is toxoplasmosis screening routinely recommended for pregnant women?**

No

**What are the options for prenatal diagnosis of toxoplasmosis?**

Serology of maternal blood (high IgG titers suggest recent infection)

Detection of the parasite

*Toxoplasma* PCR of amniotic fluid

Serology of fetal blood for *Toxoplasma* IgM—not as sensitive

**How can toxoplasmosis be diagnosed postnatally?**

Ophthalmologic, auditory, and neurologic examinations, an **LP**, and a **head CT**

Neonatal serum test for **IgM and/or IgA antibodies**

**Isolation of organism** from placental tissue, umbilical cord tissue, or infant blood

**How is congenital toxoplasmosis prevented?**

**If suspicion is high for congenital infection, spiramycin should be given until amniocentesis can be performed for toxoplasmosis PCR. Spiramycin prevents transplacental transmission of the parasite. Spiramycin, however, does not help treat or lessen the effects of congenital toxoplasmosis. If PCR of amniotic fluid is positive for *Toxoplasma*,**

pyrimethamine and sulfadiazine should be added. **Leucovorin** is given to avoid the bone marrow suppression associated with the last two of these drugs. **If PCR of amniotic fluid is negative for *Toxoplasma*, spiramycin should be continued, and additional agents are not necessary**

**How is toxoplasmosis in the newborn treated?**

With a combination of **pyrimethamine** and **sulfadiazine. Leucovorin** is given to avoid the bone marrow suppression associated with these drugs

**What is the prognosis of congenital toxoplasmosis?**

Untreated, there is a poor prognosis. Chorioretinitis can eventually lead to blindness. These infants also suffer from seizures and severe psychomotor retardation

## Rubella

**What is rubella?**

A single-stranded RNA virus of the togavirus family that is also known as **German measles**. It causes a mild, self-limited infection in adults but leads to severe disease if congenitally acquired

**What is the incidence of congenital rubella?**

Because of vaccinations, congenital rubella is extremely rare in the United States. However, it is slightly more common in the developing world

**When is congenital rubella infection most likely to cause serious sequelae?**

When maternal infection occurs in the first 8 weeks of pregnancy. Infection after the first trimester has almost no risk of developing anomalies in utero

**How is rubella diagnosed in the pregnant state?**

With history and physical examination, as well as by assessing the development of positive rubella antibody titers (which peak 1–3 weeks after the development of symptoms, if there are any)

**What tools are used to diagnose congenital rubella?**

Maternal history, physical examination of the neonate, CBC, x-rays of long bones, ophthalmologic examination, auditory examination, head CT, and LP

Viral isolation from nasal secretions

| | |
|---|---|
| | Rubella-specific IgM or monthly rising IgG levels |
| **What is the difference between rubella IgM and IgG?** | Both increase after exposure; however, **IgM disappears after 1–2 months and so can distinguish acute infection from prior immunization.** IgG is present for life |
| **What are the signs and symptoms of rubella in adults?** | Most are asymptomatic, but many women present with a rash |
| **What are the major clinical manifestations of congenital rubella and how common are each?** | **Sensorineural deafness** (50–75%)<br>**Cataracts** (20–50%)<br>**Cardiac malformations** (PDA [20–50%] or pulmonary arterial hypoplasia [20–50%])<br>**Neurologic sequelae** (meningoencephalitis, behavior disorders, or MR [10–20%])<br>Growth retardation<br>Hepatosplenomegaly<br>Thrombocytopenia<br>Dermatologic manifestations (purpura, known as "blueberry muffin" lesions)<br>Hyperbilirubinemia |
| **How is congenital rubella prevented?** | Through vaccination strategies and by testing all pregnant women for immunity |
| **Should the vaccination be given during pregnancy?** | No—it is a live, attenuated virus |
| **How is congenital rubella treated?** | Supportively—there is no known treatment for rubella |

## Cytomegalovirus

| | |
|---|---|
| **What is cytomegalovirus (CMV)?** | A DNA herpes virus that is the **most common cause of perinatal infection** in the developed world |
| **What is the incidence of CMV?** | 30–60% of Americans are seropositive; 1–4% of women seroconvert during pregnancy |
| **What increases the risk of seroconversion?** | Immune compromise |
| **What is the incidence of congenital CMV?** | 40,000 infected infants are born in the United States annually |

| | |
|---|---|
| **How is CMV transmitted?** | Via respiratory droplets, saliva, urine, blood, or sexual contact. It is commonly acquired in daycare centers |
| **How is congenital CMV transmitted?** | Transplacentally or through breast milk |
| **What is the risk of transplacental transmission for a woman who was previously seropostive or who is newly infected during pregnancy?** | **A woman who was previously seropositive is at** approximately 1% risk while one infected during pregnancy is approximately 40% at risk |
| **How is maternal CMV diagnosed?** | With antibody titers—a rise in IgG or the development of IgM antibodies predicts primary infection |
| **How is congenital CMV diagnosed prenatally?** | **Amniocentesis for PCR or culture** (preferred method)<br>Ultrasound (microcephaly, hepatosplenomegaly, intracranial calcifications, etc.)<br>IgM studies of fetal blood (less sensitive) |
| **How is congenital CMV diagnosed in the neonate?** | Viral isolation from urine or saliva in the first 3 weeks of life |
| **When is congenital CMV infection most likely to cause serious sequelae?** | When infection is acquired **early in pregnancy** |
| **What percentage of infected neonates are symptomatic?** | 5–20% |
| **What is the mortality rate associated with congenital CMV infection?** | Almost 30% |
| **What are the clinical manifestations of maternal CMV infection?** | Most are **asymptomatic**; however, some women have a mononucleosis-like syndrome |
| **What are the possible clinical manifestations of congenital CMV infection?** | Most newborns are asymptomatic at birth, but eventually develop the following anomalies:<br>Hearing loss<br>Impaired speech<br>Chorioretinitis/visual impairment<br>Mental retardation<br>Microcephaly<br>Seizures<br>Paralysis or paresis<br>Death |

**What can be used for treatment of congenital CMV infection?**

Supportive—there is no treatment

Ganciclovir, CMV immune globulin, and alpha-interferon have been studied, but results are inconclusive to date and so they are not routinely recommended

**How can congenital CMV infection be prevented?**

Through good hygiene and proper precautions for health care workers; routine prenatal screening is not recommended

## Herpes Simplex Virus

**What is the incidence of herpes simplex virus (HSV)?**

Over 20% of women are seropositive for HSV

**What are the two types of HSV?**

**HSV-1:** causes most nongenital herpes infections

**HSV-2:** causes most genital herpes infections (and most neonatal infections)

**What is the incidence of congenital HSV?**

0.01–0.04%

**How is congenital HSV transmitted?**

Mostly transplacentally; however, it can also be transmitted through ascending infection

**What is the rate of transmission if the mother has primary infection or a recurrent infection?**

**In the case of primary infection the rate of transmission is** 50% while it is 4% in the case of recurrent infection

**What can be done to reduce the risk of transmission of HSV if there is an active lesion when the patient is in labor?**

**Cesarean delivery** (reduces transmission from 8% to 1%)

**What can be done to reduce the risk of needing a cesarean section in a patient with known recurrent HSV?**

Prophylaxis with acyclovir from 36 weeks until delivery *or* initiated at an episode of preterm labor or PPROM

**How is congenital HSV diagnosed?**

Viral cultures (from skin, nose, mouth, eyes, urine, blood, stool, and/or CSF)

**What complications of pregnancy can occur as a result of HSV infection?**

**Preterm labor** or **spontaneous abortion**

**What are the three major groups of clinical manifestations of congenital HSV?**

**Disease localized to the skin, eyes, and mouth (SEM)**

**Disease localized to the CNS**

**Disseminated disease**

**What are other sequelae of congenital HSV?**

Temperature instability

Respiratory distress

Poor feeding

Lethargy

Hypotension

Jaundice

DIC

Apnea

**When do symptoms of congenital HSV develop?**

Most newborns are asymptomatic and symptoms begin within the first 4 weeks of life

**What is the mortality rate associated with neonatal HSV infection?**

Close to 60%

**What is the treatment for congenital HSV infections?**

Supportive care and high-dose **IV acyclovir**

**What is the prognosis for congenital HSV?**

Disseminated infection carries a mortality rate of 57% but localized infection is generally not fatal

Encephalitis affects many of the survivors

# OTHER VIRAL INFECTIONS

## Syphilis

**What is syphilis?**

Infection with the **spirochete *Treponema pallidum***

**What is the incidence of congenital syphilis?**

Less than 40 per 100,000 live births in the United States

**How is the fetus infected with syphilis?**

**Transplacental transmission**, typically during the second half of pregnancy. Women with primary or secondary syphilis are the most likely to transmit the disease

**What are the possible sequelae of congenital syphilis?**

Fetal manifestations: stillbirth

Spontaneous abortion

Hydrops fetalis

Prematurity

Manifestations before 2 years: lesions on palms and soles

Hepatosplenomegaly

Jaundice

Anemia

Snuffles

Manifestations after 2 years: congenital anomalies

Active congenital syphilis

Hutchinson triad

**What is the Hutchinson triad?**

Hutchinson teeth (blunted upper incisors), interstitial keratitis, and eighth nerve deafness

**How is congenital syphilis diagnosed?**

Veneral Disease Research Laboratory **(VDRL)** or vapid plasmin reagin **(RPR)** are used as **screening** tests. If positive, microhemagglutination T. pallidum **(MHA-TP)** or fluorescent treponemal antibody absorbed **(FTA-ABS)** are done as **confirmatory** tests

**How is congenital syphilis prevented?**

With adequate screening and then treatment (with penicillin) of infected mothers

**How is syphilis treated?**

With IV or IM **penicillin** G

**How should a PCN-allergic pregnant woman be treated for syphilis?**

With desensitization, because alternative drugs are teratogenic

**How should a woman be followed after treatment?**

Non-treponemal antibody serologic titers should be checked at 1, 3, and 6 months, 1 year, and 2 years after treatment to ensure proper falls of levels. If they do not fall, she should be treated for reinfection

**What is the Jarisch-Herxheimer reaction?**

An **acute febrile reaction** precipitated by treatment of syphilis thought to result from the release of large amounts of treponemal lipopolysaccharide (LPS). It may precipitate **preterm labor**, **contractions**, or **non-reassuring fetal heart tracings** in pregnant women

## Varicella-Zoster Virus

**What is varicella-zoster virus?**

A double-stranded, linear, DNA herpes virus that causes both chickenpox (varicella) and shingles (zoster)

| | |
|---|---|
| **What is the incidence of VZV in pregnancy?** | 1–5 cases per 10,000 pregnancies (most women are immune secondary to prior infection) |
| **What are the clinical features of varicella in adults?** | It includes a **prodrome of fever, malaise, and myalgia** followed, 1–4 days later, by a **vesicular rash** |
| **What are the complications of varicella infection?** | **Bacterial superinfection of vesicles**<br>**Pneumonia**<br>Arthritis<br>Glomerulonephritis<br>Myocarditis<br>Ocular disease<br>Adrenal insufficiency<br>Death<br>CNS abnormalities |
| **Why is varicella in pregnancy a medical emergency?** | Because **varicella pneumonia** can develop and it is **very severe** in pregnancy |
| **What is varicella pneumonia?** | An infection that develops within a week of the varicella rash that presents as cough, dyspnea, fever, pleuritic chest pain, and/or hemoptysis. It is very severe in pregnant women as it can rapidly progress to respiratory failure |
| **What is the incidence of varicella pneumonia during pregnancy?** | It occurs in 10–30% of all VZV cases in pregnancy |
| **What are the chest x-ray (CXR) findings of varicella pneumonia?** | A **diffuse** or **miliary/nodular infiltrative pattern** usually in a **peribronchial distribution** in both lungs |
| **What is the treatment of varicella pneumonia during pregnancy?** | Supportive care and acyclovir. All women with VZV require a CXR to rule out varicella pneumonia |
| **What is the mortality rate associated with varicella in pregnancy?** | Untreated, it carries a 40% mortality rate |
| **What are the features of congenital varicella syndrome?** | **Chorioretinitis**<br>**Cortical atrophy**<br>**Dermatologic conditions**<br>**Hypoplastic lower limbs**<br>**Hydronephrosis**<br>Clubbed feet |

Optic atrophy
Failure to thrive
Cataracts
Horner syndrome
Microophthalmos
Nystagmus
Low birth weight
Mental retardation
Early death

**What is the congenital infection rate if the mother has VZV?**
25–50% if the mother develops a rash 5 days before or 2 days after birth

**When is the fetus most likely to be affected by congenital varicella syndrome?**
When the mother is infected between 8 and 20 weeks of gestation

**How can varicella infection during pregnancy be prevented in a patient with a recent exposure?**
By giving **VariZIG**, a purified human varicella zoster immune globulin if she is IgG seronegative (not previously immune)

**When should VariZIG be given?**
To the mother **within 96 hours** after viral exposure if she is IgG seronegative

To the neonate (if there is exposure) within 4 days prior or 2 days after delivery

**How should a patient with varicella be managed if she is more than 5 days from delivery?**
With close observation (for any signs/sx of varicella pneumonia) and possibly with acyclovir

**How should a pregnant woman exposed to zoster be treated?**
Reassurance—it is only contagious from direct contact with open lesions

## Parvovirus B19

**What is parvovirus B19?**
A single-stranded DNA virus

**What is the incidence of parvovirus B19 infection in pregnant women?**
3–4%

**What is the transmission rate of parvovirus B19 from an infected woman to her fetus?**
Approximately 20%—it is the highest if infection occurs between 10 and 20 weeks of gestation

**How is parvovirus diagnosed?**
Serologic testing of IgM and IgG antibodies

**Describe the major manifestations of infection with parvovirus B19**
A self-limited infection known as **erythema infectiosum** or **fifth disease** that consists of:

Dermatologic manifestations—a "slapped cheek" appearance on the face and a "lace-like" erythematous rash on the trunk and extremities

Symmetric arthropathy

Flu-like symptoms

**What are the manifestations of parvovirus B19 during pregnancy?**

**Fetal loss** or **hydrops fetalis** may ensue; however, there are no long-term developmental sequelae if a normal pregnancy ensues

**What is the risk of fetal loss?**

If infection occurs before 20 weeks, it is 11%. If infection occurs after 20 weeks, it is <1%

**What is hydrops fetalis?**

Generalized fetal edema

**What is the etiology of hydrops in the setting of congenital parvovirus infection?**

Destruction of RBC precursors leading to fetal anemia

Myocarditis leading to fetal myocardial dysfunction

**What is the risk of hydrops fetalis?**

Less than 4%

**What do the following serologic results signify?**

**Positive IgG and negative IgM:** Prior maternal immunity

**Positive IgM and negative IgG:** Acute infection

**How should an infected pregnant woman be managed?**

Prior to 20 weeks, no action is necessary. After 20 weeks, women should receive weekly ultrasounds to look for signs of hydrops for 10 weeks after infection

**What sign on ultrasound indicates severe fetal anemia?**

Elevated peak systolic velocity on the fetal middle cerebral artery dopplers

**How is severe fetal anemia secondary to parvovirus treated?**

With intrauterine fetal blood transfusion

## HIV

**What is HIV?**

An RNA retrovirus that incorporates into the host genome and affects primary T cells leading to immunocompromise

**How is HIV infection diagnosed?**

Enzyme-linked immunosorbent assay (ELISA) testing followed by a Western blot, if the ELISA is positive

**How do most pediatric HIV infections develop?**

Through mother-to-child transmission via transplacental infection (50%), peripartum infection (30%), or via breast-feeding (20%)

**What is the rate of vertical transmission in an HIV positive woman who is untreated?**

25%

**What is the rate of vertical transmission in an HIV positive woman on zidovudine (azidothymidine) ZDV (AZT) alone?**

8%

**What is the rate of vertical transmission in an HIV positive woman on HAART (highly active antiretroviral therapy)?**

1–2%

**What are the rates of perinatal HIV transmission in the United States?**

1–2%—they have been dramatically reduced via multiple public health efforts

**What increases the risk of vertical HIV transmission?**

Preterm birth

Prolonged ROM

Concurrent syphilis infection

Chorioamnionitis

**What are the two mainstays of prevention of vertical transmission?**

1. **Antiretroviral therapy**
2. **Cesarean delivery**

**Are adverse pregnancy outcomes more common in HIV infected women?**

Yes. Preterm birth and fetal growth restriction are more common, and these rates increase with a decreased CD4 count

**Which pregnant patients should be given antiretroviral therapy?**

***All* pregnant patients**, regardless of CD4 count or viral load, **should be offered antiretroviral therapy** in order to reduce the risk of transmission

**When should CD4 counts be measured during pregnancy?**

Once each trimester

**When should the viral load be measured during pregnancy?**

4 weeks after any change in therapy, monthly until viral levels are undetectable, every 3 months while the viral load remains undetectable, and then near term

**What are some of the intrapartum precautions that should be taken?**

Avoid artificial rupture of membranes (HIV transmission increased with increased time after rupture)

Use labor augmentation sooner (HIV transmission increased with longer interval to delivery)

Give IV zidovudine intrapartum

**How should the neonate of an HIV infected mother be treated?**

With oral zidovudine

**How much does cesarean delivery reduce the risk of vertical HIV transmission?**

By half

## Hepatitis

**What are the hepatitis viruses?**

A group of both DNA and RNA viruses that **invade hepatocytes**, leading to hepatocellular inflammation, scarring, and sometimes death

**What are the symptoms of acute hepatitis infection?**

Most are asymptomatic or mild. Symptoms, when present, include:

Nausea

Vomiting

Headache

Malaise

Fatigue

Right upper quadrant (RUQ) pain

**What are the signs of hepatitis infection?**

Jaundice

RUQ tenderness

Hepatomegaly

**What are the laboratory values which can be associated with hepatitis infection?**

Elevated transaminases

Elevated bilirubin

Coagulation abnormalities—increased PT and PTT (in severe cases)

Elevated ammonia (in severe cases)

**What are the major differential diagnoses of hepatitis infection in pregnancy?**

Acute fatty liver of pregnancy, severe preeclampsia, HELLP syndrome

**What is chronic hepatitis?**

Hepatic necrosis, inflammation, and scarring that eventually can lead to cirrhosis and liver failure

**How is chronic hepatitis diagnosed?**

It is usually **asymptomatic** and so it is presumptively diagnosed by elevated transaminase levels. The diagnosis can be confirmed via liver biopsy

**How is chronic hepatitis because of viral infection treated?**

With **interferon** (a cytokine with immunoregulatory effects) and **ribavirin**. Recently, some nucleoside analogues (lamivudine and adefovir dipivoxil) have been found effective in many patients. None of these medications can be used in pregnancy

## Hepatitis A

**What is hepatitis A and how is it transmitted?**

An RNA picornavirus that is transmitted by the **fecal–oral spread**. It causes about one-third of hepatitis cases in the United States and leads to infection in 1 in 1000 pregnancies in the United States

**How is hepatitis A diagnosed?**

**IgM** antibody suggests **recent infection**; **IgG** antibody suggests **prior exposure**

**How is hepatitis A prevented?**

Vaccination for high-risk women (it is an inactivated vaccine and so is safe to administer in pregnancy)

**How is hepatitis A exposure treated?**

With passive immunity via hepatitis A immune globulin

**What is the effect of hepatitis A on perinatal outcomes?**

Hepatitis A is not teratogenic; however, infection can lead to preterm birth and neonatal cholestasis

## Hepatitis B

**What is hepatitis B and how is it transmitted?**

A DNA hepadenavirus transmitted through **infected blood or bodily fluids**. Its viral genome is covered by a middle portion and then an outer shell

**What is the relationship between hepatitis B and HIV infection?**

There is often coinfection, as they have similar modes of transmission. Coinfection with HIV leads to increased liver-related disease

**What is the prevalence of hepatitis B?**

There are 1.2 million carriers in United States and 350 million carriers globally

**What percentage of those exposed to hepatitis B develop chronic infection?**

In adults: 5–10%

In infants: 70–90%

**How is hepatitis B diagnosed?**

Through antibody testing

**Describe each of the following hepatitis B antigens**

**HBsAg** Hepatitis B surface antigen; it is on the outer viral shell and circulates in the serum

**HBcAg** Hepatitis B core antigen; it is in the middle portion of the virus and does not circulate in serum although it is expressed in infected hepatocytes

**HBeAg** Hepatitis B 'e' antigen; it correlates with infectivity

**Describe the series of hepatitis B antibody responses**

The first marker of infection in **HBsAg**. Then **HBeAg** is detectable, which also denotes early infection. Both of these resolve within 3–6 months after infection. One month after infection, **IgM anti-HBc** begins to develop. It peaks at around 4 months and, within 6 months after exposure, **IgG anti-HBc is detectable**. Around the same time, **anti-HBs** develops. Persistence of HBsAg for more than 6 months is considered to be chronic infection

**How is an acute hepatitis B infection diagnosed serologically?**

**Anti-HBc IgM** and **HBSAg**

**How is chronic hepatitis B infection diagnosed serologically?**

**HBsAg without anti-HBc IgM**

**What are the major sequelae of hepatitis B infection?**

Chronic hepatitis, cirrhosis, and hepatocellular carcinoma

**What is the percentage of risk of vertical transmission in a patient that is HBeAg positive?**

90%

**What is the percentage of risk of vertical transmission in a patient that is HBeAg negative?**

<10%

**How does infection with hepatitis B affect pregnancy?**

It does not affect the pregnancy course; however, it can increase the likelihood of preterm delivery

**How does neonatal infection with hepatitis B occur?**

Through **peripartum exposure to infected maternal fluids** and through **breast-feeding.** Transplacental infection is rare

**What is the likelihood of developing disease after neonatal hepatitis B exposure?**

Most infected neonates are asymptomatic; however, **85% become chronic carriers**

**How is neonatal infection prevented?**

Through **prenatal screening** and administration of **hepatitis B immune globulin** as well as the **hepatitis vaccination** of newborns of infected mothers (vaccination is safe in pregnancy)

**Is breast-feeding safe in women with Hepatitis B?**

There is a theoretic risk of transmission; however, hepatitis B immune globulin and neonatal vaccination should eliminate this risk

## Hepatitis C

**What is hepatitis C and how is it transmitted?**

A single-stranded Flaviviridae virus that is transmitted though exposure to blood and bodily fluids

**What is the incidence of hepatitis C in pregnancy?**

Depending on the population studied, it ranges from approximately 1–5%

**How is hepatitis C diagnosed?**

**Serum antibody testing** (those seropositive for anti-HCV have chronic hepatitis)

**How does hepatitis C infection affect pregnancy?**

It has no effect on pregnancy, although it may increase the risk of cholestatic jaundice

**What is the incidence of vertical transmission of hepatitis C?**

Between 3% and 6%

**How can vertical transmission be prevented?**

There are currently no known methods to prevent transmission at birth

## Hepatitis D

**What is hepatitis D?**

A defective RNA virus that is only infectious if it coinfects with hepatitis B and is transmitted in a similar manner

**What percentage of patients infected with hepatitis B are coinfected with hepatitis D?**

Approximately 25%

**What are the sequelae of infection with hepatitis B and D?**

The same as hepatitis B, however the infection is **more severe** than infection with hepatitis B alone

## Hepatitis E

**What is hepatitis E?**

An RNA virus transmitted via contaminated water

**What are the effects of hepatitis E infection in pregnancy?**

There may be a high rate of vertical transmission and there is some evidence that infection is more severe in pregnancy

# BACTERIAL INFECTIONS

## Group B Streptococcus

**What is group B *Streptococcus* (GBS)?**

***Streptococcus agalactiae***, a gram-positive infection of the GI, upper respiratory and genital tracts. It leads to severe disease in neonates if they are infected right before or during birth

**What percentage of women are asymptomatic carriers of GBS?**

Approximately 15–30%

**Where does colonization typically occur?**

Primarily in the **rectum**, with secondary infection in the bladder, vagina, and cervix

**What are the symptoms of GBS colonization in women?**

Usually none

**How is GBS colonization diagnosed?**

Via routine screening with urine culture and rectovaginal swab. A sample is swabbed from the vagina and rectum for culture and latex agglutination or ELISA

**What is the incidence of invasive GBS infection in pregnancy?**

Because of intrapartum chemoprophylaxis, the incidence of invasive disease is low. GBS affects only approximately 1 in 4000 births in the United States

**What is the rate of maternal-neonatal transmission of GBS if left untreated?**

35–75% depending on the degree of infection

**How does symptomatic GBS infection manifest in pregnant women?**

UTI, chorioamnionitis, or postpartum wound infection, bacteremia, or endomyometritis

**What are the clinical manifestations of neonatal GBS infection?**

**Bacteremia, sepsis, pneumonia, respiratory distress, meningitis, shock**, or **death** can ensue. If the neonate survives, 33% have long-term neurodevelopmental problems

**What is the difference between early onset and late onset GBS disease?**

Early onset refers to infection before 7 days of age and it carries the highest mortality rate. Late onset disease occurs from 1 week to 3 months after birth

**What is the mortality rate associated with neonatal GBS infection?**

5%–15%

**What are the major risk factors for neonatal GBS infection that necessitate treatment in a woman who has not been screened for GBS?**

Preterm labor

GBS bacteriuria during the pregnancy

Prolonged ROM (>18 hours)

Having a neonate affected by early-onset GBS infection in a previous pregnancy

Maternal fever >38°C during labor

**What is the recommended treatment for GBS colonization?**

**IV penicillin** or ampicillin

**What are the alternatives for patients allergic to penicillin?**

Cefazolin and vancomycin. Clindamycin or erythromycin are acceptable alternatives only if culture and sensitivities have demonstrated the bacteria to be sensitive

## *Listeria Monocytogenes*

**What is *Listeria*?**

A gram-positive, aerobic bacillus that is transmitted via fecal-oral transmission

**What is commonly implicated in *Listeria* infection?**

**Infected foods** such as raw vegetables, milk, smoked fish, soft cheeses, and some processed meats

**What are the clinical manifestations of listeriosis in adults?**

Can be **asymptomatic** or it can cause a **flu-like illness**

**What are the clinical manifestations of fetal infection with *Listeria?***

Disseminated granulomatous lesions with microabscesses

Chorioamnionitis

Sepsis

Sudden abortion or stillbirth

**What is the difference between early onset and late onset *Listeria* infection?**

**Early onset disease** occurs within the first week of life and it typically presents after a **preterm** delivery with **respiratory distress**, fever, and neurologic abnormalities. **Late onset disease** occurs after the first week, and it typically presents as **meningitis**

**What is the treatment for *Listeria* infection in pregnancy?**

**Ampicillin** or trimethoprim-sulfamethoxazole or vancomycin (in PCN-allergic patients)

## Gonorrhea

**What is gonorrhea?**

Caused by *Neisseria gonorrhoeae*, it is an STI that can have serious consequences in pregnancy

**What are the possible pregnancy complications that can occur as a consequence of gonorrhea infection?**

Spontaneous abortion

Stillbirth

Preterm labor

PROM

Chorioamnionitis

Postpartum infection

**What are the possible neonatal effects of gonorrhea infection in pregnancy?**

Gonococcal ophthalmia, arthritis, and sepsis

**How is gonococcal ophthalmia prevented?**

By giving all infants prophylactic **erythromycin** or **silver nitrate** eye drops

## *Chlamydia*

**What is *Chlamydia*?**

Infection with *Chlamydia trachomatis*, an obligate intracellular bacterium

**What are the possible pregnancy complications that can occur as a consequence of chlamydial infection?**

Preterm labor, PROM, and/or postpartum endometritis

**What are the possible neonatal effects of chlamydial infection in pregnancy?**

**Conjunctivitis, pneumonia**, and/or **otitis media**

**How should pregnant women infected with *Chlamydia* be treated?**

With **erythromycin** or **azithromycin** (tetracycline should be avoided because of teratogenicity)

**How is chlamydial ophthalmia prevented?**

By giving all infants prophylactic **erythromycin** or **silver nitrate** eye drops

## UTI IN PREGNANCY

UTI is the most common medical complication of pregnancy.

**Why is pregnancy considered a high-risk condition with asymptomatic bacteriuria?**

Both hormonal and mechanical changes predispose the pregnant woman with asymptomatic bacteriuria to develop acute pyelonephritis, which is associated with preterm birth and perinatal death. Pyelonephritis in pregnancy will lead to septicemia in 10–20% and ARDS in 2% of cases

**How prevalent is asymptomatic bacteriuria in pregnancy?**

It is estimated to occur in 4–7% of pregnant patients. If left untreated, up to 40% of cases will progress to pyelonephritis

**How is this condition detected?**

Screening for asymptomatic bacteriuria using urine culture is recommended at the first prenatal visit

**How is asymptomatic bacteriuria treated?**

Any FDA category B drug such as cephalosporins, nitrofurantoin, or trimethoprim-sulfamethoxazole can be used. Quinolones (FDA category C) are generally are not used during pregnancy. 7-day courses are recommended, along with a follow-up culture to document sterile urine. Persistent bacteruria should be treated based on sensitivities. Suppressive antibiotics (most commonly nitrofurantoin) should then be considered in these patients

**How is symptomatic cystitis treated in pregnancy?**

Treatment and follow-up is similar to asymptomatic bacteriuria. Acute pyelonephritis should be treated with IV antibiotics and hospitalization. Suppressive antibiotics should be given following treatment of any pregnant patient treated for acute pyelonephritis

# Rhesus (Rh) Alloimmunization

**What is alloimmunization of pregnancy?**

It is when the fetus inherits a blood group factor from the father which the mother does not possess. Exchange of blood during fetal-maternal bleeding causes the mother to become sensitized to the foreign antigen and stimulates the **formation of maternal antibodies (alloimmunization) during that pregnancy**. These antibodies may enter the fetal circulation of her **next pregnancy** and lead to **hemolytic disease in the fetus** and neonate by sensitizing the fetal RBCs for destruction by macrophages of the fetal spleen (see Fig. 9-6)

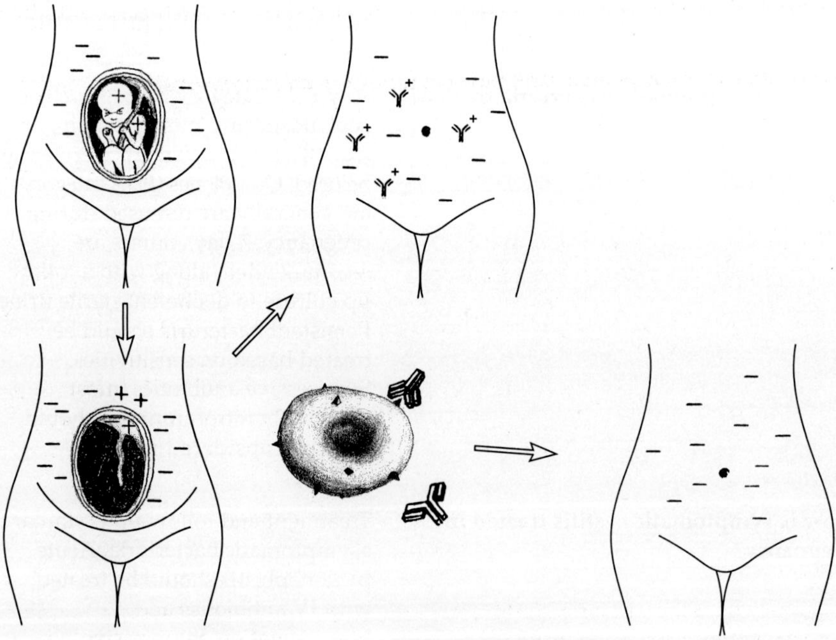

**Figure 9-6** Isoimmunization and RHOGAM treatment.

**How is erythroblastosis fetalis described?**

It is when fetal red blood cell destruction far exceeds production and severe anemia occurs. This disease is characterized by extramedullary hematopoiesis, heart failure, edema, ascites, and pericardial effusion. Hemolysis also produces heme and bilirubin, both of which are neurotoxic and may lead to kernicterus

**What is the correct nomenclature for designating a gravida's blood type?**

ABO blood type and either Rh(D+) or Rh(D–)

**What is the nomenclature of the Rh blood group system?**

The Rh blood system consists of five antigens (C, c, D, E, e). The D antigen is most commonly implicated in Rh alloimmunization and, therefore, Rh positive usually indicates the presence of the D antigen and Rh negative indicates the absence of D antigen on erythrocytes

**By what mechanisms can Rh alloimmunization occur?**

1. **Transplacental fetomaternal hemorrhage during any pregnancy (most common)**
2. Injection with needles contaminated by Rh(D+) blood
3. Inadvertent transfusion of Rh(D+) blood

**What is the most common scenario for fetomaternal hemorrhage?**

**Uncomplicated vaginal delivery** in 15–50% of births. A minimum volume of 0.1 mL of fetal blood entering the maternal circulation can result in alloimmunization

**What are several less common situations where fetomaternal hemorrhage can occur?**

Cesarean delivery, multifetal gestation, bleeding placenta previa or abruption, manual removal of the placenta, and intrauterine manipulation, first-trimester spontaneous and induced abortion, threatened abortion and ectopic pregnancy, obstetrical procedures such as chorionic villus sampling, pregnancy termination, amniocentesis, and external cephalic version

**When should a blood and Rh(D) typing and antibody screen be performed?**

**Always at the first visit!** These tests should also be repeated with every subsequent pregnancy. The American

Association of Blood Banks also recommends repeated **antibody screening before administration of anti-D immune globulin at 28 weeks of gestation, postpartum**, and at the time of any event in pregnancy

**What test is the most sensitive test for determining antibody titers and diagnosing Rh(D) alloimmunization? How does it work?**

**Indirect Coomb's test**. Incubation of a known specimen of Rh(D+) RBCs with maternal serum is the first step in the indirect Coomb's test. Maternal anti-Rh(D) antibodies, if present, will adhere to the RBCs. The RBCs are then washed and suspended in serum containing antihuman globulin (Coomb's serum). Red cells coated with maternal anti-Rh(D) will be agglutinated by the antihuman globulin, which is referred to as a positive indirect Coomb's test

**What titer levels are considered critical for significant risk of severe erythroblastosis fetalis and hydrops?**

Critical titers may vary from laboratory to laboratory. In general, the critical titer that poses a significant risk for erythroblastosis fetalis and hydrops is 1:16 to 1:32

**What is the direct Coomb's test?**

It is similar to the indirect Coomb's test and is done after birth to detect the presence of maternal antibody on the neonate's RBCs. It is performed by placing the infant's RBCs in Coomb's serum; maternal antibody is present if the cells are agglutinated

**Who should be given anti-D immune globulin (RhoGAM)?**

It is not effective once alloimmunization to the Rh(D) antigen has occurred. Therefore, it is essential that it be given to an **Rh(D−) woman whose fetus is or may be Rh(D+) whenever there is a risk of fetomaternal hemorrhage**

**How does RhoGAM prevent alloimmunization?**

It is an IgG that will attach to the Rh antigen and prevent an immune response by the mother (see Fig. 9-6)

**How are sensitized Rh(–) patients evaluated?**

There are three options once the gravida reaches the critical titer:

1. MCA doppler can be performed weekly. MCA doppler is sensitive in diagnosing moderate to severe

hemolytic disease. Once the fetus reaches a value indicating moderate to severe anemia, cordocentesis with transfusion is indicated.

2. Amniocentesis can be performed with two indicated tests: PCR on the fetal amniocytes will determine the fetal blood type. If the fetus is Rh(–), no additional testing is indicated. Indirect measurement of hemolytic disease can be determined by measuring bilirubin concentration in the amniotic fluid using spectrophotometry at a wavelength of delta-OD 450. The absorbance measurements indicate the degree of fetal anemia. Measurements in zone III and high range of zone II indicate a need for cordocentesis with transfusion.
3. Cordocentesis can be performed initially to determine fetal blood type and hemoglobin concentration. However, this procedure can have up to a 1% risk of fetal loss per procedure

**What is the management of the unsensitized Rh(–) pregnancy (the Rh(–) patient who has a negative antibody screen)?**

1. All pregnant women should undergo type and antibody screening for the ABO and Rh group at the first prenatal visit
2. Another antibody screen is obtained at 28 weeks of gestation to detect women who have become alloimmunized in the interval since the first screen
3. Anti-D immune globulin should be administered early in the third trimester, 300 μg at 28 weeks of gestation
4. Anti-D immune globulin is effective for 12 weeks, and if the gravida received an injection at 28 weeks' gestation, she should have a repeat injection at 40 weeks' gestation

**What are additional indications to give 300 μg anti-D immune globulin to any Rh(D–) woman whose fetus is or may be Rh(D+)?**

**Whenever there is increased risk of fetomaternal hemorrhage such as** spontaneous abortion, ectopic pregnancy, invasive procedures such as amniocentesis, chorionic villus sampling and cord blood sampling, antepartum hemorrhage, external cephalic version

**What is the Kleihauer-Betke test and when should it be used?**

It is a test to quantify the amount of fetal RBCs in the maternal circulation in circumstance where excessive fetomaternal hemorrhage has occurred and Rh sensitization is positive for persistent antibody after initial administration of RhIgG. Additional doses of RhIgG is given according to the amount of excess hemorrhage

**What is the role of postpartum administration of anti-G immune globulin?**

It is recommended to administer 300 μg of anti-D immune globulin within 72 hours of delivery of an Rh (D+) infant

**What should one do if anti-D immune globulin is inadvertently omitted after delivery?**

It is still recommended to give it as soon as possible. Partial protection is afforded with administration within 13 days of the birth, and there may be an effect as late as 28 days after delivery

**How are sensitized Rh(–) patients (positive Rh antibody screen on initial visit) evaluated?**

It depends on whether the patient has a history of an affected fetus in a previous pregnancy.

**No history of a previous pregnancy affected by Rh isoimmunization:**

1. Antibody screen and titers at 0, 20 weeks' EGA, and then every 4 weeks
2. Determine the paternal Rh(D) type and if Rh(D+), determine zygosity
3. Amniocentesis should be performed if titers reach critical levels (1:32)
4. Doppler ultrasound of the MCA should be performed every 2 weeks beginning at 24 weeks. High peak velocity blood flows correlates with severe fetal anemia

**History of a previous pregnancy affected by Rh isoimmunization:**

1. Maternal titers are not helpful in following the degree of fetal anemia after the first affected gestation
2. Determine the paternal Rh(D) type and if Rh(D+), determine zygosity
3. In cases of a heterozygous paternal phenotype, perform amniocentesis at 15 weeks of gestation to determine the fetal Rh(D) status
4. If the father is a homozygote or the fetus is Rh(D+), begin MCA doppler velocity assessment at 18 weeks of gestation. Repeat at 1–2 week intervals

**How is the severity of disease predicted in fetuses in which isoimmunization has occurred?**

Bilirubin present in amniotic fluid derives from fetal pulmonary and tracheal effluents and correlates with the degree of fetal hemolysis. Amniotic fluid is analyzed by spectrophotometer, which measure the light absorbance by bilrirubin. Absorbance measurements are plotted on a **Liley curve**, which predicts the severity of disease

# Fetal Growth Abnormalities

## FETAL GROWTH RESTRICTION

**What are other common terms to describe fetuses with disproportionately small growth?**

Small for gestational age (SGA); intrauterine growth restriction (IUGR); low birth weight (LBW); and fetal growth restriction (FGR)

**How is FGR commonly defined?**

It is defined as **estimated fetal weight (ESW) at or below the 10th percentile for gestational age**. This definition is controversial because it does not make a distinction among fetuses who are constitutionally small, growth restricted and small, and growth restricted but not small. In addition, birth weight is also related to maternal height, parity, paternal height, and the fetus's sex

**FGR or LBW is associated with increased perinatal mortality. At what percentile is this risk greatest?**

Weights below the third percentile for gestational age

**Abnormal fetal growth may be classified as symmetrical or asymmetrical. What is meant by these terms?**

**In symmetric FGR**, all fetal organs including the brain are proportionally small because of abnormalities in early fetal cellular hyperplasia. There is cellular hypoplasia or a reduction in the total number of cells. This comprises 20–30% of all growth-restricted fetuses

**In asymmetrical FGR**, there is a relatively greater decrease in abdominal size than head circumference. This is thought to occur from redistribution of blood from non-vital organs (liver, abdominal viscera) to vital organs (heart, brain). There is redistribution away from the kidneys in asymmetrical growth restriction which may give lower AFIs and oligohydramnios. This comprises 70–80% of growth-restricted fetuses

**What are the several causative factors for both symmetric and asymmetric FGR?**

**Symmetric:** early insults such as chromosomal abnormalities, early teratogenic exposure, and early exposure to TORCH infections

**Asymmetric:** maternal conditions such as hypertension, vasculopathies, diabetes with vascular disease, and placental abnormalities

**FGR may be caused by fetal, maternal, or placental factors. What are several fetal etiologies that cause FGR?**

Genetics, congenital anomalies, multi-fetal pregnancy

**What are some genetic diseases or syndromes that typically manifest with FGR?**

Trisomy 21 (Down syndrome), Trisomy 18 (Edwards syndrome), Trisomy 13 (Patau syndrome), cri-du-chat syndrome, Turner syndrome,

Fanconi syndrome, skeletal dysplasias

**Abnormal placental conditions cause FGR because of mismatch between fetal nutritional or respiratory demands and placental supply. What are some placental etiologies?**

Chorioangioma or hemangioma of the placenta, placenta previa, placental mosaicism, single umbilical artery, velamentous umbilical cord insertion, placenta biloba

**Several maternal conditions affect the microcirculation causing fetal hypoxemia, vasoconstriction, or a reduction in fetal perfusion, thus causing FGR. What are these common maternal etiologies?**

Hypertension, both chronic and acute (as in preeclampsia), cyanotic heart disease, and severe anemia (as with sickle cell anemia), renal insufficiency, systemic lupus erythematosus, thrombophilias (acquired such as antiphospholipid antibody syndrome and inherited), chronic anemia, and pregestational diabetes

**What other maternal etiologies cause FGR?**

Infections (rubella, toxoplasmosis, cytomegalovirus, varicella-zoster, malaria)

Teratogens (trimethadione, phenytoin, methotrexate, and warfarin)

Poor nutrition

Substance abuse (cocaine, alcohol)

Socioeconomic factors (race, pregnancy at the extremes of reproductive life, and previous delivery of an FGR neonate)

**What are some maternal complications associated with an FGR pregnancy?**

Complications because of underlying disease, preeclampsia, premature labor, cesarean delivery

**What are some fetal complications associated with an FGR pregnancy?**

Stillbirth, hypoxia and acidosis, malformations

**What are some neonatal complications associated with an FGR pregnancy or complications found in small-for-gestational age infants?**

Difficult cardiopulmonary transition: perinatal asphyxia, meconium aspiration, or persistent pulmonary hypertension

Complications with prematurity: neonatal death, necrotizing enterocolitis, and respiratory distress syndrome

Impaired thermoregulation

Hypoglycemia

Polycythemia and hyperviscosity

Impaired immune function

**What are the long-term complications for the child of an FGR pregnancy?**

Lower IQ, learning and behavior problems, major neurologic handicaps

**How is the diagnosis of FGR determined?**

**Patient history, clinical assessment of fundal height, and sonographic evaluation of the fetus, placenta, and amniotic fluid** is necessary

**What sonographic measurements are diagnostic and predictive of FGR?**

**Estimation of fetal weight** is the single best morphometric test for identifying fetuses whose birth weight is likely to be below the 10th percentile for gestational age (FGR)

**What is oligohydramnios and what role does it have in the diagnosis of FGR?**

Oligohydramnios may be a consequence of FGR and refers to amniotic fluid volume that is less than expected for gestational age. It occurs when there is diminished fetal urine production, and in FGR this may be because of hypoxia-induced redistribution of blood flow to vital organs at the expense of less vital organs, such as the kidney. Severe oligohydramnios is associated with high perinatal mortality

**(15–80% of fetuses with FGR do not have decreased amniotic fluid volume)**

**What is the role of doppler assessment of the umbilical arteries in evaluating FGR?**

They are not useful for screening and diagnosis of the small fetus. They are useful for identifying the small fetus that is at risk for adverse perinatal outcome (non-reasssuring fetal heart rate patterns, cesarean delivery, preterm birth, neonatal intensive care admission, asphyxia)

## FETAL MACROSOMIA

**What is the definition of fetal macrosomia and large-for-gestational age (LGA)?**

**Macrosomia** implies growth beyond a specific threshold, usually 4000 g or 4500 g, regardless of gestational age. However, maternal and fetal morbidity rises sharply with birth weights >4500 g

**Large-for-gestational age** implies a birth weight equal to or greater than the 90th percentile for a given gestational age

**What is the incidence of fetal macrosomia?**

The worldwide prevalence of the birth of infants ≥4000 g is approximately 9%, with wide variations between countries. 1.5% of all infants weigh >4500 g

**What are maternal and fetal complications associated with macrosomia?**

**Maternal:** protracted labor, cesarean delivery, genital tract lacerations, postpartum hemorrhage, uterine rupture

**Fetal: shoulder dystocia**, brachial plexus injuries, fractures of the clavicle, asphyxia

**Neonatal:** increased risk of depressed 5-minute APGAR scores, increased risk of admission to the NICU, jaundice, hypoglycemia

**Long-term:** obesity

**What are risk factors for macrosomia?**

In decreasing order of importance:

Prior history of macrosomia

Maternal prepregnancy weight

Maternal weight gain during pregnancy

Multiparity

Male fetus

Gestational age >40 weeks

Ethnicity

Maternal birth weight, height, age

Positive 50 g glucose screen with a negative result on the 3-hour glucose tolerance test

**What pregnancy-related disease is an independent factor for and highly associated with macrosomia?**

Pregestational diabetes and gestational diabetes

**Which genetic and congenital syndromes are associated with macrosomia?**

Beckwith-Wiedemann syndrome (pancreatic islet cell hyperplasia)

Fragile X syndrome

**How is macrosomia diagnosed?**

An accurate diagnosis of macrosomia can only be made after weighing the newborn. However, prenatal

| | |
|---|---|
| | diagnosis of fetal macrosomia is best diagnosed by evaluation of maternal risk factors, clinical examination (Leopold maneuvers), and ultrasound measurements |
| **Are there any available interventions for treating fetal macrosomia?** | For mothers without diabetes, there are no reported interventions<br>For diabetic mothers, addition of insulin to diet therapy may treat early macrosomia |
| **Is prophylactic cesarean delivery indicated for pregnant women suspected to have macrosomic fetuses?** | Prophylactic cesarean delivery to prevent shoulder dystocia may be considered for an ESW >5000 g in nondiabetic women and >4500 g in women with diabetes (induction of labor for macrosomia is also not recommended) |
| **When should elective cesarean delivery be considered?** | For women whose previous delivery was complicated by shoulder dystocia, particularly when a brachial plexus injury occurred |

# Multi-fetal Gestation

| | |
|---|---|
| **What is the incidence of *spontaneous* twins and multiple births in the United States?** | Twins: 1:80<br>Triplets: 1:8000 |
| **How has the incidence of multifetal gestation changed over time?** | Since 1980 there has been a 65% increase in the frequency of twins and a 500% increase in triplet and high-order births |
| **What is causing this increasing trend in multi-fetal gestation?** | Increased use of ART and ovulation-induction agents |
| **What is the role of maternal age in increased multi-fetal pregnancy?** | The rate of multiples increases with increasing age. This is most likely the result of older women undergoing antiretroviral therapy (ART) and higher levels of FSH in advancing age |
| **What is the significance of multi-fetal gestation on fetal morbidity and mortality?** | It causes a significant effect on preterm delivery and low birth weight of newborns |

They account for 17% of all preterm births (before 37 weeks of gestation)

**How significant is the impact of multi-fetal gestation on maternal morbidity and mortality?**

It increases maternal morbidity and mortality significantly, as well as hospital costs. Women with multiple gestations are six times more likely to be hospitalized with complications. Hospital costs are on an average 40% greater compared to women with single gestations. Neonatal intensive care unit (NICU) admissions are significantly more frequent and are of longer duration. Multi-fetal gestations contribute to maternal conditions such as preeclampsia and gestational diabetes

**What is meant by monozygosity and dizygosity?**

**Monozygotic (identical or maternal) twins** form from a fertilization of a single ovum that subsequently divides into two separate individuals. **Dizygotic (nonidentical or fraternal) twins** result from fertilization of two separate ova by two separate sperm during a single ovulatory cycle

**Monozygotes can either be monoamnionic/monochorionic or diamnionic/monochorionic depending upon the timing of division of embryos**

**When does division of the embryo occur in these two types of twins?**

**Conjoined twins:** division after 13 days post-fertilization results in conjoined twins where the twins share a single cavity and have one placenta, one chorion, one amnion, and one shared umbilical cord

**Monoamnionic/monochorionic placentation** occurs with division after amnion formation (between days 8 and 12 postfertilization). These gestations have a single placenta and are at increased risk of cord entanglement during the pregnancy

**Diamnionic/monochorionic placentation** occurs with division (after trophoblast differentiation and before amnion formation between days 4 and 8 postfertilization). Twins are in separate cavities and have one placenta, one chorion, two amnions, and two umbilical cords. These gestations are at increased risk for twin-to-twin transfusion syndrome (TTTS) (see Fig. 9-7).

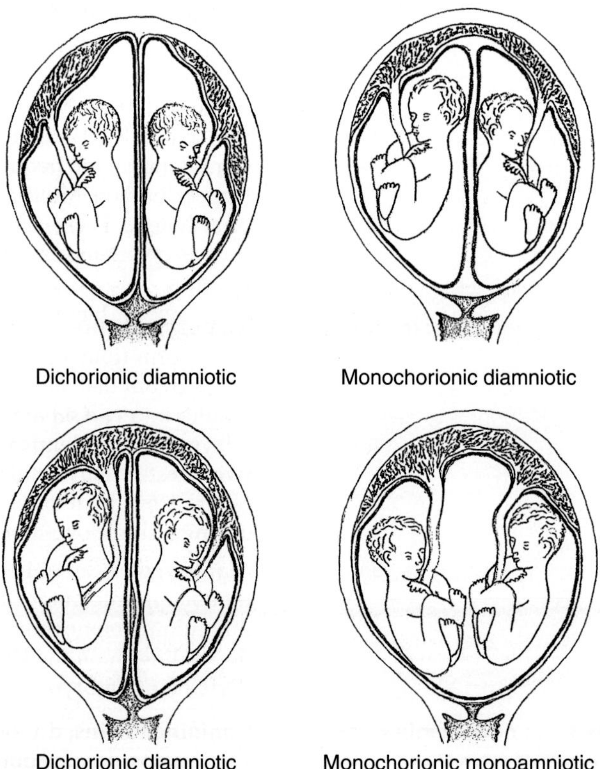


**Figure 9-7** Twin pregnancies.

| | |
|---|---|
| **What type of twinning may occur in dizygotic twins? Explain these types of twins** | Dichorionic/diamnionic separate or fused development. In both types, division of embryos occurs before differentiation of the trophoblast (within 3 days of fertilization). In fused development, the chorions may fuse. Sexes may be different in dizygotic twins |
| **What percentage of same sex twins with monochorionic placentas are identical?** | 100% |
| **What is twin-to-twin transfusion syndrome?** | TTTS is a syndrome in which there is unequal flow of blood across the shared placenta, typically resulting |

in one twin who is smaller (donor twin) and has decreased amniotic fluid and another twin (recipient twin) who is larger with excess amniotic fluid. Perinatal mortality associated with TTTS is high, and twins who survive are at risk of severe cardiac, brain, or developmental disorders

**What are several complications of pregnancy that are increased in multi-fetal gestation?**

Spontaneous preterm delivery, intrauterine growth restriction, small for gestational age (SGA), gestational diabetes, hypertension, preeclampsia, pulmonary embolism, pulmonary edema, and acute fatty liver (which is marked by severe coagulopathy, hypoglycemia, and hyperammonemia) are increased among multi-fetal gestations

**What is the association between multi-fetal gestation and cerebral palsy?**

There is a three-fold greater risk of cerebral palsy. Causes that may contribute to this risk include low birth weight, congenital anomalies, cord entanglement, preterm delivery, and abnormal vascular connections

**What technique is used to reduce the number of fetuses in a multi-fetal gestation?**

Fetal reduction or selective fetal termination

**Preterm delivery is a common and serious complication of multiple births. What are some methods to predict pre-term delivery?**

Cervical length measurement by ultrasound and the presence of fetal fibronectin in cervical-vaginal fluids can predict those at highest risk for preterm delivery

**How may a multiple gestation pregnancy be prolonged?**

While there are no proven methods to delay delivery in multi-fetal pregnancies, a prophylactic cerclage may benefit those with proven cervical insufficiency, decreasing strenuous activity levels, and closer monitoring may have small benefits in these gestations

**How is preterm labor managed in multiple gestation?**

Judicious use of tocolytics is recommended with the administration of antenatal corticosteroids to accelerate fetal lung maturity

# Abnormal Labor and Delivery

## DYSTOCIA

**What is dystocia and what is its incidence?**

Abnormal labor; occurs in approximately 25% of nulliparous women

**What are the risk factors for abnormal labor?**

Advanced maternal age

Non-reassuring fetal heart tracing

Epidural anesthesia

Macrosomia

Occiput posterior position

Nulliparity

Short stature

High station with full dilatation

Chorioamnionitis

Post-term pregnancy

Obesity

**What are the three major categories of causes of dystocia?**

Problems with the three "P"s: **power**, **passage**, and **passenger**

**What is meant by abnormal power?**

Inadequate or uncoordinated contractions

**What is meant by abnormal passage?**

Abnormal size or shape of maternal pelvis leading to **cephalopelvic disproportion** (a disproportion between the fetal head and maternal pelvis)

**What is meant by abnormal passenger?**

Malposition, malpresentation, macrosomia, or multiple gestations

**What are the two major categories of failure to progress?**

**Protraction disorders**—slower than normal progress

**Arrest disorders**—complete cessation of progress

**Name and describe two of the major causes of failure to progress**

**Uterine hypocontractility:** the most common cause of failure to progress; refers to uterine activity that is not strong enough or is not coordinated enough to dilate the cervix; quantified as uterine contractions <200 Montevideo units

**Epidural anesthesia:** leads to an increased duration of the first and second stages of labor and an increased incidence of fetal malposition

**What are the criteria for the diagnosis of abnormal labor in each of these categories?**

| | Nullipara | Multipara |
|---|---|---|
| **Duration of labor:** | >24.7 hours | >18.8 hours |
| **Protracted dilation:** | <1.2 cm/hr | <1.5 cm/hr |
| **Arrest of descent** (with epidural): | >3 hours | >2 hours |
| **Arrest of descent** (without epidural): | >2 hours | >1 hour |

**When is an arrest of dilation diagnosed?**

Cessation of dilation after 4 cm or more despite adequate uterine contractions (>200 Montevideo units for 2 hours or more)

**How is poor progression in the first stage of labor managed?**

With an **amniotomy** (if membranes are intact) and/or **oxytocin** (for hypocontractile uterine activity)

**If protraction persists despite these interventions, how should the patient be managed?**

Cesarean delivery—she is in active phase arrest

**What is a prolonged latent phase?**

A latent phase (in the first stage of labor) of over 20 hours for a nullipara or 14 hours for a multipara

**What are the risks associated with a prolonged latent phase?**

Increased risks of cesarean delivery

Newborn requiring NICU admission

Thick meconium

Depressed apgars

**What are the risk factors for poor progression in the second stage of labor?**

Nulliparity

Diabetes

Macrosomia

Epidural anesthesia

Use of oxytocin

Chorioamnionitis

**How is poor progression in the second stage of labor managed?**

Fetal surveillance and expectant management or active pushing by the patient

**How is a hypocontractile uterus treated?**

With oxytocin

**What is assisted vaginal delivery?**

Also known as operative vaginal delivery, it involves the use of forceps or a vacuum device

| | |
|---|---|
| **What fetal position is most associated with abnormal labor?** | Occiput posterior |
| **How is occiput posterior position managed?** | Most spontaneously rotate. If it doesn't, it can be managed with manual/instrumental rotation to occiput anterior, operative vaginal delivery, or spontaneous delivery in the occiput posterior position |
| **What types of abnormal presentations are possible and what are the relative incidences of each?** | Face (~1/700)<br>Brow (~1/1400)<br>Breech (~1/30)<br>Compound (~1/1500) |
| **Describe face presentation** | The fetal neck is sharply extended, causing the face to lead into the birth canal |
| **What are the risk factors for face presentation?** | Cephalopelvic disproportion<br>Macrosomia<br>Contracted maternal pelvis<br>Platypelloid pelvis<br>Multiparity<br>Abnormal fetal head (e.g., anencephaly) |
| **What are the three types of breech presentation?** | **Frank breech:** fetus has hips flexed and knees extended (feet near head)<br>**Complete breech:** fetus has hips and knees flexed<br>**Footling/incomplete breech:** fetus has one or both feet present below the buttocks (see Fig. 9-8) |
| **How common is breech presentation?** | Approximately 3–4% of fetuses at term are breech (increased rates at earlier gestational ages) |
| **What are some of the factors that affect presentation?** | Uterine shape (fibroids, placenta previa, poly/oligohydramnios, müllerian anomaly, etc.)<br>Fetal shape (anomalies such as anencephaly)<br>Fetal mobility (asphyxia, impaired growth, fetal structural malformation, fetal chromosomal anomaly, etc.) |
| **How is breech presentation diagnosed?** | With abdominal palpation and ultrasound |

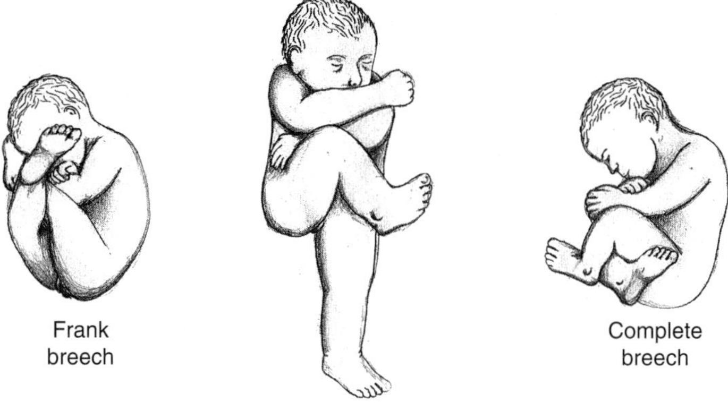


**Figure 9-8** Breech presentations.

**What are the options for management of a breech presentation near term?**
External cephalic version
Cesarean delivery
Vaginal delivery (rarely done)

**What is external cephalic version?**
A procedure that externally rotates the fetus from the breech presentation to the cephalic presentation

**When is external cephalic version done?**
After 36 weeks

**What is the success rate of external cephalic version?**
Approximately 65%

**What is a transverse lie?**
When the fetus's longitudinal axis is perpendicular to the long axis of the uterus

**What are the two types of transverse lie?**
Back down: fetal back facing toward the cervix
Back up: fetal back facing away from the cervix

**What is the incidence of transverse lie?**
1 in 300 deliveries. Many more are transverse early in gestation, but convert spontaneously before term

**What are the options for the intrapartum management of transverse lie?**
Cesarean delivery
External cephalic version

**What potential problems can be associated with transverse lie?**
Placenta previa
Prolapsed umbilical cord
Fetal trauma
Prematurity

## ABNORMAL FETAL TESTING

| | |
|---|---|
| **What causes non-reassuring fetal testing?** | Fetal hypoxia or acidosis, which in turn can be caused by:<br>Maternal diseases (e.g., hypotension, hypoventilation)<br>Placental problems (e.g., insufficiency, abruption)<br>Uterine factors (e.g., hyperstimulation, uterine rupture)<br>Fetal factors (e.g., umbilical cord prolapse, arrhythmia, infection) |
| **What is the fetal response to transient hypoxia?** | Initially, slowing of the fetal heart rate resulting in decelerations |
| **What are the fetal responses to prolonged hypoxia?** | Persistent bradycardia<br>Repetitive late decelerations<br>Loss of heart rate variability<br>Loss of fetal biophysical activities (low BPP) (see Fig. 9-9) |
| **What is a reassuring fetal heart rate pattern?** | Rate between 110 and 160 beats per minute (bpm) with accelerations<br>No decelerations<br>Variability between 6 and 25 bpm |
| **Fetal acidosis is suggested by what findings on a fetal heart tracing?** | Decelerations: **prolonged** (>2 minutes and <10 minutes) decelerations, **late** decelerations, or periodic **severe variable** decelerations<br>Minimal (<5 bpm) **or absent long-term variability**<br>**Tachycardia** (>160 bpm for more than 10 minutes) or bradycardia (<110 bpm for more than 10 minutes) |
| **How is fetal acidosis directly assessed?** | Blood is sampled from fetal presenting part |
| **What is the most common cause of fetal tachycardia?** | Maternal tachycardia |
| **What are some other causes of fetal tachycardia?** | Maternal fever<br>Fetal anemia<br>Asphyxia<br>Infection<br>Autoimmune disorders |

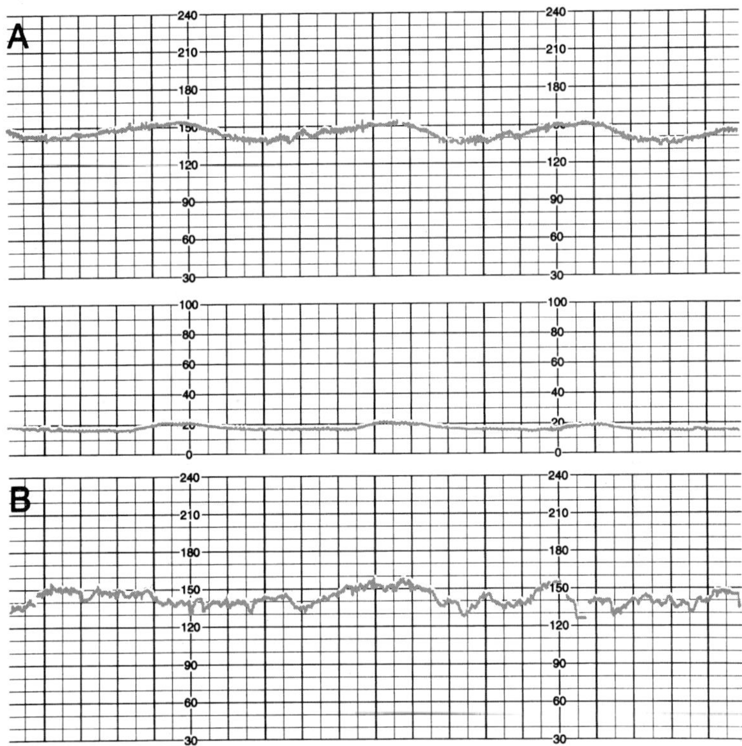


**Figure 9-9** Antepartum fetal heart rate tracings at 28 weeks' gestation in woman with diabetic ketoacidosis. A. During maternal and fetal acidemia B. Return of normal accelerations. (Reproduced, with permission, from Cunnigham FG et al: *Williams Obstetrics*, 22nd ed. New York: McGraw-Hill, 2005:378.)

Adrenergic medications

Fetal cardiac arrhythmia (e.g., sinoventricular tachycardia [SVT])

**What is fetal bradycardia?**

A baseline FHR <110 bpm

**What are some of the causes of fetal bradycardia?**

Physiologic (short episodes—because of transient compression of the fetal head/umbilical cord)

Maternal hypotension

Local anesthesia (e.g., paracervical block)

Uteroplacental insufficiency (e.g., placental abruption, uterine rupture, cord prolapse)

Fetal cardiac arrhythmia

**What are the different classifications of fetal heart rate variability?**

Absent

Minimal (<5 bpm)

Moderate (6–25 bpm)

Marked (>25 bpm)

**What is suggested by a sinusoidal pattern on electronic fetal monitoring (EFM)?**

Fetal anemia, hypoxia, or exposure to sedative hypnotics

**How can chronic fetal stress be manifested?**

**Oligohydramnios** (AFI <5 cm or maximum vertical pocket <2 cm), decrease in BPP score, intrauterine growth restriction, or abnormal umbilical artery doppler assessment

**During hypoxic stress, where is fetal blood preferentially shunted?**

Brain, heart, adrenals, and placenta

**How is feto-placental perfusion assessed with doppler ultrasound?**

Systolic versus end diastolic flow velocity (**S/D flow**) in the umbilical vessels, middle cerebral artery, and ductus venosus

**What is a normal umbilical artery S/D ratio?**

It is gestational age-dependent.
At term, <3

**What is a high umbilical artery S/D ratio associated with?**

Placental insufficiency

**What are the three types of decelerations?**

Early, late, and variable

**Describe early decelerations**

A gradual decrease from baseline that mirrors a contraction with the nadir of the heart rate at the same time as the peak of the contraction

**What do early decelerations signify?**

A vagal response from **compression of the fetal head** during uterine ctx; they are **normal**

**Describe variable decelerations**

A **rapid decline** of more than 15 beats from the baseline. **The shape and timing of the deceleration is variable. They may or may not occur with contractions**

**What do variable decelerations signify?**

Usually **cord compression** (can be relieved by changing the mother's position)

**How are variable decelerations managed?**

If mild or moderate: expectant management

If severe and periodic: move mother to left or right lateral decubitus position; consider stopping oxytocin

| | |
|---|---|
| | and starting amnioinfusion to alleviate cord pressure |
| **What is an amnioinfusion?** | Catheter administration of sterile saline into the uterine cavity |
| **Describe late decelerations** | A gradual decrease from baseline with an onset, nadir, and recovery after the beginning, peak, and end of a contraction |
| **What do late decelerations signify?** | Fetal hypoxia |
| **How are late decelerations managed?** | Move mother to left or right lateral position<br>Supplemental $O_2$<br>Stop oxytocin (and potentially start tocolytics)<br>Increase IV hydration<br>Monitor maternal BP to ensure maternal hypotension is not the cause<br>Fetal blood sampling to assess for acidosis (if available) |
| **What are the indications for operative delivery because of fetal distress?** | Fetal acidosis as determined by fetal scalp sampling<br>Persistent late decelerations or repetitive severe variable decelerations in a tracing without reassuring features (i.e., accelerations) |

## MECONIUM

| | |
|---|---|
| **What is meconium?** | **Fetal feces** released into the amniotic fluid |
| **How often is meconium noted before or during delivery?** | 10–15% of births |
| **What are some of the causes of meconium passage in utero?** | Placental insufficiency<br>Cord compression<br>Infection |
| **What is meconium aspiration syndrome (MAS)?** | A **chemical pneumonitis** caused by inhalation of meconium into the fetal tracheobronchial tree during the antepartum or intrapartum period |
| **What are some of the potential complications of MAS?** | Respiratory distress, persistent pulmonary hypertension, death |

## POST-TERM PREGNANCY

**What is the definition of post-term pregnancy?**
Also called prolonged pregnancy; a pregnancy **beyond 42 weeks** gestation

**What is the incidence of post-term pregnancy?**
Approximately 7–10% in the United States

**What are factors associated with post-term pregnancy?**
**Incorrect dating**
**Primiparity**
**Prior post-term pregnancy**
Fetal congenital anomaly
Placental sulfatase deficiency

**What are the risks to the fetus in post-term pregnancy?**
Perinatal death
Intrauterine infection
Macrosomia and associated risks
Asphyxia
Fetoplacental insufficiency
Anencephaly
Fetal dysmaturity syndrome

**What is fetal dysmaturity syndrome?**
Also known as **postmaturity syndrome**, it is placental insufficiency resulting in wrinkly, peeling skin (especially on palms and soles); long, thin body—wasting of subcutaneous tissue; alert appearance with open eyes; long nails

**What are the fetal risks of post-term pregnancy?**
Oligohydramnios (and subsequent umbilical cord compression)
Non-reassuring fetal heart tracing
Meconium aspiration
Complications at birth (hypoglycemia, seizures, respiratory insufficiency)
Long-term neurologic sequelae

**What are the maternal risks of post-term pregnancy?**
Labor dystocia
Macrosomia-related perineal injury
Increased rate of cesarean delivery

**How should post-term pregnancies be monitored?**
With antenatal fetal monitoring (either via **NST and AFI**, **BPP**, or **oxytocin challenge test**) twice

weekly beginning at 41 weeks gestation

**When should delivery be entertained?**

**At 41 weeks of gestation if the cervix is favorable**

**After 42 completed weeks** or earlier if there is evidence of **fetal compromise** or **oligohydramnios**

**What factors must be considered when deciding whether to induce?**

Results of antepartum fetal assessment

Favorability of the cervix

Gestational age

Maternal preference

**Are there any long-term consequences of post-term pregnancy?**

No

# Teratogens

**What is the definition of a teratogen?**

An agent that acts during the embryonic or fetal development to produce structural abnormalities in the fetus

**What percentage of congenital abnormalities are caused by teratogens?**

Approximately 10%

**What properties of drugs allow their toxic effects on fetuses to occur?**

**Lipid-soluble molecules readily cross the placenta** compared to water-soluble substances

Molecules bound to carrier proteins are less likely to cross the placenta

**What is meant by embryopathy versus fetopathy?**

Embryopathy refers to exposure to a teratogen within the first 8 weeks, whereas fetopathy refers to exposure after 8 weeks

**What is the general effect of teratogens on each of the three developmental periods of gestation?**

Gestation is divided into three periods known as:

1. **Preimplantation period**—the period from fertilization to implantation or bilaminar disk formation. An insult causing damage to a large

number of cells at this period usually causes death of the embryo (all or nothing phenomenon)

2. **Embryonic period**—the period from the second through the eighth week following conception. This period is the critical stage of organ development (see Fig. 9-10) and is most crucial in regards to structural malformations
3. **Fetal period**—the period where maturation and functional development continue after 9 weeks. Certain organs, such as the brain, remain vulnerable to teratogens during this period

**What are the FDA Pregnancy Drug Categories?**

Category A: safety has been established using human studies

Category B: presumed safety based on animal studies

Category C: uncertain safety; though animals studies show an adverse effect, there are no human studies

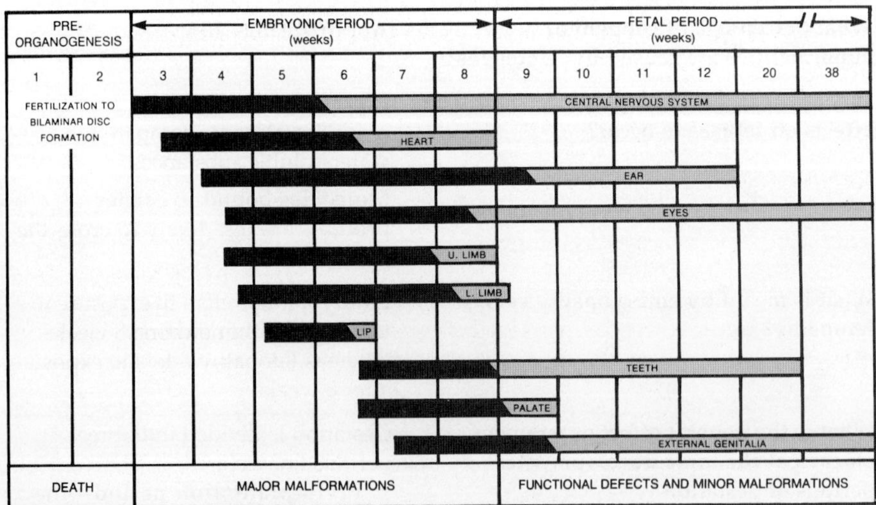


**Figure 9-10** Illustrates the critical development period of each organ system.

Category D: unsafe—evidence of risk that may in certain clinical circumstances by justifiable

Category X: highly unsafe—risk outweighs any possible benefit

**What are the major abnormalities associated with each known teratogen?**

See the following table.

| Teratogen | Syndrome and/or Well-Known Effects of the Teratogen | Other Comments |
|---|---|---|
| Alcohol | **Fetal alcohol syndrome:** congenital heart and brain defects, failure to thrive, developmental delay, mental retardation, ADHD, craniofacial anomalies (absent/hypoplastic philtrum, broad upper lip, micrognathia, microphthalmia, short palpebral tissues, short nose). **Growth restriction** before and after birth | A safe threshold dose for alcohol has not been established. Fetuses of women who consume six drinks/day are at 40% risk of having characteristics of fetal alcohol syndrome |
| Androgens and testosterone derivatives (i.e., danazol) | Virilization of females; advanced genital development in males | Effects are dose-dependent and related to the time of exposure during the developmental period |
| Phenytoin | **Fetal hydantoin syndrome:** craniofacial anomalies (upturned nose, mild midfacial hypoplasia, thin philtrum, facial clefts), fingernail hypoplasia, growth deficiency, developmental delay, cardiac defects | Syndrome results from accumulation of free oxide radicals in fetal tissues |
| Carbamazepine | Fetal hydantoin syndrome, spina bifida, fingernail hypoplasia, IUGR | |
| Valproate | Neural-tube defects | Lowers fetal folate levels |
| Phenobarbital | Clefts, cardiac anomalies, urinary tract malformations | Lowers fetal folate levels |
| Trimethadione, parametha-dione | Cleft palate, V-shaped eyebrows, microcephaly, growth deficiency, mental retardation, speech disturbance, cardiac defects | 70% of newborns affected by this drug |
| Warfarin | *Exposure between 6–9 weeks*: nasal and midface hypoplasia, stippled vertebral and femoral epiphyses, phenotypically identical to chondrodysplasia punctata | Fetal malformations are significant when doses exceeding 5 mg are taken during the first semester. The |

(*Continued*)

| Teratogen | Syndrome and/or Well-Known Effects of the Teratogen | Other Comments |
|---|---|---|
| | *Exposure between second and third trimester*: hemorrhage, organ scarring, agenesis of the corpus callosum, Dandy-Walker malformation, optic atrophy, blindness, mental retardation | incidence of spontaneous abortion is 72% |
| ACE inhibitors | Renal ischemia, renal tubular dysgenesis, anuria, oligohydramnios, lung hypoplasia, limb contractures, hypoperfusion, growth restriction, limb shortening | These changes mostly occur during the fetal period, ACE inhibitor fetopathy. Enalapril is the most teratogenic of the ACE inhibitors |
| Retinol-vitamin A | No conclusive data available for dose toxicity and birth defects | Vitamin A doses higher than 5000 IU should be avoided |
| Isotretinoin | First trimester use: high rate of fetal loss<br>Strongly associated malformations include bilateral microtia, agenesis or stenosis of the external ear canal, cleft palate, abnormal facial bones/calvarium, cardiac defects, hydrocephalus. | No safe first trimester exposure period or dose |
| Diethylstilbestrol (DES) | Clear-cell adenocarcinoma of the cervix and vagina and abnormalities of the female genital tract (T-shaped uterus) | |
| Cyclophosphamide | Absent or hypoplastic digits on the hands and feet, cleft palate, single coronary artery, imperforate anus, fetal growth restriction with microcephaly | Should be avoided in the first trimester but can be given in the second and third trimester |
| Methotrexate | Growth restriction, craniosynostosis, failure of calvarial ossification, hypoplastic supraorbital ridges, micrognathia, and severe limb deformities | Drug alters folate metabolism. Used as an abortifacient. Should not exceed a dose >10 mg/week Contraindicated for treatment of psoriasis |
| Tetracyclines | Yellow-brown discoloration of teeth, hypoplasia of tooth enamel | Effects occur if drug is used in second or third trimester. Should only be used for tx of maternal syphilis in penicillin-allergic women |

(*Continued*)

| Teratogen | Syndrome and/or Well-Known Effects of the Teratogen | Other Comments |
|---|---|---|
| Aminoglycosides | Nephrotoxicity and ototoxicity in preterm newborns treated with gentamicin or streptomycin | No confirmation regarding congenital defects from prenatal exposure |
| Streptomycin, kanamycin | Hearing loss, eighth nerve damage | No ototoxicity has been reported with use of gentamicin or vancomycin |
| Lead | Increased abortion rates, stillbirths | |
| Tobacco | Dose-dependent intrauterine fetal growth reduction, spontaneous abortion, preterm delivery, placenta previa, cleft lip/palate, hydrocephaly, microcephaly, omphalocele, gastroschisis, and hand abnormalities, sudden infant death syndrome (SIDS) | Cessation of smoking throughout and after pregnancy should be strongly advised |
| Cocaine | Placental abruption, porencephaly, subependymal and periventricular cysts, ileal atresia, cardiac anomalies, urinary tract defects, and visceral infarcts | |
| Thalidomide | Upper limb reduction, lower limb reduction, gall bladder aplasia, duodenal atresia | Excellent example shows timing of drug exposure and type of birth defect |
| Methyl mercury | Ranges from developmental delay to microcephaly and severe brain damage | Not a drug but a major pollutant found in fish. Pregnant women should abstain from seafood thought to be exposed to mercury |
| Marijuana | Possible low birth weight; otherwise, no evidence of association with human anomalies | |
| Amphetamines | Symmetrical fetal growth restriction, SIDS | |
| Heroin | Fetal-growth restriction, perinatal death, small head circumference, developmental delays, SIDS | 40–80% of newborns have typical heroin withdrawal symptoms |
| Lithium | Ebstein anomaly, diabetes insipidus, hypothyroidism, and hypoglycemia | |

**Can heparin be used for anticoagulation in pregnant women?**

Yes. Heparin does not cross the placenta because of its large negative charge and thus does not have any adverse fetal effects. Low-molecular weight heparins also do not cross the placenta

**Has paternal exposure to these drugs been found to be teratogenic?**

There is no evidence for this

SECTION IV

# Women's Health Issues

CHAPTER 10

# Issues in Women's Health

## DOMESTIC VIOLENCE

**Describe the epidemiology of domestic violence?**

When violence occurs within the household, 90–95% of the victims are women. Annually, nearly 5 million women are victims of domestic or intimate partner violence and **one-fifth of American women will be abused by an intimate partner within their lifetime**

**Domestic or intimate partner violence perpetuated against women in family or intimate relationships typically follows a predictable cycle. Describe the three stages of the cycle of violence**

The three phases of the cycle include the following: **Tension-building phase**—usually contains intense arguing and blaming
**Battering phase**—characterized by verbal threats, physical battering, sexual abuse, or assault with weapons
**Honeymoon phase**—is characterized by the abuser's attempt to apologize, deny, or offer gift compensation for previous violence. With time, the tension-building phase gets longer and more frequent, and the honeymoon phase gets shorter and less frequent

**What are four major social risk factors for domestic violence?**

Although domestic violence spans all socioeconomic groups, **poverty, unemployment, alcohol, and substance abuse** tend to be highly associated with a history of domestic violence

**How do battered women often present for medical care?**

Women who are being battered present for medical care with a wide variety of complaints, ranging from **sexual dysfunction** (decreased interest or arousal, dyspareunia, etc) and **persistent somatic complaints** (headaches, abdominal pain, sleep or eating disorders) to **psychiatric illnesses** (depression, post-traumatic stress disorder [PTSD], or multiple personality disorder). Because there is no pathognomonic presentation of domestic violence, many cases go undiagnosed

*Other factors that should trigger practitioners to inquire regarding possible violence in the home include apparent **noncompliance, frequent emergency room visits, or frequently cancelled appointments**

**What screening questions can be asked of all women to increase the likelihood of diagnosing domestic violence despite its various presentations?**

Women presenting for routine preventative care or urgent care visits should be routinely screened for domestic violence regardless of their socioeconomic background

**Stage 1 screening** should be directed at specific behaviors. Sample questions include:

Has anyone close to you ever threatened to hurt you?

Has anyone ever hit, kicked, choked, or hurt you physically?

Has anyone, even your partner, ever forced you to have sex against your will?

Are you afraid of your partner?

**What questions should be asked after violence has been determined to be present in a household?**

Stage 2 screening should **assess safety and lethality of violence and develop a safety plan.** Patients who are unsafe at home should be offered shelter.

Has your partner ever threatened to kill you or your children?

Are there weapons in the house?

Does your partner abuse drugs or alcohol?

Is it safe for you to go home?

Are your children safe at home?

**What agencies should be utilized in the referral of a patient who is a victim of domestic violence?**

Contact information for local police and emergency departments, women's shelters, rape crisis centers, counseling services, self-help, and advocacy agencies should be given to battered women

## SEXUAL ASSAULT

**What is sexual assault?**

Sexual assault is the performance of genital, anal, or oral penetration by one person on another without the person's consent

**Describe the epidemiology of sexual assault?**

Although some authors estimate that less than 50% of sexual assaults are reported, **nearly 1 million women are sexually assaulted annually.**

Furthermore, 20% of adult women, 15% of college-age women, and 12% of adolescents have been sexually assaulted in their lifetime

**Sexual assault can happen under a variety of conditions and relationships. Describe four special variants of sexual assault**

**Marital rape** is forced sexual acts within a marital relationship without the consent of a partner. **Acquaintance rape** is sexual assault committed by someone known to the victim. **Incest** involves sexual assault perpetuated by a family member. **Date rape** is sexual assault occurring in the context of a dating relationship

**What is statutory rape?**

Statutory rape occurs when an adult has intercourse with a minor, whose age makes him or her legally incapable of consenting to sexual intercourse. Many states mandate physician reporting of statutory rape. Legal definitions for a minor, or someone at the age of consent, vary depending on jurisdiction

**What is child sexual abuse?**

Child sexual abuse is any contact between a child and an adult where the child is being used for sexual stimulation of the adult. This type of behavior must be immediately reported to child protection services

**Date rape drugs diminish a woman's ability either to consent to sexual activity or remember an assault. What drugs are considered date rape drugs?**

Many of the **benzodiazepines**, because of their sedative/hypnotic properties and their propensity to cause amnesia can be considered to be date rape drugs. Currently, **flunitrazepam (Rohypnol) and gamma-hydroxybutyrate (GHB)** are the two most frequently used date rape drugs; however, ketamine, chloral hydrate, and MDMA (Ecstasy) have the potential to be abused in this manner

**What is the Rape Trauma Syndrome (RTS) and how does it differ from PTSD?**

**Rape Trauma Syndrome is a biphasic PTSD-like condition that occurs within hours to days after a sexual assault and can persist for months to years**. In the acute or disorganization stage, which occurs over 2 weeks following a sexual assault and can have a cyclical relapsing-remitting presentation, the victim's coping mechanisms are impaired leading to either an emotionally labile, expressive catharsis or a controlled, emotional detachment. In the late or reorganization phase, minimal symptoms of PTSD emerge, but do not disrupt the victim's life as in PTSD. During this phase, some victims experience nightmares, flashbacks, feelings of alienation and isolation, depression, and anxiety

**After obtaining informed consent to do a careful history and full, chaperoned physical examination, what specimen will be collected from the patient to look for DNA evidence to identify the perpetrator?**

Victim's clothing

Air-dried swabs and smears from the oropharynx, vagina, and rectum

Cervical mucus for a Pap smear

Washings from the skin and vagina

Combed specimen from scalp and pubic hair with control samples of the victim's hair from each site

Fingernail scrapings and clippings

Whole blood samples

Saliva samples

The patient should be counseled regarding the ability to photograph any physical findings. The consent process for taking pictures should include a discussion of the disposition and confidentiality surrounding these photographs

**What substances contained within the collected specimen will be used as evidence of sexual assault and to identify the perpetrator?**

Motile and nonmotile sperm and hair to provide evidence of sexual assault and for DNA

Acid phosphatase to provide evidence of sexual assault

**The following are conditions and their prophylactic treatments the victim should receive immediately after verifying the patient's allergy history:**

| Condition | Treatment |
|---|---|
| *Chlamydia* | Azithromycin (1 g PO) or Doxycycline (100 mg, PO, bid × 7 days) |
| Gonorrhea | Ceftriaxone (125 mg, IM) |
| Trichomoniasis | Metronidazole (2 g, PO × 1 or 500 mg bid, PO × 7 days) |
| Hepatitis B | Hepatitis B immune globulin and Hepatitis B vaccine (0, 1, and 6 months) |
| HIV | Low risk (basic regimen): ZDV (TDF, d4T or ddI) and 3TC or FTC<br>High risk: basic regimen and either LPV/RTV, SQV/RTV, NFV, ATV ± RTV, IDV ± RTV, or FPV ± RTV |
| Pregnancy | Yuzpe (100 mcg ethinyl estradiol, 0.5 mg levonorgestrel): Q12H × 2<br>Plan B (0.75 mg levonorgestrel): Q12H × 2 doses<br>Mifepristone (RU 486): 600 mg, PO |

ZDV, zidovudine; TDF, tenofovir; d4T, stavudine; ddI, didanosine; 3TC, lamivudine; FTC, emtricitabine; LPV, lopinavir; RTV, ritonavir; SQV, saquinavir; NFV, nefinavir; ATV, atazanavir; IDV, indinavir; FPV, fosamprenavir

## ETHICS AND LAW

**Two forms of advanced directives include the living will and a durable power of attorney for health care. These structures allow patients to state their preferences for future medical treatment in the event of loss of capacity because of medical illness. How does the living will differ from the power of attorney?**

The living will offers a competent adult patient a means to express her wishes and offer informed consent governing the use of life-sustaining treatments in writing in advance of a medical condition that leads to incapacity or incompetence. However, in making a power of attorney, the patient appoints a surrogate decision maker to stand in her place and express her wishes or give informed consent in the event of incapacity or incompetence

**The doctrine of informed consent requires physicians to obtain the patient's permission for treatment, operations, or some diagnostic procedures. What conditions need to be met in order to validate the patient's offering of consent?**

A valid informed consent must be voluntarily granted by a competent patient who has full comprehension of the risk, benefits, alternatives, and consequences of the relevant, available diagnostic or treatment options

**Under what circumstances is the requirement of informed consent waived?**

Informed consent is often not required before administering treatment or performing lifesaving procedures in a medical emergency, preventing suicide, or attending to minors in the absence of a parent

**In general, the information disclosed by a patient during a physician consultation is strictly confidential, and thus should not be revealed without the patient's consent, unless disclosure is required by law. Under what circumstances is the maintenance of strict patient confidentiality not required?**

Patient confidentiality can be broken under the following circumstances:

When a patient discloses an intention to inflict serious bodily harm on herself or another person

In the event of a life-threatening emergency

When a reportable, communicable disease has been diagnosed

However, in these and other cases, disclosure is permitted only to those for whom it is medically or legally necessary

**Laws governing malpractice are formed by two mechanisms, from legislative action or from judicial opinion rendered during precedent cases. Under which type of law do most malpractice claims proceed?**

Most malpractice claims proceed under the body of law defined by judicial opinion derived from precedent cases, or common law. A dynamic body of law, common law is constantly changing and thus continually redefining the grounds for potential litigation

**What are the four principles that must be proven in order to establish medical liability in a negligence suit?**

Medical liability requires the plaintiff to demonstrate the presence of duty, breach of duty, causation, and consequent damages. Causation is defined as the link between the alleged breach of duty and an injury and must be supported by proof of causation. Damages constitute demonstrable injuries and can either be purely economic (e.g., lost wages) or noneconomic (e.g., pain and suffering)

**Identify the elements needed to prove malpractice in a wrongful birth and wrongful conception claim**

In a wrongful birth claim, a clinician interviewing a pregnant couple (duty) omits the family history and fails to recognize a serious disability that has a hereditary or genetic basis (breach of duty). Consequently, a baby with appreciable disabilities is born (damages) to parents who would have sought termination, but for the clinician's failure which prevented proper counseling. In a wrongful conception claim, a clinician treating a nonpregnant couple (duty) fails to provide histologic evidence of sterilization during a tubal ligation or provides improper contraceptive counseling or techniques (breach of duty). Consequently, a normal but unwanted child is born (damages) to the couple seeking sterilization or effective contraception

SECTION V

# Review Questions and Answers

CHAPTER 11

# Review Questions and Answers

(1) At which of the following time periods of zygotic division does the formation of dichorionic, diamnionic twins occur following fertilization? Answer: d

(a) >264 hours

(b) >120 and ≤240 hours

(c) >72 and ≤120 hours

(d) ≤72 hours

(2) Which surgical procedure is most commonly performed in the second trimester of pregnancy? Answer: d

(a) Ovarian cystectomy

(b) Cholecystectomy

(c) Laparoscopy

(d) Appendectomy

(3) A 21-year-old female presents to the emergency room (ER) stating that she "was raped." Which medications should she be given for prevention of sexually transmitted diseases (STDs) in this situation? Answer: a

(a) Ceftriaxone, azithromycin, and metronidazole

(b) Ceftriaxone plus cefixime

(c) Ceftriaxone plus azithromycin

(d) Ceftriaxone plus penicillin

(4) **Maternal obesity is a risk factor for all of the fetal complications *except*:**

Answer: c

(a) **fetal macrosomia**

(b) **neural-tube defects**

(c) **dizygotic twinning**

(d) **stillbirth**

(5) **Your pregnant patient has mitral stenosis and is New York Heart Association functional class II. Which of the following sets of vaccinations, cultures, and antibiotics is indicated during her pregnancy?**

Answer: b

(a) **Influenza, pneumococcal, intrapartum bacterial endocarditis prophylaxis**

(b) **Influenza, pneumococcal, group B streptococcal vaginal and rectal culture at 36 weeks**

(c) **Influenza, pneumococcal, intrapartum bacterial endocarditis prophylaxis, group B streptococcal vaginal and rectal culture at 36 weeks**

(d) **Influenza and pneumococcal vaccine**

(6) **Your patient states that she is comfortable at rest but begins to experience shortness of breath and chest pain after walking three blocks. What New York Heart Association classification would you assign her?**

Answer: b

(a) **I**

(b) **II**

(c) **III**

(d) **IV**

(7) **Which of the following analgesics is a non–histamine-releasing narcotic and therefore should be used for asthmatics?**

Answer: c

(a) **Fentanyl**

(b) **Codeine**

(c) Morphine

(d) Meperidine

(8) Your current patient is pregnant and has a history of deep vein thrombosis (DVT) in her previous pregnancy. How should she be managed during this pregnancy? Answer: c

(a) Low-dose aspirin

(b) Careful observation

(c) Mini-dose subcutaneous heparin or LMWH

(d) Full prophylactic dose subcutaneous heparin or LMWH

(9) Your patient is 18 weeks pregnant and presents with idiopathic hematuria. Which of the following outcomes is she at increased risk of developing? Answer: a

(a) Preeclampsia

(b) Pyelonephritis

(c) Chronic renal disease

(d) Preterm labor

(10) Which of the following pregnancy complications is most common in women with chronic renal insufficiency? Answer: b

(a) Fetal growth restriction

(b) Anemia

(c) Preeclampsia

(d) Preterm delivery

(11) During a first trimester surgical abortion, signs of complete evacuation include all of the following except: Answer: d

(a) Gritty sensation

(b) Contraction around the uterus

(c) Bubbles in the cannula and hose

(d) Bleeding from the os

(12) **Typically, postabortal infections present:** Answer: b

(a) **within the first 24–36 hours**

(b) **within the first 48–96 hours**

(c) **within the first 6 days**

(d) **after at least 1 week post-procedure**

(13) **During a suction dilation and curettage (D & C), the surgeons note a midline perforation. If the uterus is not completely evacuated, all of the following options may be indicated except:** Answer: a

(a) **continue with the same procedure**

(b) **exploratory laparotomy**

(c) **perform ultrasound**

(d) **exploratory laparoscopy**

(14) **The method of abortion at 15 weeks' gestation with the least psychologic and emotional impact on the patient is:** Answer: c

(a) **intra-amniotic hypertonic saline**

(b) **intra-amniotic prostaglandin**

(c) **dilation and evacuation**

(d) **prostaglandin vaginal suppositories**

(e) **abdominal hysterectomy**

(15) **The most common complication arising from a first-trimester surgical pregnancy termination is:** Answer: d

(a) **uterine perforation**

(b) **cervical trauma**

(c) **retained products of conception**

(d) **pelvic infection**

(e) **vaginal laceration**

(16) A 21-year-old G0, with a history of irregular menses presents for her first gynecologic examination. Pelvic examination reveals fullness in the right adnexa. The examination is otherwise unremarkable. You obtain a transvaginal ultrasound which reveals a thin-walled 4-cm unilocular, clear fluid-appearing cystic structure in the right ovary. How do you manage this patient?

(a) Send tumor markers

(b) Follow-up sonogram in 3–6 months

(c) Drainage of the cyst via transvaginal approach

(d) Laparoscopy and cystectomy

Answer: b

(17) An 18-year-old female presents to the ER with acute right-sided pain. She reports nausea and vomiting and states that her pain is unrelenting when it is present, though it seems to "come and go" over the last few hours. Her examination is significant for involuntary rebound and guarding. You obtain a transvaginal ultrasound, which reveals an adnexal mass consistent with a 7-cm unilocular structure with both hyperechoic and hypoechoic components. How do you manage this patient?

(a) Call general surgery consult for suspected appendicitis

(b) Paracentesis of adnexal structure

(c) Laparoscopy and oophorectomy

(d) Laparoscopy and cystectomy

Answer: d

(18) A 41-year-old G3P3 presents to the ER with complaints of unrelenting lower abdominal pain. She denies nausea and vomiting but reports subjective fevers. In the ER, she is febrile to 100.9. Pelvic examination reveals a mobile 12-week size uterus with point tenderness midline in the lower abdomen, no cervical motion tenderness, no discharge. Urinalysis (UA) is significant for few white cells with many squamous cells. You obtain an ultrasound which reveals a multimyomatous uterus with a subserosal anterior myoma of 6-cm size with internal components suggestive of calcification and necrosis; adnexal structures are within normal limits. What is this patient's diagnosis?

(a) PID

(b) Cystitis

(c) Degenerating fibroid

(d) Appendicitis

Answer: c

(19) How would you manage the patient above?

(a) Admission and IV antibiotics

(b) Discharge home and PO antibiotics

(c) Discharge home with NSAIDs

(d) Admission and myomectomy

(e) Admission and hysterectomy

Answer: c

(20) How does progesterone affect various organ systems during pregnancy?

(a) Lowers diastolic blood pressure less than systolic

(b) Increases lower esophageal sphincter tone causing painful spasms

Answer: d

(c) Decreases the central respiratory drive resulting in dyspnea of pregnancy

(d) Reduces ureteral tone, decreases peristalsis, and relaxes the bladder wall

(21) Why is there an increase in total $T_4$ and $T_3$ concentrations in pregnancy? Answer: b

(a) Pregnancy is a state of physiologic stress with upregulation of all hormones

(b) β-hCG stimulates TSH receptors

(c) Liver production of binding globulins is decreased

(d) Fetal production results in increased maternal concentrations

(22) Which of the following hemodynamic values remains unchanged in pregnancy? Answer: d

(a) Pulmonary vascular resistance

(b) Colloid osmotic pressure

(c) Pulmonary capillary pressure

(d) Systemic vascular resistance

(23) Which of the following is not a cause of DVT in pregnancy? Answer: d

(a) Decreased protein S

(b) Resistance to protein C

(c) Increased factor I (fibrinogen), II, V, VII, VIII, X, and XII

(d) Compression of the left iliac vein by the right iliac artery

(24) Which of the following complications in pregnancy is increased in women with a female fetus? Answer: d

(a) Hepatitis

(b) Cholelithiasis

(c) Reflux esophagitis

(d) Hyperemesis gravidarum

**(25) Your patient is pregnant and is found to be positive for hepatitis C. Which of the following outcomes is associated with hepatitis C?** Answer: c

**(a) Abruptio placentae**

**(b) Fetal growth restriction**

**(c) Vertical transmission of hepatitis C**

**(d) Preterm birth**

**(26) Which class of gestational diabetes in *not* at increased risk for unexplained stillbirth?** Answer: a

**(a) A1**

**(b) A2**

**(c) B**

**(d) C**

**(27) What fetal malformation is most strongly associated with diabetes?** Answer: c

**(a) Neural-tube defects**

**(b) Congenital heart defects**

**(c) Caudal regression**

**(d) Renal agenesis**

**(28) What is the most common etiology of pregnancy-associated osteoporosis?** Answer: d

**(a) Bed rest**

**(b) Corticosteroids**

**(c) Heparin therapy**

**(d) Idiopathic**

**(29) A pregnant patient presents with symptoms and signs of thyrotoxic storm. All of the following medications are indicated *except*:** Answer: b

**(a) potassium iodide**

**(b) magnesium sulfate**

**(c) dexamethasone**

**(d) propylthiouracil**

**(30) Your patient has a history of epilepsy and is also found to be pregnant. She refuses to take antiepileptic medications. Of which of the following complications are fetuses at an increased risk?** Answer: c

**(a) Fetal growth restriction**

**(b) Congenital malformation**

**(c) Seizure disorder**

**(d) Perinatal death**

**(31) What is the most common cause of female sexual dysfunction?** Answer: b

**(a) Vaginismus**

**(b) Inhibited sexual desire**

**(c) Arousal disorder**

**(d) Anorgasmia**

**(32) Which antidepressant listed below is the least likely to cause sexual dysfunction?** Answer: c

**(a) Prozac**

**(b) Zoloft**

**(c) Wellbutrin**

**(d) Effexor**

**(33) An 18-year-old female with no history of STIs and who has had two sexual partners presents to her gynecologists' office for her last dose of HPV vaccine. She asks how often she needs to have a Pap smear. The correct response is:** Answer: c

**(a) every 3 years**

**(b) every 5 years**

**(c) annually**

**(d) never again—she is now immune to HPV**

**(34) A 62-year-old G2P2002 presented for her gynecologic visit and was found to have high-grade squamous intraepithelial lesions (HSIL). A colposcopy was performed and found to be negative; however, the squamocolumnar junction was unable to be visualized. What is the next appropriate step in management?**

Answer: a

**(a) Conization**

**(b) Repeat Pap smear within 3 months**

**(c) Endocervical curettage**

**(d) Biopsy of cervical tissue**

**(35) The above patient underwent conization via loop electrosurgical excision procedure (LEEP), which was found to be negative. Which of the following follow-up management is the most appropriate?**

Answer: a

**(a) Repeat Pap smear in 4–6 months**

**(b) Repeat Pap smear in 1 year**

**(c) Repeat colposcopy in 6 months**

**(d) Repeat conization in 6 months**

**(36) A 37-year-old female is diagnosed with invasive squamous cell carcinoma of the cervix. She is found to have minimal microscopic stromal invasion that is confined to the cervix. What are the most appropriate treatment options? (Choose all that apply.)**

Answer: a or b

**(a) Conization**

**(b) Simple hysterectomy**

**(c) Radical hysterectomy**

**(d) Radiotherapy**

**(e) Combination chemotherapy**

**(37) All of the following increase during pregnancy *except*:**

Answer: c

**(a) tidal volume**

**(b) minute ventilation**

(c) total lung capacity

(d) alveolar partial pressure of oxygen

(38) What screening test is listed with the appropriate condition? Answer: a

(a) Maternal serum alpha fetal protein and neural tube defects

(b) Urine dip and gestational diabetes

(c) Magnetic resonance imaging and cleft lip

(d) Percutaneous umbilical blood sampling and Rh isoimmunization

(39) What diagnostic test is listed with the appropriate condition? Answer: b

(a) Maternal serum alpha fetal protein: aneuploidy

(b) Amniocentesis: Down syndrome

(c) Glucose challenge test: gestational diabetes

(d) Biophysical profile: fetal lung maturity

(40) All of the following cause persistent or increasing levels of β-hCG *except*: Answer: d

(a) retained products of conception

(b) trophoblastic disease

(c) choriocarcinoma

(d) complete spontaneous abortion

(41) All of the following drugs can be used for the treatment of migraine headaches during pregnancy except: Answer: d

(a) propranolol

(b) meperidine

(c) amitriptyline

(d) ergonovine

**(42) What is the best treatment for syphilis in a penicillin-allergic patient during pregnancy?**

Answer: a

**(a) Penicillin desensitization**

**(b) Tetracycline**

**(c) Ceftriaxone**

**(d) Erythromycin**

**(43) Your pregnant patient presents with chlamydial cervicitis. Which of the following treatments is appropriate?**

Answer: d

**(a) Tetracycline, 500 mg PO qid × 7 days**

**(b) Ciprofloxacin, 500 mg PO bid × 14 days**

**(c) Erythromycin estolate, 250 mg PO qid × 4 days**

**(d) Erythromycin base, 500 mg PO qid × 7 days**

**(44) How does breast-feeding affect the risk of HIV transmission?**

Answer: a

**(a) Increases**

**(b) Decreases**

**(c) Unaffected**

**(d) Unknown**

**(45) Which of the following is increased in pregnancies complicated by sickle-cell trait?**

Answer: a

**(a) UTI**

**(b) Low birth weight**

**(c) Perinatal mortality**

**(d) Spontaneous abortion**

(46) A 65-year-old female presents to her gynecologist with complaints of progressive vulvar itching and perineal pain. On examination, there is diffuse atrophy with one raised, whitish area on the posterior aspect of the vulva. What is the most appropriate first step in her management?

Answer: d

(a) Trial of low-dose corticosteroid cream

(b) Trial of high-dose corticosteroid cream

(c) Trial of topical antifungal cream

(d) Vulvar biopsy of the affected area

(47) The biopsy results for the above patient demonstrate vulvar intraepithelial neoplasia II (VIN II). What is the most appropriate treatment for her?

Answer: b

(a) Chemotherapy

(b) Complete local excision

(c) Wide excision with laser ablation

(d) Chemotherapy followed by localized radiation

(48) A 72-year-old female presents to her gynecologist with pruritus and soreness of the vulva. On inspection, there are multiple well-demarcated white hyperkeratotic areas on a bright red background. What is the most likely diagnosis?

Answer: c

(a) Squamous cell carcinoma of the vulva

(b) Basal cell carcinoma of the vulva

(c) Paget disease of the vulva

(d) Vulvar melanoma

**(49) A 17-year-old female presents to her gynecologist with complaints of cramping lower abdominal pain that begins with menstruation. She also admits to mild nausea and diarrhea around the same time. Her physical examination is unremarkable. What should be used as first-line therapy?**

Answer: a

**(a) NSAIDs**

**(b) Oral contraceptive pills**

**(c) Presacral neurectomy**

**(d) Antispasmodic agents**

**(50) A 28-year-old female presents with increasing pelvic pain with menstruation that is not relieved with NSAIDs. Physical examination reveals some uterine immobility as well as tender nodularities in the posterior cul-de-sac. What is the most likely diagnosis?**

Answer: b

**(a) Primary dysmenorrhea**

**(b) Endometriosis**

**(c) Leiomyomas**

**(d) Adenomyosis**

**(51) Match each of the following terms to their correct description**

Answers 1-c, 2-a, 3-b

| | |
|---|---|
| **(1) Prolonged, irregular menstrual bleeding** | **(a) Menorrhagia** |
| **(2) Prolonged, regular menstrual bleeding** | **(b) Metrorrhagia** |
| **(3) Irregular menstrual bleeding** | **(c) Menometrorrhagia** |

**(52) What is the fetal lie, presentation, and position if the head is down, flexed, and the fetal back is near the left maternal pelvis? Additionally, on sterile vaginal examination a diamond fontanel is noted near the right ischial spine, a triangular fontanel is the leading edge, and the sagittal suture is not parallel with the floor**

Answer: a

**(a) Longitudinal lie and left occiput anterior (LOA)**

**(b) Longitudinal lie and right occiput anterior (ROA)**

**(c) Transverse lie and left occiput anterior (LOA)**

**(d) Transverse lie and right occiput anterior (ROA)**

**(53) On examination, the sagittal suture is deflected toward the sacrum, which allows more of the parietal bone to be palpated anteriorly. What is the term that describes this physical finding?**

Answer: d

**(a) Transverse diagonal**

**(b) Posterior diagonal**

**(c) Posterior asynclitism**

**(d) Anterior asynclitism**

**(54) How is zero station determined on sterile vaginal examination?**

Answer: b

**(a) The leading fetal edge is flush with the introitus**

**(b) The leading fetal edge is parallel with the maternal ischial spines**

**(c) The leading fetal edge is engaged in the maternal pelvis**

**(d) The leading fetal edge is engaged in a fully dilated cervix**

**(55) A multigravid mother has a history of previous group B streptococcus (GBS)-negative pregnancies, a GBS-positive urinary tract infection during the current pregnancy, and a negative GBS culture at 36 weeks. She presents to labor and delivery with spontaneous rupture of membranes and contractions every 5 minutes. Which of the following is indicated?**

**(a) Immediate urinalysis for signs of current infection**

**(b) Immediate urine culture and rectal swab for identification of GBS status**

**(c) Empiric treatment for unknown GBS status**

**(d) Antibiotics immediately due to history of GBS colonization**

Answer: d

**(56) A group B *Streptococcus*-positive G2P1 with a penicillin allergy presents at 38 weeks with loss of fluid for 3 hours and contractions every 5 minutes. What is the next step in management?**

**(a) Place the mother and infant on cardiac monitors**

**(b) Assess for rupture of membranes**

**(c) Begin ampicillin prophylaxis**

**(d) Desensitize patient to penicillin**

Answer: b

**(57) How often is meconium noted during labor and what does it signify?**

**(a) Rarely, and only in the presence of anoxic brain injury**

**(b) Often, without any significance**

**(c) Half of the time with variable outcomes**

**(d) Occasionally, and it is suggestive of some degree of fetal stress**

Answer: d

(58) Your patient, a 21-year-old G2P1 with a prior cesarean delivery and currently with a singleton gestation, is found to have placenta previa. Which of the following is not associated with an increased incidence of placenta previa?

Answer: d

(a) Advanced maternal age

(b) Grand multiparity

(c) Prior cesarean delivery

(d) Singleton gestation

(59) Your patient presents at 30 weeks with complaints of vaginal bleeding. There is currently no active vaginal bleeding. She is admitted to a labor room for evaluation. A fetal heart strip is obtained and reveals an FHR of 130 bpm with no accelerations or decelerations. An ultrasound is obtained and reveals a partial previa. What is the next step in management?

Answer: a

(a) Observation in labor and delivery (L&D)

(b) Assessment of fetal lung maturity

(c) Cesarean delivery

(d) Gentle cervical examination to assess dilation and amnionic membrane status

(60) During the third stage of labor, your patient's uterus inverts and the placenta becomes detached from the uterus. Which of the following is the next best step in management?

Answer: b

(a) Prompt oxytocin administration

(b) Attempt to manually replace the uterus

(c) Prompt hysterectomy

(d) Administration of inhalation anesthetics prior to manual replacement

**(61) A 62-year-old postmenopausal woman presents to your office with episodic vaginal bleeding over the past 3 months. You are most suspicious of:**

**(a) perimenopausal spotting**

**(b) adrenal hyperplasia**

**(c) cancer**

**(d) fibroids**

Answer: c

**(62) A 26-year-old female presents with 8 months of irregular bleeding. Bleeding occurs at markedly irregular intervals and varies in its quantity. A progesterone challenge test demonstrates withdrawal bleeding. Which of the following laboratory tests are indicated for the evaluation of dysfunctional uterine bleeding in this woman? (Mark all that apply.)**

**(a) CBC**

**(b) Coagulation profile**

**(c) Endocrine profile (TSH, LH, FSH, prolactin)**

**(d) Endometrial biopsy**

Answer: a, b, and c

**(63) A 45-year-old woman presents to her gynecologist with complaints of amenorrhea for 7 months. She denies any symptoms of vasomotor instability. Her lab work reveals a negative β-hCG and a decreased LH and FSH. What is the most likely cause of her amenorrhea?**

**(a) Menopause**

**(b) Hypothalamic-pituitary dysfunction**

**(c) Outflow obstruction**

**(d) Pregnancy**

Answer: b

(64) A patient with amenorrhea does not have withdrawal bleeding after a progesterone challenge test. What is the next test that is indicated?

Answer: a

(a) An estrogen-progesterone test

(b) Head CT

(c) Hysteroscopy

(d) Laparoscopy

(65) Which of the following lower genital tract organisms in *not* associated with increased puerperal infection?

Answer: a

(a) *Trichomonas vaginalis*

(b) Group B *Streptococcus*

(c) *Gardnerella vaginalis*

(d) *Mycoplasma hominis*

(66) What uterotonic is not appropriate to administer a woman with preeclampsia?

Answer: c

(a) Oxytocin (Pitocin)

(b) Carboprost (Hemabate)

(c) Methylergonovine (Methergine)

(d) Misoprostol (Cytotec)

(67) All of the following mothers are advised to breast-feed *except* those with:

Answer: a

(a) HIV with a low viral count

(b) Fluctuant and indurated mastitis

(c) Current hepatitis A infection

(d) Hepatitis B following infant vaccination and IgG administration

(68) When does serum hCG return to normal (non-detectable levels) after delivery?

Answer: c

(a) Within hours

(b) Within days

(c) Within weeks

(d) Within months

**(69) When does menstruation begin in a postpartum woman?** Answer: d

**(a) Average duration is about 20 weeks postpartum in a breast-feeding woman**

**(b) Average duration is about 8 weeks postpartum in a breast-feeding woman**

**(c) Average duration is about 20 weeks in a postpartum nonlactating woman**

**(d) Average duration is about 8 weeks postpartum in a non-lactating woman**

**(70) What is the most likely diagnosis in a woman with frequency, urgency, pyuria, dysuria, and a sterile urine culture?** Answer: a

**(a) *Neisseria gonorrhoeae* urethritis**

**(b) *Chlamydia trachomatis* urethritis**

**(c) *Escherichia coli* cystitis**

**(d) Group B *Streptococcus* cystitis**

**(71) What is the treatment for condylomata accuminata during pregnancy?** Answer: d

**(a) Interferon**

**(b) 5-Fluorouracil**

**(c) Podophyllin resin**

**(d) Trichloroacetic acid**

**(72) What is the "gold standard" for the diagnosis of genital herpesvirus in adults?** Answer: d

**(a) ELISA or serology**

**(b) DNA probes**

**(c) Tissue culture**

**(d) Cervical smear cytologic examination**

(73) What is the major cause of menopause-related bone loss? Answer: c

(a) Decline in calcium production

(b) Decline in calcium absorption

(c) Decline in estrogen levels

(d) Rise in LH and FSH levels

(74) When following up on the results of a DEXA scan for one of your postmenopausal patients, you notice her bone mineral density (BMD) is 1.5 standard deviations below the mean. Her diagnosis is: Answer: b

(a) normal age-related bone loss

(b) osteopenia

(c) osteoporosis

(d) osteomalacia

(75) For a patient with osteoporosis, which of the following lab abnormalities would you expect? Answer: d

(a) High calcium, low phosphorus, low PTH

(b) Low calcium, high phosphorus, high PTH

(c) Low calcium, low phosphorus, low PTH

(d) No lab abnormalities

(76) A 22-year-old G1P0 presents with uterine bleeding at 8 weeks' gestation. On physical examination, her cervix is found to be dilated to 2 cm. Vaginal ultrasound reveals the products of conception in the uterine cavity. What is her diagnosis? Answer: b

(a) Complete abortion

(b) Inevitable abortion

(c) Incomplete abortion

(d) Missed abortion

(77) A 28-year-old G3P1011 at 10 weeks' gestation presents to the ER with uterine bleeding. Her cervix is found to be closed and her β-hCG is at an appropriate level for the stated gestational age. Ultrasound reveals a nonviable fetus in the uterine cavity. What is her diagnosis?

(a) Complete abortion

(b) Inevitable abortion

(c) Incomplete abortion

(d) Missed abortion

Answer: d

(78) For the above patient, which of the following management options are appropriate?

(a) Surgical management

(b) Medical management

(c) Expectant management

(d) Any of the above

Answer: d

(79) A 21-year-old female with a history of PID presents to the ER with right-sided pelvic pain and vaginal bleeding. She is hemodynamically stable. Her LMP was 8 weeks ago and her urine β-hCG is positive. What is the next appropriate step in management?

(a) Serum β-hCG

(b) Transvaginal ultrasound

(c) Immediate laparoscopy

(d) Immediate laparotomy

Answer: b

(80) The above patient has a nondiagnostic ultrasound. Her serum β-hCG is found to be 1000. What is the next step in management?

(a) Repeat β-hCG in 24 hours

(b) Repeat β-hCG in 72 hours

(c) Repeat transvaginal ultrasound in 24 hours

(d) Immediate laparoscopy

Answer: b

(81) A 16-year-old G1P1 presents to her obstetrician 2 weeks postpartum with increased vaginal bleeding. Which of the following steps should be used in management? (Choose all that apply.)

(a) D and C

(b) Serum β-hCG level

(c) CXR

(d) Expectant management

Answers: a, b, and c

(82) A 42-year-old G3P3 presents with 12 weeks of amenorrhea, nausea, vomiting, and mild tremors. Ultrasound reveals a heterogeneous intrauterine mass with theca lutein cysts that appear like a snowstorm. What is the most likely diagnosis?

(a) Early intrauterine pregnancy

(b) Perimenopause

(c) Partial mole

(d) Complete mole

Answer: d

(83) A G3P3 female presents 2 months postpartum with irregular vaginal bleeding. Physical examination reveals an enlarged uterus with bilateral ovarian cysts. Ultrasonographic evaluation reveals an enlarging, heterogeneous, hypervascular mass in the uterus with areas of hemorrhage and necrosis. What is the most likely diagnosis?

(a) Pregnancy

(b) Partial mole

(c) Complete mole

(d) Choriocarcinoma

Answer: d

(84) What is the difference between gestational hypertension and preeclampsia?

Answer: a

(a) Proteinuria is present in preeclampsia, and it is absent in gestational hypertension

(b) Patient has a history of hypertension in gestational hypertension

(c) Patient exhibits sustained elevated blood pressures in preeclampsia

(d) Patient reports lower extremity pitting edema

(85) What is the cure for preeclampsia?

Answer: b

(a) Magnesium sulfate

(b) Delivery

(c) Nifedipine

(d) Diazepam

(86) What is not a complication of placenta previa?

Answer: c

(a) Maternal hemorrhage

(b) Placenta accret

(c) Gestational diabetes

(d) Preterm premature rupture of the membranes (PPROM)

(87) What intrapartum obstetrical maneuvers are used to treat a shoulder dystocia?

Answer: a

(a) McRoberts maneuver

(b) Fundal pressure

(c) Decreasing anesthesia to facilitate maternal effort

(d) Placing the mother in the left lateral decubitus position

(88) An 18-year-old woman with no prenatal care presents to labor and delivery in labor. After delivery, her neonatal infant is found to have sensorineural deafness,

Answer: b

cataracts, PDA, hepatosplenomegaly, hyperbilirubinemia, and blue purpura that appear like a blueberry muffin. What congenital infection is the most likely culprit?

(a) *Toxoplasma*

(b) Rubella

(c) Cytomegalovirus

(d) Syphilis

(89) Which of the following are modalities of mother-to-child HIV transmission? Answer: d

(a) Transplacental infection

(b) Peripartum infection

(c) Breast-feeding

(d) All of the above

(90) A 29-year-old G1P0 female presents to L & D at 33 weeks' gestation in preterm labor. Her GBS status is unknown and she has no known drug allergies. What is the best management for this patient? Answer: a

(a) Penicillin

(b) Clindamycin

(c) Erythromycin

(d) No antibiotics are required

(91) A 23-year-old G1P0 at 39 weeks gestation presents to L & D with painful contractions every 3 minutes. She has a history of HSV-2, and on sterile speculum examination she is found to have an active lesion on the right labia. Which of the following is an appropriate next step in management? Answer: a

(a) Cesarean section

(b) Treatment with acyclovir

(c) Careful delivery with pediatrics present at birth

(d) All of the above

**(92) A 29-year-old G1P0 presents to L & D after 3 hours of painful contractions occurring every 3 minutes. Her initial cervical examination on the floor was 5/80%/–2. Two hours later, no change is noted. An IUPC is placed and her contractions are found to have 250 Montevideo units over the next 2 hours. What is the most appropriate diagnosis?**

**(a) Normal latent labor**

**(b) Arrest of labor**

**(c) Protraction of labor**

**(d) Inadequate contractions**

Answer: b

**(93) An ultrasound is preformed at a 28-week prenatal visit, the fetus is found to be in breech presentation with its hips and knees flexed. What type of breech presentation is this?**

**(a) Frank breech**

**(b) Complete breech**

**(c) Footling breech**

Answer: b

**(94) For the above patient, which of the following are appropriate management options?**

**(a) Cesarean delivery**

**(b) External cephalic version**

**(c) Vaginal delivery**

**(d) All of the above**

Answer: a and b

**(95) A G2P1001 is in active labor with her last cervical examination 2 hours prior of 3/90%/–1. You begin to notice decelerations on the monitor. The decelerations rapidly drop approximately 20 bpm below baseline, quickly return to baseline, and appear unrelated to uterine contractions. What causes this type of deceleration?**

**(a) Fetal scalp compression**

**(b) Uteroplacental insufficiency**

Answer: c

(c) Umbilical cord compression

(d) Fetal acidosis

(96) The amniotic membranes in the above patient are artificially ruptured in order to accelerate labor. The fluid is noted to be clear with a slightly greenish tint. What is the fetus at risk of? Answer: d

(a) Renal failure

(b) Conjunctivitis

(c) Toxoplasmosis

(d) Chemical pneumonitis

(97) Which method is used to reliably diagnose fetal alcohol syndrome prenatally? Answer: a

(a) Cannot be diagnosed prenatally

(b) Ultrasound

(c) Amniocentesis

(d) History of heavy alcohol consumption

(98) A neonate who was born preterm is found to have hyperbilirubinemia. Which antibiotic was most likely given to the mother near delivery? Answer: d

(a) Cephalosporins

(b) Macrolides

(c) Penicillins

(d) Sulfonamides

(99) Which of the following antiviral drugs used to treat HIV infection is teratogenic? Answer: d

(a) Zidovudine

(b) Amprenavir

(c) Didanosine (DDI)

(d) None of the above

(100) The "double-bubble" sign is an ultrasonographic finding of which of the following anomalies? Answer: c

(a) Aqueductal stenosis

(b) Cystic hygroma

(c) Duodenal atresia

(d) Two-vessel umbilical cord

(101) A 23 year old GO presents to your office for an annual exam. Her Pap comes back as ASCUS. She has never had any other abnormal Pap smears. Which of the following management options could you do? Answer: d

(a) Repeat Pap in 6–12 months

(b) Send a reflex HPV and triage based on those results

(c) Send patient directly to colposcopy

(d) All of the above

(102) A 32 year old female presents to the ED with vaginal bleeding. Her LMP was 4 weeks ago and her βhCG is 1200. An ultrasound is done and no intrauterine pregnancy is seen. Her cevix is closed and the bleeding resolves. Which of the following management options is most appropriate? Answer: b

(a) Immediate laparoscopy for a presumed ectopic pregnancy

(b) Repeat serum βhCG in 48 hours

(c) Discharge home with prenatal follow up in 4 weeks

(d) Dilation & curretage for missed abortion

(103) Which of the following characteristics on US is most suspicious for malignancy when evaluating an ovarian mass? Answer: c

(a) Size < 6 cm

(b) Unilocular mass

(c) Complex mass

(d) Minimal flow on Doppler

(104) A 33 year old GIPO presents to L & D in labor. She progresses to the second stage of labor and pushes for 3 hours with an epidural. The decision is made to apply a vacuum as the fetal station is +3. The vacuum pops off 3 times. Which of the following management options is most appropriate? Answer: c

(a) Reapply to vacuum and reattempt delivery

(b) Apply forceps

(c) Immediate cesarean delivery

(d) All of the above are appropriate

(105) A 28-year-old patient presents to you with symptoms of a leiomyoma. Which set of symptoms is most consistent with a leiomyoma? Answer: b

(a) Hirsutism, acne, amenorrhea, virulization

(b) Pelvic pain, dyspareunia, urinary incontinence, menorrhagia

(c) Dysmenorrhea, dyspareunia, infertility, painful defecation

(106) What disease is most associated with the symptoms listed under option (c) in the above question? Answer: b

(a) Pelvic inflammatory disease

(b) Endometriosis

(c) Uterine sarcoma

(107) A distraught couple visits your office, upset at not being able to conceive after 1 year of regular, unprotected intercourse. The female is a nulligravid, takes no medication, and denies any medical illnesses. The husband reports that he is healthy as well and has never fathered a child before. What is the most appropriate initial step in the evaluation of this couple?

Answer: d

(a) Basal body temperature charting

(b) Postcoital test

(c) Semen analysis, including sperm antibodies

(d) History and physical examination of both partners

(e) Laparoscopy

(108) A 25-year-old woman presents to the ER immediately after being rescued from a motor vehicle accident. She states that she is pregnant and ultrasound reveals an 18-week-old fetus. A fetal heart rate is appreciated. The patient looks stable on physical examination and has sustained cuts and scrapes on her arms, face, and legs. Her clothes and exposed skin are soiled. The cervix remains long and closed. While reading her medical record, you notice that her MMR, varicella, and tetanus are not up to date. Which shot is the most appropriate to give at this time?

Answer: d

(a) Measles

(b) Mumps

(c) Rubella

(d) Tetanus

(e) Varicella

**(109) Your patient presents at 30 weeks of pregnancy and requests an elective cesarean delivery. While discussing why she wants this procedure, you describe to her the complications that can arise from a cesarean delivery. Of all the following complications, which one has the highest association with cesarean delivery?**

Answer: e

**(a) Bladder injuries**

**(b) DVT**

**(c) Aspiration pneumonia**

**(d) Wound infections**

**(e) Postpartum endometritis**

**(110) Which of the following can be visualized on a sonogram during the first trimester?**

Answer: d

**(a) Diencephalon**

**(b) Mesencephalon**

**(c) Prosencephalon**

**(d) Rhombencephalon**

**(e) Telencephalon**

**(111) A 44-year-old woman is diagnosed with epithelial ovarian cancer. She is found to have cancer that is limited to one ovary with extension to the uterus and fallopian tubes. What ovarian cancer stage should be assigned to this patient?**

Answer: c

**(a) Stage 1**

**(b) Stage IIA**

**(c) Stage IIB**

**(d) Stage IIC**

**(e) Stage III**

**(112) A 34-year-old woman had a colposcopic examination with a negative biopsy result. Her endocervical canal curettage result returned positive. What is the next appropriate step in management?** Answer: e

**(a) Observe for the next 4–6 months**

**(b) No follow-up is needed**

**(c) Repeat colposcopic examination in the next 2–3 months**

**(d) Vaginal hysterectomy**

**(e) Perform conization of the cervix**

**(113) Which of the following sets contain the most important risk factors for cervical cancer?** Answer: d

**(a) The use of oral contraceptives**

**(b) Family history of cervical cancer**

**(c) Marriage at an early age and having HSV-1**

**(d) History of smoking, multiple sex partners, and first intercourse in the adolescent years**

**(e) Multiparous woman with marriage at a late age**

**(114) Which of the following sets describe the clinical appearance of lichen sclerosis?** Answer: c

**(a) Moist, thick, white, scaly plaques**

**(b) Nontender ulcerative lesions**

**(c) White, thin, atrophic-appearing plaques**

**(d) Excoriated, thickened, and erythematous epithelium**

(115) A 31-year-old woman presents to you with complaints of intense vaginal itching and frothy discharge with malodorous odor. Pelvic examination reveals greenish-gray discharge with numerous "strawberry-like" punctate marks on the cervix. What is the proper treatment for this patient?

(a) Fluconzazole

(b) Estrogen cream

(c) Metronidazole

(d) Penicillin

(e) Doxcycline

Answer: c

(116) A 62-year-old woman presents to your office with complaints of a 6-month history of intense and painful vulvar itching. She also states that she can feel a "small lump." She denies any vaginal bleeding. Her past medical, surgical, and family histories are unremarkable. Examination of the vulva reveals a small fleshy outgrowth on her left labia majora. A biopsy is performed and pathology reveals squamous cell carcinoma in situ. Which of the following statements is most appropriate in the management of this patient?

(a) Postoperative radiation is recommended

(b) Careful observation for the next 6 months to see if the growth enlarges or remains the same is recommended

(c) Colposcopy of the vagina and cervix should be done postoperatively

(d) Total vulvectomy is recommended

(e) Groin dissection is necessary

Answer: c

**(117) A 30-year-old woman presents to the office with complaints of intense itching in the vulva and axillae. She states that she can feel small bumps in these areas and that they appeared suddenly when the weather became hot and humid. She asks for some kind of treatment as the itching prevents her from sleeping well. On examination there are multiple, smooth, flesh-colored papules with excoriations around the vulva and bilateral axillae. There is small whitish vaginal discharge and wet mount reveals epithelial cells, with no hyphae or clue cells. What is the most likely diagnosis?**

**(a) Fox-Fordyce disease**

**(b) Behcet disease**

**(c) Contact dermatitis**

**(d) Folliculitis**

Answer: a

**(118) A 21-year-old female visits you complaining of a 1-month history of pyuria and dyspareunia. She is newly married and returned from her honeymoon 2 weeks ago. She is concerned that this will affect her marriage. What is the most likely cause of her discomfort?**

**(a) *Trichomonas***

**(b) *Candida***

**(c) *E. coli***

**(d) Lactobacillus**

**(e) Inadequate vaginal lubrication**

Answer: c

**(119) A 23-year-old female comes to your office with complaints of intense vaginal itching over the past 4 days that has been getting progressively worse. She states that she had been in good health until 1 week ago when she was treated with ampicillin for a urinary tract infection. Her past**

Answer: b

medical history is unremarkable, and she believes she is in a monogamous sexual relationship with her partner. What is the most appropriate step in management?

(a) Repeat urinalysis to rule out urinary tract infection

(b) Perform a pelvic examination and evaluate the discharge

(c) Reassure the patient that it is a natural response to the antibiotics and will diminish over time

(d) Prescribe antifungals for presumed candidiasis

(e) Perform a Pap smear

(120) Which of the following is the most common cause of precocious puberty in females? Answer: c

(a) Adrenal tumor

(b) Ovarian tumor

(c) Idiopathic

(d) Functional ovarian cyst

(121) Your 23-year-old female patient has mild endometriosis. Her symptoms include irregular menses with no pelvic pain. Which of the following is the best treatment for her? Answer: d

(a) Oral estrogen

(b) GnRH agonists

(c) Danazol

(d) Oral contraceptive pills

(e) Medroxyprogesterone acetate

(122) A 35-year-old African-American woman presents to your office with complaints of increasingly heavy and prolonged menstrual periods over the past year. She also describes feeling a "fullness" in her pelvic area. In addition, she reports having mild dyspareunia. She is happily married to her husband and they have two children. They are considering having another child in the future. Presently, she uses oral contraceptive pills for birth control.

In addition to her chief complaint, she reports feeling "more tired" and having difficulty sleeping. She has associated this with her job, as she is a vice-president for a consulting company and work has been more stressful recently. Her past medical history is unremarkable and she takes no prescription medications.

What is the next most appropriate step in management? Answer: c

(a) Reassurance that her symptoms will resolve when her job-related stress subsides

(b) Obtain LH and FSH levels

(c) Obtain an ultrasound

(d) Obtain cultures for *Chlamydia* and gonorrhea

(e) Perform an exploratory laparoscopy

(123) For the above scenario, what is the most likely diagnosis? Answer: d

(a) Endometriosis

(b) Polycystic ovarian syndrome

(c) Pelvic inflammatory disease

(d) Uterine leiomyoma

(e) Endometrial cancer

**(124) Considering that the patient in the above question is considering having another child in the future, which of the following statements is true for this patient?** Answer: e

**(a) A myomectomy should be performed as soon as possible to allow as much time as possible for uterine healing prior to the stress of pregnancy**

**(b) An open-surgery myomectomy is a common cause of infertility because of the formation of postoperative adhesions**

**(c) Following a myomectomy, cesarean delivery is required to avoid uterine rupture**

**(d) Myomectomy is expected to increase this patient's fertility rate by 50% in 1–2 years**

**(e) Uterine artery embolization (UAE) has been shown to diminish bleeding symptoms and recovery time, but it is not recommended for women who desire children in the future**

**(125) A 36-year-old woman has heavy, painless bleeding every 4–5 months. She comes to your office asking for contraceptives. An examination of her cervix is normal and her Pap smear is class I. What is the most appropriate procedure?** Answer: d

**(a) Oral estrogen only**

**(b) Bilateral-salpingo-oophorectomy**

**(c) Cyclic oral contraceptive agents**

**(d) Fractional dilation and curettage (D & C)**

**(e) Conization of the cervix**

(126) A 26-year-old female visits your office for a routine gynecologic examination. She has no complaints and is in good health. Her menstrual periods began when she was 12 years old and are regular with a 28-day interval and duration of 5 days. She is single but sexually active and uses oral contraceptive pills and barrier contraception. During the pelvic examination, you palpate a mass on the right side. An ultrasound is performed and reveals a complex, cystic tumor approximately 5 cm in diameter in the right ovary. There is no free fluid in the peritoneum and there is no family history of cancer. What is the most appropriate step in her treatment?

Answer: e

(a) Laparoscopy and cystectomy

(b) Hormonal treatment with progesterone

(c) Pelvic examination in 6 months

(d) Ovariectomy of the right ovary

(e) Sonogram surveillance over the next two menstrual cycles

(127) Which of the following ovarian tumors is most sensitive to radiation therapy?

Answer: b

(a) Gonadoblastoma

(b) Dysgerminoma

(c) Choriocarcinoma

(d) Serous cystadenocarcinoma

(128) Which neoplasm is most sensitive to chemotherapy?

Answer: e

(a) Ovarian dysgerminoma

(b) Uterine sarcoma

(c) Ovarian serous carcinoma

(d) Fallopian tube cancer

(e) Gestational trophoblastic disease

**(129) The release of clear or blood-tinged vaginal discharge, whether spontaneously or pressure induced, followed by shrinkage of an adnexal mass and relief of cramping pain is pathognomonic for which neoplasm?**

**(a) Fallopian tube cancer**

**(b) Ovarian cystadenocarcinoma**

**(c) Epithelial ovarian cancer**

**(d) Dermoid cyst**

**(e) Krukenberg tumor**

Answer: a

**(130) Herniation of the peritoneum between the uterosacral ligaments through the pouch of Douglas into the rectovaginal septum represents which of the following defects?**

**(a) Uterine prolapse**

**(b) Rectocele**

**(c) Enterocele**

**(d) Urethrocele**

**(e) Cystocele**

**(f) Retrodisplacement of the uterus**

Answer: b

**(131) A 65-year-old menopausal woman visits your office with complaints of urinary difficulty and discomfort in the vagina. She complains that the feeling in her vagina is like she is "sitting on an egg." What is the appropriate therapy?**

**(a) Remove the foreign body**

**(b) Perform a hysterectomy**

**(c) Recommend a pessary**

**(d) Reassurance**

Answer: b or c (Depending on patient's preference. However, b is preferred if there is other uterine pathology, whereas c is preferred for those who want to avoid surgery.)

(132) A 26-year-old multiparous patient at 33 weeks' estimated gestational age reports significant abdominal pain of 40-minutes duration. The pain is improved when sitting up and was not associated with exertion. The patient has a history of alcohol dependence and had just finished eating a spiced curry tomato dish. On presentation, her vital signs and physical examination are within normal limits. Which of the following lab values is abnormal?

Answer: a

(a) Amylase 300 U/dL

(b) White blood cells 13,000 per $mm^3$

(c) Fibrinogen 500 mg/dL

(d) Alkaline phosphatase 17 U/L

(133) An obese 22-year-old woman has a history of irregular periods. She was placed on oral contraceptive pills and after two normal cycles she has begun to miss her period again. Her BhCG is zero. What is the next course of action?

Answer: d

(a) Begin metformin so as to better control the metabolic derangements associated with polycystic ovarian syndrome

(b) Check FSH and LH levels for possible premature ovarian failure

(c) Do a transvaginal ultrasound to look for ovarian cysts

(d) Change the oral contraceptive to a monophasic instead of a triphasic

(134) A 19-year-old, obese, Type A1 diabetic at 30 weeks of pregnancy complains of nausea, dizziness, and shortness of breath when lying down. Her vital signs and physical examination are within normal limits, urine dip reveals trace protein. What is the next step in her treatment?

Answer: d

(a) Urgent biophysical ultrasound with evaluation of the fetus for macrosomic presentation and likely labor dystocia

(b) Lower-extremity doppler and electrocardiogram for possible DVT and pulmonary embolism

(c) Neurologic evaluation with attention paid to signs of end-organ damage related to preeclampsia

(d) Request that the patient sleep on her left side so as to assume a left lateral displacement of the gravid uterus and schedule the patient for clinic visit the following day

(135) After completing an abdominal x-ray, a woman discovers that she is several weeks pregnant. She is concerned regarding the status of the fetus. Which of the following is accurate?

Answer: c

(a) Organogenesis is completed by the 15th week

(b) The bulk of neural development occurs during the third trimester

(c) Preimplantation exposure to radiation typically results in a spontaneous abortion

(d) Radiation exposure of less than 5 rads has been associated with neurologic defects

(136) A 26-year-old Type I diabetic class B reports decreased fetal movement. She is at 37 weeks' estimated gestational age and has had poor glycemic control throughout pregnancy. The manual estimated fetal weight is 2000 grams and the fundal height is somewhat less than the estimated gestational age. What type of screening should be performed to assess fetal well-being and placental sufficiency?

(a) Non-stress test followed by abdominal ultrasound to assess for presentation, amniotic fluid, and placental location

(b) Biophysical profile

(c) Amniocentesis with analysis for fetal lung maturity

(d) Cordocentesis with analysis of pH, lactic acid, and immunoglobulins

Answer: a and c

(137) An obese 38-year-old with chronic hypertension and Type II diabetes is found to be 6 weeks pregnant. Her medications include: an ACE inhibitor, beta-blocker, thiazide diuretic, metformin, folic acid, and a multivitamin. Which of the following medications (choose all that apply) are safe in pregnancy?

(a) Insulin

(b) ACE inhibitors

(c) Glyburide

(d) Thiazide

Answer: a and c

(138) An Rh(–) mother has just undergone a normal spontaneous vaginal delivery with significant postpartum hemorrhage attributed to atony. What test would assist in determining how much RhoGam should be administered postpartum?

(a) Quantitative titer analysis of maternal circulating antibodies

(b) Flow cytometry to determine which isoforms the mother has developed

Answer: c

(c) Kleihauer-Betke serum stain

(d) Indirect Coombs test

(139) A woman with gestational diabetes class A1 and poor glycemic control requests a repeat cesarean delivery. Fetal lung maturity (FLM) at 37 weeks shows a lecithin/ sphingomyelin ratio of 2.2/ and phosphatdylglycerol negative. Following delivery, the infant develops respiratory distress syndrome (RDS). What about the patient's history would suggest that the infant was at risk for RDS?

Answer: d

(a) Two or more types of fetal lung maturity tests should be used when determining the risk of RDS

(b) Elective cesarean delivery should only take place after 39 weeks

(c) The amniocentesis was likely contaminated with blood, resulting in a false L/S ratio

(d) Surfactant function and production is adversely affected by increased fetal insulin and maternal diabetes

(140) A 36-year-old female presents with a single, firm, well-delineated, round, nontender nodule in her left upper breast. When her gynecologist palpates, it is very mobile with respect to its surrounding tissue. What is the most likely diagnosis of this mass?

Answer: d

(a) Ductal carcinoma in situ

(b) Papillary cystadenocarcinoma

(c) Breast cyst

(d) Adenocarcinoma

**(141) Tubal patency or "pelvic factor" in evaluation of infertility is best accomplished by:**

Answer: a

**(a) Hysterosalpingogram (HSG)**

**(b) Hysteroscopy**

**(c) Pelvic magnetic resonance imaging (MRI)**

**(d) Transvaginal ultrasound**

**(e) Pelvic CT scan**

**(142) You are seeing your 35-year-old patient, who has sought your help several times prior for vague but persistent gynecologic concerns. She currently complains of pelvic discomfort. You have evaluated her in the past for the same concern and found no gynecologic or gastrointestinal etiology. As you continue to ask her more questions, she begins to cry and reveals that she was sexually abused as a child.**

**Which of the following statements aboutsexual abuse is most statistically accurate?**

Answer: b

**(a) Her abuser was someone she did not know well**

**(b) Her abuser was a member of her family**

**(c) Approximately 5% of women have experienced childhood sexual abuse**

**(d) The abuse took place at a daycare center**

**(e) She was abused between the ages of 2 and 10**

**(143) Through chromosome analysis, you find that your patient has a sex genotype of XO. What is the proper therapeutic regimen for this patient?**

Answer: e

**(a) Androgens and cortisol**

**(b) Cortisol and human growth hormone**

(c) Small doses of estrogen in early childhood

(d) Progesterone, estrogen, and cortisol

(e) Androgens, human growth hormones, small doses of estrogen, and later progesterone

**(144)** In evaluating an infertile couple, the postcoital test is performed to assess which of the following? Answer: a

(a) Interaction of sperm with cervical mucus prior to ovulation

(b) Interaction of sperm with cervical mucus anytime during the cycle

(c) Interaction of sperm with cervical mucus during ovulation.

(d) Interaction of sperm with cervical in midluteal phase

**(145)** All of the following may be direct causes of female infertility except: Answer: a

(a) previous uncomplicated abortion

(b) endometriosis

(c) pelvic inflammatory disease (PID)

(d) hyperprolactinemia

(e) polycystic ovarian syndrome (PCOS)

**(146)** What is the most common presenting fracture in osteoporosis? Answer: a

(a) Vertebral compression fracture

(b) Wrist fracture

(c) Tibial fracture

(d) Femoral head fracture

(e) Femoral neck fracture

(147) What is the gold standard for the diagnosis of osteoporosis?

Answer: d

(a) Plain x-ray of the thoracic spine

(b) Qualitative ultrasound densitometry

(c) Peripheral dual x-ray absorptiometry (DXA)

(d) Central (DXA)

(e) A quantitated computed tomography (QCT)

(148) A 52-year-old woman has been experiencing signs of menopause, including increasing hot flushes during the day and night, difficulty sleeping, emotional lability, and anxiety. She denies any other complaints or medical illnesses. Her last period was approximately 12 months ago. Her vital signs are all within normal range. Her pelvic examination reveals atrophic external genitalia, a small anteverted uterus, and no adnexal masses. The rest of her examination is normal.

Answer: d

What is the most effective treatment option for this patient?

(a) Progestin alone

(b) Estrogen alone (ERT)

(c) Antidepressants

(d) Estrogen with progestin (hormone replacement therapy [HRT])

(149) If this patient also complained of vaginal dryness and pain during intercourse, reasonable treatment options would include?

Answer: d

(a) Topical estrogen cream

(b) An estrogen ring (Estring)

(c) Vaginal moisturizers

(d) All of the above

**(150) According to the World Health Organization (WHO), osteoporosis is defined as:**

**(a) BMD between 1.5 and 2.0 standard deviations below the mean for young normal adults (T score)**

**(b) BMD is between 1.5 and 2.0 standard deviations below the mean for age-matched adults (Z score)**

**(c) BMD is less than 2.5 standard deviations below the mean for young normal adults (T score)**

**(d) BMD is less than 2.5 standard deviations below the mean for age-matched adults (Z score)**

Answer: c

# Suggested Readings and Sources of Information

Beckmann C, Ling FW, Smith RP, Barzansky BM, Herbert W, and Laube DW. *Obstetrics and Gynecology.* 5th ed. Philadelphia, PA: Lippincott Williams & Wilkins; 2005.

Berek, Jonathan S. *Berek and Novak's Gynecology (Novak's Textbook Gynecology).* 14th ed. Philadelphia, PA: Lippincott Williams & Wilkins; 2006.

Cunningham FG, Leveno KJ, Bloom SL, Hauth JC, Gilstrap LC III, and Wenstrom KD. *Williams Obstetrics.* 22nd ed. New York, NY: McGraw-Hill Companies; 2005.

Decherney AH, Nathan L, Goodwin TM, Laufer N. *Current Diagnosis & Treatment.* 10th ed. New York, NY: McGraw-Hill Companies; 2007

www.ACOG.org (Medical Students are eligible for Free Membership)

www.UpToDate.com

# Index

Page numbers followed by *f* or *t* indicate figures or tables, respectively.

**I**